CARDIOVASCULAR EFFECTS OF MOOD-ALTERING DRUGS

Cardiovascular Effects of Mood-Altering Drugs

Barry Stimmel, M.D.
Associate Dean
Associate Professor of Medicine (Cardiology)
Associate Professor of Medical Education
The Mount Sinai School of Medicine
of The City University of New York
New York, New York

Raven Press ▪ New York

Raven Press, 1140 Avenue of the Americas, New York, New York 10036

Made in the United States of America

Library of Congress Cataloging in Publication Data

Stimmel, Barry, 1939–
Cardiovascular effects of mood-altering drugs.
Includes bibliographical references and index.
1. Cardiovascular system—Drug effects.
2. Psychotropic drugs. I. Title.
RM345.S75 615′.71 77–91582
ISBN 0-89004-287-X

Preface

In compensation for the almost daily frustrations and frequent failures experienced by the scientific investigators, there must come certain satisfactions. The most rewarding of these is inherent in the compulsive pleasure of seeking and searching which occasionally culminates in the thrill of perceiving a little corner of the universe into which no one has previously been privileged to glimpse.

Solomon A. Berson, M.D.
1918–1972

Since antiquity people have endowed certain persons and substances with magical healing powers. Although a number of these substances were later found to have specific medicinal properties, the greater majority consisted of naturally occurring hallucinogens and stimulants. Through the centuries the shaman or witch doctor has been slowly but inevitably replaced by the physician-scientist and the homeopathic remedies by a vast array of synthetic drugs. The armamentarium of today's physician is indeed impressive. Still, as in primitive times, a large proportion of drugs is administered specifically to relieve anxiety or alter mood.

The effectiveness and usefulness of modern mood-altering drugs have resulted in a prominent focus on their psychotropic actions, with insufficient attention directed to the systemic effects of these agents, most notably on the cardiovascular system. Many persons taking psychotropic drugs under a physician's prescription are suffering from cardiovascular disease, and an equal number may be at risk for the development of heart disease with continued and frequent ingestion of some of these mood-altering substances. Knowledge of the effects of these drugs on the cardiovascular system therefore becomes of considerable importance. This book is written to provide such knowledge to physicians prescribing these medications, treating persons abusing drugs or giving advice to patients concerning the consumption of the readily available social drugs, alcohol, nicotine, caffeine, and marijuana.

This volume consists of a review of the effects of mood-altering drugs on the heart and vasculature. The basic pharmacologic actions of these agents are not discussed in great detail, as this information is readily available in a number of other books. Focus is on the specific effects of these agents on the cardiovascular system in healthy persons, as well as in those with cardiac disease. Since an increasing number of individuals receiving psychotropic drugs also have cardiovascular disease and are taking multiple medications, attention is paid to possible drug interactions between these agents and other cardiac medications. Wherever possible, tables and illustrations are used to simplify the material presented and to make summaries readily available. It should be emphasized that the purpose of this book is not to discourage the appropriate use of these agents but rather to make the physician aware of their physiologic and, in some cases, pathologic effects on the heart and blood vessels, so that advice concerning their use may be tempered with a competent knowledge of their cardiovascular actions.

DEDICATION

To Alexander

Acknowledgments

As with most scientific reviews, this publication was greatly facilitated by the past contributions of other investigators whose works are amply referenced in the text. Particular help was provided by several who were kind enough to allow reproduction of their previously published material. Acknowledgment can be found in the appropriate chapters.

I am grateful to Dr. Stephen Geller who provided illustrations of the pathological specimens. Dr. Spencer Shaw's critical advice concerning the material dealing with cardiovascular effects secondary to alcohol was quite helpful. My wife Barbara, in her role as psychotherapist, provided additional insight for the chapter on the effects of stress on the cardiovascular system. Dr. Ephraim Donoso deserves special mention as the one who initially encouraged my taking pen in hand to integrate the superficially discordant fields of psychopharmacology and cardiology.

Finally, the timely publication of this book would not have been possible without the aid of Ms. Mary Kennedy who worked above and beyond the call of duty so that the originally agreed upon schedule could be maintained.

Contents

Chapter 1

Psychotropic Drug Use: Defining the Problem

The use of plant substances to alter moods or to provide medicinal relief extends so deeply into antiquity that the precise dates of their appearance remain uncertain (1). Perhaps thousands of years ago an awareness of the change occurring when fruits or berries were mixed with water and left in the sun resulted in the production of mead, one of the earliest alcoholic beverages. Similar chronologic estimates have been made with respect to the appearance of opiate and cannabis use. By 4000 B.C., alcoholic beverages in the form of beer and wine were commonly consumed not only for pleasure but also as medications of great value (2). An ancient clay tablet from the Sumarian city of Nippur, dated approximately 3000 B.C., described drugs containing wine to be effective in many disorders.

The Sumarians also cultivated the poppy for its opium (2,3). The term *gil,* indicating happiness and joy, was applied to this plant. Cultivation of the poppy seed spread eastward to Persia and westward to Egypt by the Babylonians. Hesiod, in the 8th century B.C., described the city of Mekône (poppy town) known for cultivating this flower (4). The writings of Hippocrates (460–377 B.C.) contain treatises on the medicinal value of the poppy as hypnotic, analgesic, cathartic, and styptic (5).

The appreciation of hallucinogenic substances also occurred early in civilization. The actions of cannabis (marijuana) were described in a Chinese treatise on pharmacology (approximately 2700 B.C.) that lauded its medicinal value (6). In the second millenium B.C., the Hindu scriptures, the *Atharva veda,* described use of this drug, as well as serpentina, the parent compound of reserpine (7). Although the Greeks were predominantly wine drinkers rather than marijuana smokers, the writings of Herodotus mention the psychotropic effects of marijuana smoke.

Exploration of the new world by the Europeans resulted in a rediscovery by the West of hallucinogens in the indigenous plant life. The leaves of the abundantly cultivated cannabis, coca, and tobacco plants were quickly heralded by these explorers for their psychotropic potential. Such substances, of course, were not really discovered at this time as the native populations had long since appreciated their value. Coca leaves, for example, have been found in tombs of Indian mummies dated circa 600 A.D. Throughout the ensuing centuries, derivatives of natural mood-altering substances continued to be consumed by people all over the world, with the possible exception of the Eskimos, whose environs were too cold for a fertile climate for plant growth. The 19th and 20th centuries, however, were highlighted by great gains in scientific knowledge, including the use of chemical techniques to synthesize potent pharmacologic agents.

In Germany in 1805, Serturner, separating meconic acid from opium, produced morphine from the alkaline base. The isolation of narcotine and codeine rapidly followed. The hypodermic syringe, perfected by Rynd and Wood in the 1850s, provided a more potent vehicle for obtaining relief from anxiety and pain. It is sad yet true that Mrs. Wood was one of the first to realize the potential danger of the hypodermic by becoming a parenteral opium addict (7,8). Heroin was synthesized from morphine in 1874 by Wright; it was not until 1898, however, when Dreser began to investigate the potential of this drug that it became known to the public (9). The degree of enthusiasm for heroin can best be illustrated by the campaign of the Ebhart-Bayer Pharmaceutical Company, which initiated an international market for its distribution and sale (10). Enthusiasm for this drug spread to this country, with endorsement by the American Medical Association (AMA) of heroin for general use and as a specific substitute for morphine in 1906. Several years later, the hazards associated with inappropriate heroin use became increasingly clear. As a result, Congress, realizing that the liabilities of heroin exceeded its therapeutic advantage, passed legislation in 1924 prohibiting its manufacture or importation.

Erythroxylone, extracted from the coca leaf in 1858, was subsequently refined by Niemann to the alkaline base cocaine. The pharmacologic effects of cocaine were first studied by Von Anrep in 1880, followed shortly by a comprehensive review of the action of the drug on the central nervous system by Aschenbrandt and Freud (6). Freud was an enthusiast of cocaine, anticipating widespread medicinal use including treatment for disorders of the digestive tract, cachexia, morphine and alcohol addiction, and asthma. It was also thought to be an excellent stimulant, aphrodisiac, and local anesthetic. After Koller's confirmation of the effectiveness of cocaine as a local anesthetic, the drug gained wide popularity in minor surgical procedures. By the early 20th century, cocaine was hailed as a miracle drug with a distribution

TABLE 1. *Drug store prescriptions for sedative-hypnotic tranquilizer drugs*[a]

Drug	1971	1973	Change (%)	1976	Change (%)
Barbiturates	38,225	32,573	−14.8	18,461	−43.3
Nonbarbiturates	106,528	123,396	15.8	113,226	− 8.2
Total	144,753	155,969	7.7	131,687	−15.5

[a] NPA: number of prescriptions in thousands. (Adapted from Fitzgerald et al., ref. 45.)

so ubiquitous it even appeared as a prominent ingredient in Coca Cola®. But this was not the only available cocaine-containing beverage; as late as 1909, there were 69 cola drinks containing cocaine as a prominent ingredient. The producers of Coca Cola had in fact removed cocaine from their drink around 1906, replacing it with caffeine (11). During the next 15 years, adverse publicity concerning the ability of cocaine to foment social unrest became a topic of increasing concern. This resulted in passage of legislation by a number of states restricting or prohibiting its use. When the Harrison Act was passed in 1914, the availability of this drug decreased precipitously.

The second major group of stimulants, the amphetamines, was synthesized in 1887. They did not become popular in clinical medicine until 1932, however, when the AMA Council on Pharmacy designated 1-phenyl 2-aminopropane amphetamine as an effective therapeutic agent (12). Smith, Kline and French Laboratories received the patent rights introducing the Benzedrene® nasal inhaler several years later, initiating widespread physician use of these drugs (13).

The first synthetic sedative, chloral hydrate, was developed by Liebig in 1932. Thirty-two years later, in 1864, Baeyer synthesized barbituric acid. It was not until 1903, however, that the first hypnotic barbiturate barbital (Veronal®) was introduced to clinical medicine (14). Widespread use of the barbiturates continued unabated, replaced only in popularity by the benzodiazepines, following the synthesis of chlordiazepoxide in 1958 (Table 1). In the mid-1900s, the clinical development of the phenothiazines (first synthesized in 1883), the synthesis of the hallucinogens in pharmaceutical as well as clandestine laboratories, and the development of the monoamine oxidase (MAO) inhibitors, followed shortly by the tricyclic antidepressants, completed the basic categories of available synthetic, mood-altering drugs.

CURRENT USE OF MOOD-ALTERING AGENTS

Approximately 90% of presently available prescription drugs were unknown when the Food and Drug and Cosmetic Act became law more than 40 years ago. Since then, the pharmaceutical industry has increased its annual operating expenses from $300 million to $7 billion, with enough drugs being produced to provide every man, woman, and child in this country with

5.7 prescriptions per year (15). An impressive number of these drugs has been produced specifically to provide more effective relief of anxiety and depression. Indeed, the effectiveness of many of these drugs is undisputed. Following the introduction of new psychotropic agents, the number of persons in mental hospitals decreased from a peak of 559,000 in 1955 to the present level of approximately 200,000. Many of these individuals have not only been able to return to their communities but have become productive and self-sufficient. Unfortunately, the efficacy of these drugs has led to widespread and perhaps excessive use in an attempt to provide rapid relief of anxiety.

At present, public consumption of mood-altering agents is nothing less than phenomenal. Studies indicate that during a year, 25 to 35% of adult Americans have used a licit psychotropic agent; a random sampling of persons on the street showed 14% to have used such a drug, excluding alcohol, within the previous 24 hours (16). The prevalence of psychotropic drug use at any time has been estimated to approach a magnitude of approximately one-half of our population, with one person in three using some psychotrope at least once during a 12-month period (17). Abelson and Fishburne (18) have found nonmedical use of sedatives, tranquilizers, or stimulants by adults, aged 18 to 25, to approximate 12, 9, and 17%, respectively. A survey by Johnston (19) of sedative and hypnotic use among high school seniors has shown that approximately 17% of these students reported nonmedical use of both barbiturates and tranquilizers in 1975 and 1976, with more than 4% likely to have used these drugs within any given 30-day period. Data from the National Marijuana Commission Survey have shown 56% of adults and 20% of youths surveyed to have had experience with one or more psychotropic over-the-counter (OTC) medication, with 70% having taken one or more of such drugs within the past year (20). Comparable data from other Western countries indicate that America is not at all unique in the consumption of mood-altering drugs and, indeed, places in a middle position among nine countries surveyed (21).

Illicit Drug Use

The prevalence of illicit purchase and use of drugs is extremely difficult to determine with any accuracy. Although probably not as widespread as nonmedical use of prescription or OTC agents, illicit use is certainly substantial. In 1962, it was estimated that of the 9 billion doses of amphetamines and barbiturates produced nationally, approximately 50% appeared on the black market (13).

Abuse of inhalants through sniffing of glue or aerosols first appeared in the media in 1959 and was considered to be prominent through the 1960s. Subsequent to 1967, approximately four deaths per month were recorded by the Food and Drug Administration (FDA). Hallucinogenic use started to gain popularity at this time and had become epidemic among high-risk groups by 1970. Fortunately, the prevalence of this type of drug use appears to have diminished during the past several years.

Currently, more than one million persons have been estimated to smoke marijuana on a regular basis; and this is undoubtedly a conservative figure (22). Marijuana use remains a phenomenon of importance among younger age groups; the proportion of adults over age 30 using this drug is small. Indeed, Abelson and Fishburne (18) have noted 53% of adults between the ages of 18 and 25 to have admitted to marijuana use, with one-half of these persons using this drug within the past month. Cocaine use, also difficult to determine with any degree of accuracy, has been reported in 2 to 13% of young adults.

The use of heroin, although not as widespread as that of other agents, was of sufficient importance in New York City several years ago to be considered one of the leading causes of death in young men between the ages of 15 and 35 (23). Estimates of the number of heroin users nationwide at the end of 1974 have been as high as 724,000 (20). Although these figures are only estimates, data obtained from admissions to treatment programs and hepatitis case reports for this period recorded as 10-fold increase in heroin use. Equally as important as current prevalence is the potential for heroin use to develop in a conducive environment. Robins (24), in a survey of 571 Vietnam veterans, found only 3% to become addicted after return to the United States. However, 35% of these men used heroin while in Vietnam, reemphasizing the effectiveness of this drug to relieve anxiety.

Acceptable Habits

Other substances are readily available that, when consumed in moderation, are associated with minimal sanction; in reality, however, they are potent drugs. Surveys of alcohol use have found up to two-thirds of the population to be consumers, with heavy use reported in 12% (25). Excessive alcohol use presents a considerable social as well as medical problem to approximately 9 million Americans (26). In New York City, this agent has been reported to be responsible for six times as many deaths as those occurring from illicit heroin use, as well as an unknown number of associated social and physical affirmaties (27). Nationally, mortality due to alcoholism accounts for 7% of all male deaths. A few prospective studies have revealed the magnitude of the detrimental effects of excessive alcohol use. In a survey of 240 inner-city youths followed for a period of 25 years, Robins and Guze (28) found almost one-half of these individuals to have had their lives interrupted in some way by alcohol.

Nicotine, also recognized as a major health hazard, is believed to be consumed by 30 to 46% of the population, despite persistent warnings of the detrimental effects of this drug on each pack of cigarettes. Although the number of smoking adults decreased by 10% between 1965 and 1975, an impressive 46.9 million persons still have this habit. In addition, the number of smoking teenagers, aged 13 to 19, has unfortunately increased from 14 to 20% during this period (29). Caffeine-containing drinks are consumed by the majority of the population of all ages, with the possible effects of excessive intake, such as nervousness, irritability, anxiety, palpitations, and epigastric distress, just beginning to be realized.

Populations at Special Risk

Although the use of psychotropic drugs can be found among all age groups, certain persons are at particular risk with respect to frequency of use or development of adverse reactions. Infants, for example, may not be capable of effective biotransformation of many drugs, leading to a greater potential for toxicity with accidental drug overdose. Pregnant women are another high-risk group because of the effects that drug ingestion might have on the developing fetus. With respect to the effects of mood-altering drugs on the cardiovascular system, however, the three main groups at special risk are: (a) the elderly, (b) persons with preexisting cardiovascular disease, and (c) diabetics.

The Elderly

The elderly frequently take multiple medications for physical ailments and are probably the largest consumers of drugs in our country. A large proportion of the 225 million prescriptions written annually for persons 55 years of age or older are for mood-altering drugs (30,31). A survey conducted by the National Institute on Drug Abuse (NIDA) (32) on legal drugs used by the elderly showed sedatives, tranquilizers, and antidepressants to be second only to cardiovascular drugs in frequency of prescription drug use, being present in 14.6 and 39.3%, respectively, of all persons surveyed. If analgesic medications taken for chronic arthritic conditions are included, then mood-altering medications represent 24% of all prescription drugs consumed by this population. Since 80 to 86% of persons over age 65 are estimated to be suffering from at least one chronic medical condition (33), treatment is likely to involve the prescription of multiple medications, which increases the risk of clinically important drug interactions. The considerable prevalence of cardiovascular disease in the elderly further enhances the risk of an untoward interaction. Finally, as discussed in the following chapter, physiologic changes accompanying the aging process are associated with an incidence of adverse drug reactions in persons 60 to 70 years of age twice that seen in persons 30 to 40 years old.

Ambulatory use of prescription psychotropic medication by the elderly is considerable; however, the magnitude of the problem with respect to those elderly confined in nursing homes is even greater. Although at any time only 5% of the elderly live in nursing homes, approximately 25% of deaths in this population in 1972 occurred in these institutions or during a brief hospital admission from a long-term care facility (33a). Among the nursing home population, multiple medical conditions coexist, with mental disability being prominent. Large doses of psychotropic medications are frequently used, with persons carrying a medical diagnosis sometimes receiving more of these drugs than those with primary psychiatric problems (33a). The ingestion of multiple medications by people who may not be completely rational, in an environment with a less-than-optimal staffing pattern, can provide a fertile environment for serious drug interactions or the appearance of specific side-effects that may go undetected for prolonged periods of time. It is not by accident that the association of sudden death and phenothiazine therapy (Chapter 7) was first noticed after a retrospective review of deaths in state hospitals.

Elderly individuals reporting psychotropic drug use as compared to those recording no such use are found to have a poorer quality of life relationship, poorer health, and a greater degree of physical disability, suggesting a propensity toward misuse or abuse of mood-altering drugs. It is not surprising, therefore, that alcohol use in this population may be considerable and associated with a greater potential for toxicity than in younger persons. Surveys have shown 10 to 15% of elderly medical outpatients to have serious problems secondary to alcohol consumption (34). Admissions to inpatient medical services record up to 16% of men over age 60 to have alcohol-related problems (35). A prevalence of excessive drinking has been noted in nonmedical admissions to inpatient psychiatric services in up to 28% of individuals over 60 years of age (36). Of this group, 80% presented with overt alcoholism. Since the overwhelming majority of elderly persons consuming psychotropic medications do so under a physician's prescription rather than by purchase of OTC drugs, a knowledge of the possible drug interactions among alcohol, other psychotropic medications, and drugs used for the treatment of cardiovascular disease is of special importance.

Persons With Cardiovascular Disease

Many persons with cardiovascular disease also consume a considerable number of mood-altering substances. This consumption may be part of the medical treatment to help alleviate anxiety or ingrained in their daily activities, such as smoking and drinking alcohol or caffeine-containing beverages. Many of the currently available prescription psychotropes are known to effect the cardiovascular system, with several having clearly demonstrable effects on the electrocardiogram. Inappropriate use of these drugs or an unawareness of their interactions with commonly prescribed cardiac medications may place the patient at unnecessary risk. Certain substances shown to be a risk factor in coronary and peripheral vascular disease, such as nicotine, may be particularly hazardous in the cardiac patient. Persons recovering from a myocardial infarction frequently express anxiety about the safety of drinking alcohol or coffee. Similarly, persons at high risk for the development of coronary heart disease frequently request guidance with respect to continuing these habits, mandating physician familiarity with the cardiovascular effects of these substances.

Diabetics

Diabetes is a disease that can be found in all parts of the world, affecting an estimated 200 million persons consisting of a metabolic and a vascular disturbance, both of which can be adversely influenced by consumption of mood-altering substances.

Many psychotropes can influence glucose metabolism (Table 2). In addition, clinically important drug interactions can occur with the use of these agents and antidiabetic medications. Physician knowledge of these interactions becomes quite important when managing diabetics in need of psychotropic drugs.

The vascular disease seen in diabetics consists of accelerated development of atherosclerosis and formation of widespread microangiopathic lesions, particularly in the retinal or renal cuculations. The prevalence of coronary artery disease is augmented in diabetics with a frequency of more than twice that of the nondiabetic population (37). The predisposition to coronary artery disease is such that the normal frequency difference seen between

TABLE 2. *Selected potential mood-altering drug interactions in the diabetic*

Drug	Effect
Alcohol	Production of hypoglycemia with tendency to ketoacidosis Enhances ketosis and lactic acidosis in persons receiving phenformin Decreases half-life of tolbutamide Decreases myocardial function Antabuse® reaction may be provoked by chlorpropamide
Amphetamines	May produce hypoglycemic response (47)
Caffeine	May impair glucose tolerance with elevation of blood glucose (48)
Lithium carbonate	May enhance hyperglycemia (49)
Marijuana	May impair glucose tolerance (50)
MAO inhibitors	May enhance or prolong hypoglycemia and response to insulin and oral agents (51)
Phenothiazines	Enhances hyperglycemia (52,53)
Propoxyphene	May decrease blood sugar (54)

men and premenopausal women is eliminated. Myocardial function assessed by systolic time intervals has been found to be impaired even in asymptomatic diabetics (38). Myocardial infarction tends to present atypically, with up to 30% of diabetics experiencing little or no pain even with infarcts of considerable size (39). Mortality rates are high, with approximately 50% of diabetics dying from coronary artery disease, a rate nearly double that of the nondiabetic population (40).

Of all the potential dangers inherent in psychotropic drug use by diabetics (Table 2), the two drugs associated with the greatest risk are nicotine and alcohol. The association of nicotine with coronary artery disease and peripheral vascular disease has been well established (Chapter 14). Cigarette smoking by the diabetic further increases this risk. The acceleration of the atherosclerotic process results in a greater tendency toward clinical development of angina, myocardial infarction, or intermittent claudication, which may progress to lower limb ischemia or even gangrene of the feet or toes.

Alcohol consumption can also present the diabetic with considerable metabolic problems and adversely affect cardiovascular performance. Alcohol, in the presence of fasting or glycogen depletion, can produce considerable hypoglycemia which, in the diabetic, may lead to ketoacidosis. In persons on phenformin (41,42), alcohol has also been associated with the production of lactic acidosis (43). The effect of alcohol on the hepatic microsomal system may result in interaction with the oral hypoglycemics, with a marked decrease in half-life of tolbutamide (44). Concomitant use of alcohol and chlorpropamide can result in a systemic reaction similar to that seen with Antabuse® (45).

Recently, Rubler et al. (46) presented evidence of impaired myocardial performance, as determined by systolic time intervals, in diabetics without known preexisting heart disease following ingestion of small doses of alcohol. The myocardial depression could be measured at 30 and 60 min postdrinking and was not observed in a group of control subjects. Alcohol consumption in the diabetic can be associated with both metabolic and vascular alterations and should, therefore, be undertaken judiciously.

THE PHYSICIAN'S ROLE

The physician has had a primary role in fostering consumption of mood-altering medications. In 1962, the FDA estimated that enough amphetamines were produced to supply every man, woman, and child with 35 5-mg doses (55). Although a good portion of these drugs may have appeared on the illicit market, physician use, personally as well as professionally, may be considerable. Indeed, a survey of amphetamine use by medical students in 1966 revealed 35% to have taken amphetamines at least once (56). By 1970, the Physician's Desk Reference listed 40 companies producing 65 amphetamine or amphetamine-like preparations available as single drugs or in combination with analgesics, tranquilizers, or hormones (57). Over the past several years action has been taken to restrict physician prescription of these agents on both state and federal levels.

The distribution of barbiturates in the 1960s was so widespread to supply each individual in the United States with 24 100-mg doses (58). Although physician prescription of barbiturates has been decreasing during the past several years (Table 1), in 1976, approximately 18.5 million prescriptions, representing 228 million tablets, were still being written (59). Accompanying the decrease in prescription of barbiturates, there has been a steady increase in the use of the benzodiazepines, which reached a peak in 1973 when more than 156 million prescriptions were written for these agents, as well as for the nonbarbiturate sedatives, at a cost in excess of $200 million (59,60).

The use of chlorpromazine has become of increasing importance in the armamentarium of effective mood-altering agents. Smith, Kline and French reported their net sales to increase from $53 million in 1953 to $347 million in 1970, largely because of Thorazine® and its derivatives (61). The increasing availability and documented effectiveness of tricyclic antidepressants have also resulted in an escalation in prescription of these drugs, with more than 24 million prescriptions being written in 1973 (62).

The profiles of physicians prescribing psychotropic medications reveal three medical specialties—family/general practice, internal medicine, and psychiatry/neurology—to be responsible for the majority of prescriptions, which is not proportionate to their representation in private practice (63). A study from the National Disease and Therapeutic Index for 1974 (64) found the average internist to employ 25.6 drugs per day in treatment of patients, with the use of tranquilizing agents ranking second only to the diuretics. General practitioners, representing 25% of all office-based physicians in 1976, prescribed 46% of all prescriptions written for Nembutal®. Psychiatrists, representing only 7% of office-based physicians, were responsible for 42% of all prescriptions for Noludar®. It is difficult to transform these data into prescriptions per capita; however, such a calculation has been made by the Addiction Research Foundation in Ontario where an average of five prescriptions per capita is dispensed annually, with almost 25% of these prescriptions written for psychotropic substances. The amount of pills prescribed was considerable, with each prescription averaging just under 1 month's supply of drug (65).

Psychotropic drugs usually are not prescribed for patients with a diagnosis of a specific mental disorder but rather to alleviate anxiety or tension. Indeed, physicians lose some of their customary scientific objectiveness when prescribing mood-altering agents. Sapira, (66), in an evaluation of the degree to which physicians endorse the disease concept in their everyday practice, studied prescribing habits in patients receiving antihypertensive medication as compared to patients receiving psychotropic drugs. Evaluative criteria consisted of the degree of utilization of six measures, which included adequate diagnosis prior to prescription, chart documentation of the evidence leading to this diagnosis, and recording of prescribed medication on a problem sheet used for interclinic or interdisciplinary communication. Although only four of the six measures reviewed were found in records of patients receiving antihypertensive medication, the disease concept was not endorsed by the use of any of the six measures in records of persons receiving psychotropic medications.

The potential dangers inherent in too-frequent prescription of such drugs are considerable. The National Prescription Audit (NPA) provides annual projections on the volume of drugs sold by retail pharmacies, recording average prescription size, daily consumption prescribed, and duration of therapy. Based on a sample of 800 participating retail drug stores, prescription projections are made with respect to national medication use. In 1976, the data from the NPA suggested that physicians regularly prescribed hypnotic drugs for significantly longer periods than the effective duration of these agents (63). Since tolerance to the hypnotic actions of these drugs develops quickly, at times not accompanied by a concomitant increase in the amount needed for a toxic reaction, a danger of accidental overdose in those who self-adjust their medication becomes real. Data from emergency rooms regarding sedative and hypnotic abuse have shown that approximately 40 to 60% of those individuals admitted as a result of nonmedical sedative or hypnotic use receive their medications from a physician. Recent evidence has also appeared in the lay press suggesting that inappropriate prescription of psychotropic drugs may not always be inadvertent, with 2% of California physicians estimated to be responsible for an abundant illegal street supply of drugs (67).

SUMMARY

The use of mood-altering drugs, whether physician-prescribed, self-administered, or consumed in excess specifically to provide an escape from reality, is prevalent among all segments of our society, with certain populations, such as the elderly or individuals with preexisting cardiac disease, being at special risk. Physicians are primary providers of these drugs and, in addition, are frequently turned to for advice concerning consumption of caffeine-containing beverages, alcohol, and nicotine. All too often, psychotropic medications are prescribed without the same degree of diligence exercised in prescribing other therapeutic agents, with insufficient attention paid to the potential risks of these drugs and the possibility of adverse drug interactions. Similarly, since most physicians are exposed only minimally to illicit drug use, they are frequently ignorant of the adverse medical complications secondary to illicit use or intentional overdose with these agents.

In the chapters to follow, the effects of mood-altering drugs on the cardiovascular system are described in some detail. Attention is paid to these effects on the healthy, the elderly, and persons with cardiovascular disease. Treatment of drug overdose and cardiac complications of the more frequently abused agents is also discussed in some detail. It should be reemphasized that the intent of this book is neither to discourage the appropriate use of psychotropic agents nor to advocate the "temperance" philosophy of total abstinence from coffee, alcohol, and other stimulants. Rather, the objective is to increase the awareness of the physician and the physician-to-be of the action of these drugs on the cardiovascular system in order to encourage judicious prescription in all patients, especially in those with disease of the heart and vasculature.

REFERENCES

1. Lewin, L. (1931): *Narcotic and Stimulating Drugs. Their Use and Abuse,* translated by P. H. H. Wirth. Dutton, New York.
2. Leake, C. D., and Silverman, M. (1966): *Alcoholic Beverages in Clinical Medicine.* Yearbook Medical Publishers, Chicago.
3. Anslinger, H. J., and Tompkins, W. F. (1953): *The Traffic in Narcotics.* Funk and Wagnalls, New York.
4. Kritikos, P. G., and Papadaki, S. N. (1967): The history of the poppy and of opium and their expansion in antiquity in the eastern Mediterranean area. *Bull. Narc.,* 19:17.
5. *Oeuvres complètes d'Hippocrate,* chapter 12, pp. 1840–1849. Littré, Paris.
6. Byck, R. (editor) (1974): *Cocaine Papers: Sigmund Freud.* Stonehill Publishing, New York.
7. Howard-Jones, N. (1947): A critical study of the origins and early development of hypodermic medication. *J. Hist. Med.,* 2:201.
8. Terry, C. E., and Pellens, M. (1928): *The Opium Problem.* Committee on Drug Addiction, Bureau of Social Hygiene, New York.
9. United Nations Department of Social Affairs (1953): *Bull. Narc.,* 5:3.
10. McCoy, A. W. (1972): *The Politics of Heroin in Southeast Asia.* Harper and Row, New York.
11. Grinspoon, L., and Bakalar, J. B. (1976): *Cocaine: A Drug and its Social Evolution.* Basic Books, New York.
12. Leake, C. D. (1958): *The Amphetamines: Their Action and Uses.* Charles C Thomas, Springfield, Illinois.
13. Walsh, J. (1964): Psychotropic drugs. *Science,* 145:1418.
14. Harvey, S. C. (1975): Hypnotics and sedatives. In: *The Pharmacological Basis of Therapeutics,* edited by L. S. Goodman and A. Gilman, p. 109. MacMillan, New York.
15. Kennedy, D. (1978): Why our drug laws need to be changed. *The Sciences,* 18:11.
16. Parry, H. (1968): The use of psychoactive drugs by U.S. adults. *Public Health Serv. Rep.,* 83:799.
17. Parry, H. J., Balter, M. B., Mellinger, G. D., et al. (1973): National patterns of psychotherapeutic drug use. *Arch. Gen. Psychiatry,* 28:769.
18. Abelson, H., and Fishburne, P. (1976): Nonmedical use of psychoactive substances: 1975/6 nationwide study among youth and adults. Response Analysis Corp., Princeton.
19. Johnston, L. (1976): Monitoring the future study: Drug use among high school seniors in 1975, 1976. NIDA research grant DA 01411.
20. Greene, M., Nightingale, S. L., and Dupont, R. (1975): Evolving patterns of drug abuse. *Ann. Intern. Med.,* 83:402.
21. Balter, M. B., Levine, J., and Manheimer, D. (1974): Cross national study of the extent of antianxiety/sedative drug uses. *N. Engl. J. Med.,* 290:769.

22. McGlothlin, W. H. (1973): Marijuana use, distribution and control. In: *Drug Dealers, Taking Action,* edited by R. H. Blum, p. 31. Jossey Bass, San Francisco.
23. Halpern, M. (1971): Fatalities from narcotic addition in New York City. Incidence, circumstances and pathologic findings. *Hum. Pathol.,* 3:13.
24. Robins, L. (1977): Estimating addiction rates and locating target populations. In: *The Epidemiology of Heroin and Other Narcotics,* edited by J. D. Rittenhouse, p. 25. NIDA Research Monograph 16. U.S. Government Printing Office, Washington, D.C.
25. Calhalan, D., Cisin, I. H., and Crossley, H. M. (1969): American drinking practices: A national survey of drinking behavior and attitudes. Rutgers University Center, Alcohol Study Monograph No. 6, New Brunswick, New Jersey.
26. Berry, R. E., and Boland, J. P. (1975): *The Economic Cost of Alcohol Abuse.* New York Free Press, New York.
27. Baden, M. (1972): Alcoholism as related to drug addiction—A medical examiner's view. In: *Drug Abuse—Current Concepts and Research,* edited by W. Keup, p. 64. Charles C Thomas, Springfield, Illinois.
28. Robins, L. N., and Guze, S. B. (1976): Drinking practices and problems in urban ghetto populations. Presented at Recent Advances in Studies of Alcoholism, National Center for Prevention and Control of Alcoholism, National Institute of Mental Health, Washington, D.C.
29. Morbidity and Mortality Weekly Report (1977): Center for Disease Control, Atlanta, 26:160, 1977.
30. Pascarelli, E. F., and Fisher, W. (1974): Drug dependence in the elderly. *Int. J. Aging Hum. Dev.,* 5:347.
31. Swanson, D. W., Weddige, R. L., and Morse, R. M. (1973): Abuse of prescription drugs. *Mayo Clin. Proc.,* 48:359.
32. NIDA Services Research Report (1977): A study of legal drug use by older Americans. U.S. Dept. Health, Education and Welfare. U.S. Government Printing Office, Washington, D.C.
33. Lenhart, D. G. (1976): The use of medications in the elderly population. *Nurs. Clin. North Am.,* 11:135.
33a. Kane, R. L., and Kane, R. A. (1978): Care of the aged: Old problems in need of new solutions. *Science,* 200:913.
34. Schuckit, M. A. (1977): Geriatric alcoholism and drug abuse. *Geriontologist,* 17:168.
35. Schuckit, M. A., and Miller, P. L. (1975): Alcoholism in elderly men. A survey of a general medical ward. *Ann. N.Y. Acad. Sci.,* 273:558.
36. Simon, A. (1968): Alcoholism in the geriatric mentally ill. *Geriatrics,* 23:125.
37. Stearns, S., Schlesinger, M. D., and Rudy, A. (1967): Incidence and clinical significance of coronary artery disease in diabetes mellitus. *Arch. Intern. Med.,* 80:463.
38. Ahmed, S. S., Jaferi, G. A., Narang, R. M., et al. (1975): Preclinical abnormality of left ventricular function in diabetes mellitus. *Am. Heart J.,* 89:153.
39. Editorial (1978): Cardiac deaths in diabetes *Lancet,* 2:1241.
40. Bradley, R. F. (1970): Cardiovascular disease. In: *Joslin's Diabetes Mellitus,* edited by A. Marble, P. White, R. Bradley, et al., p. 417. Philadelphia, Pennsylvania.
41. Jenkins, D. W., Eckel, R. E., and Craig, U. W. (1971): Alcoholic ketoacidosis. *JAMA,* 217:177.
42. Davidson, M. B., Bozarth, W. R., Challoner, D. R., et al. (1966): Phenformin, hypoglycemia and lactic acidosis. *N. Engl. J. Med.,* 275:886.
43. Kreisberg, R. A., Owen, W. C., and Siegal, A. M. (1972): Hyperlacticacidemia in man: Ethanol phenformin synergism. *J. Clin. Endocrinol.,* 34:29.
44. Kater, R. M. H., Roggin, G., Tobon, F., et al. (1969): Increased rate of clearance of drugs from the circulation of alcoholics. *Am. J. Med. Sci.,* 258:35.
45. Fitzgerald, M. G., Gaddie, R., Malins, J. M., et al. (1962): Alcohol sensitivity in diabetics receiving chlorpropamide. *Diabetes,* 11:40.
46. Rubler, S., Sajadi, R. M., Araoye, M. A., et al (1978): Noninvasive estimation of myocardial performance in patients with diabetes. *Diabetes,* 27:127.

47. Sirtori, C., Hurwitz, A., and Azarnoff, D. L. (1971): Hyperinsulinemia secondary to chronic administration of mazindol and d amphetamine. *Am. J. Med. Sci.,* 261:341.
48. Jankelson, O. M., Beaser, S. B., Howard, F. M., et al. (1967): Effect of coffee on glucose tolerance and circulating insulin. *Lancet,* 1:527.
49. Van Der Velde, C. D., and Gordon, M. W. (1969): Manic depressive illness, diabetes mellitus and lithium carbonate. *Arch. Gen. Psychiatry,* 21:478.
50. Podolsky, S., Pattavina, C. G., and Amaral, M. A. (1971): Effect of marijuana on the glucose tolerance test. *Ann. N.Y. Acad. Sci.,* 191:54.
51. Adnitt, P. I. (1968): Hypoglycemic action of monoamine oxidase inhibitors (MAOI's). *Diabetes,* 17:628.
52. Korenyi, C., and Lowenstein, B. (1968): Chlorpromazine induced diabetes. *Dis. Nerv. Syst.,* 29:827.
53. Arneson, G. A. (1964): Phenothiazine derivatives and glucose metabolism. *J. Neuropsychiatry,* 5:181.
54. Wiederholt, I. C., Genco, M., and Foley, J. M. (1967): Recurrent episodes of hypoglycemia induced by propoxyphene. *Neurology,* 17:703.
55. Connell, D. H. (1966): Clinical manifestations and treatment of amphetamine dependence. *JAMA,* 196:718.
56. Smith, S., and Blackly, P. (1966): Amphetamine usage by medical students. *J. Med. Educ.,* 41:167.
57. Edison, G. R. (1971): Amphetamines: A dangerous illusion. *Ann. Intern. Med.,* 74:605.
58. American Medical Association Committee on Alcoholism and Addiction Council of Mental Health. *JAMA,* 193:673.
59. Cooper, J. R. (1977): *Sedative-Hypnotic Drugs: Risks and Benefits.* National Institute on Drug Abuse. U.S. Dept. of Health, Education and Welfare, pp. 65, 78, 80.
60. Blackwell, B. (1973): Psychotropic drugs in use today. The role of diazepam in medical practice. *JAMA,* 225:1637.
61. Swazey, J. P. (1974): Chlorpromazine in psychiatry. A study of therapeutic innovation. MIT Press, Cambridge, Massachusetts.
62. National Disease and Therapeutic Disease Index: Listing for October 1973, September 1974. IMS America, Ambler, Pennsylvania.
63. Cooper, J. R. (1977): *Sedative-Hypnotic Drugs: Risks and Benefits.* National Institute on Drug Abuse, U.S. Dept. of Health, Education and Welfare, pp. 78–592.
64. National Disease and Therapeutic Index Specialty Profile: Internal Medicine 1974. IMS America, Ambler, Pennsylvania.
65. Cooperstock, R. (1976): Psychotropic drug use in women. *Can. Med. Assoc. J.,* 115:760.
66. Sapira, J. D. (1978): Contemporary use of disease concept. *JAMA,* 239:1634.
67. Reasons, G., and Goodman, M. (1978): California's new drug pushers. A series of articles reprinted from the Los Angeles Times, March, 1978. Los Angeles Times, Los Angeles.

Chapter 2

Pharmacologic Considerations

CLASSIFICATION

Although the use of mood-altering substances can be traced to antiquity, only in modern times has an attempt been made to logically classify these drugs to better understand their actions. Over the years, several schemata of varying degrees of complexity have been formulated. The simplest, most frequently used by the public is a division of these agents into licit or illicit. With this categorization, a relationship is perceived to exist between illicit agents and the severity of the social, psychologic, and medical effects associated with their use. In reality, however, the complications observed are usually due not to the pharmacologic action of the drug but rather to the impurities associated with formulation of the "street" product and inappropriate techniques of administration. This results in adulteration, contamination, and inappropriate consumption, frequently followed by the appearance of adverse effects. Since the terms illicit and licit are more appropriate to a moral rather than a scientific arena, their value is quite limited, restricted mainly to enforcers of public policy.

Another classification separates mood-altering substances into those (a) consumed so frequently as to be considered nonmedications (coffee, tea, alcohol, and nicotine), (b) purchased as over-the-counter (OTC) agents, generally considered to have little or no adverse effects; (c) requiring a physician's prescription and thereby recognized to be more potent, and (d) associated with such severe adverse effects to be prohibited by society and available only through illicit channels. This division is also of little value. Frequently, those drugs considered "nonmedications" are associated with as many or more adverse effects than those requiring prescriptions.

Potential for Dependence

A more scientific categorization defines mood-altering substances as addicting or nonaddicting. The confusion associated with these terms leaves much to be desired as scientific, legal, and popular definitions of addiction and dependence differ considerably. In 1967, the Expert Committee on Addiction Producing Drugs of the World Health Organization (1), in an attempt to provide a uniformity of terms, recommended that the term dependence be substituted for addiction.

Dependence is an adaptive state characterized by behavioral and other physiologic responses, including (a) a compulsion to continually take a drug to experience its pleasurable effects and/or to prevent withdrawal symptoms, and (b) the appearance of disturbances (withdrawal symptoms) when the drug is discontinued abruptly. Dependence may be physical or psychologic, or both. Physical dependence occurs as a consequence of exposure to a drug, resulting in physiologic changes that necessitate the continued presence of the drug to maintain normal function. Psychologic dependence may be associated with a similar requirement of drug presence, but there are no objective homeostatic changes upon discontinuing the agent, the changes observed being subjective rather than objective. Tolerance often associated with dependence is a state of decreased responsiveness to the pharmacologic effect of a drug that has been chronically administered. This is manifested by the need to increase the dose of a drug over time to sustain its initial effects. Dependence can exist in the absence of tolerance, and tolerance may vary considerably within wide limits.

All mood-altering drugs by definition are consumed by individuals to lessen anxiety and produce pleasurable effects. Since such effects produce positive reinforcement, all psychotropic agents may to some extent produce dependency (Table 1). Different drugs, however, exhibit the features of dependence to varying degrees. Alcohol, barbiturates, most nonbarbiturate hypnotics and sedatives, and narcotics are associated with the components of dependence to such a marked degree as to severely impair individual functioning with excessive chronic use.

Amphetamines and some of the more potent hallucinogens produce both

TABLE 1. *Types of dependence-producing drugs*[a]

Alcohol Sedative-hypnotic Minor tranquilizer	Includes barbiturates and other drugs with sedative effects, e.g., chloral hydrate, chlordiazepoxide, diazepam, meprobamate, methaqualone
Amphetamines	
Cannabis	Includes all preparations of *Cannabis sativa*
Cocaine group	Includes coca leaves
Hallucinogens	
Khat	Includes preparations of *Cathaedulis forssk*
Opiates and opioids	Includes narcotics with morphine-like effects
Volatile solvents	

[a] Adapted from ref. 21.

psychologic dependence and tolerance. Actual physical dependence, however, is usually not found or is minimal, and withdrawal from these drugs is associated with little or no physiologic syndromes. Milder stimulants, such as nicotine and caffeine, can produce a mild physical dependence, a mild degree of tolerance, and, not infrequently, a marked psychologic dependence, which can result in considerable discomfort and behavioral changes when these medications are withheld. Cocaine may be associated with a hypersensitivity in chronic users, a low degree of tolerance, and a mild physical dependence. A marked psychologic dependence, however, may exist.

Marijuana can be associated with a considerable degree of psychologic dependence with little tolerance and no physical dependence. The use of narcotic antagonists can result in tolerance and physical dependence that may vary in degree, depending on the ability of the drug to produce an agonist as well as an antagonist effect.

Site of Action on the Nervous System

Another useful classification categorizes mood-altering drugs in accordance with their pharmacologic similarities as well as their site of action on the nervous system (Table 2). This format can separate mood-altering drugs into two primary categories: (a) those exhibiting generalized central nervous system (CNS) effects, and (b) those with effects localized to specific brain areas. This scheme is more helpful than classification of general groups of agents as it can explain the predominant effect of a drug at conventional therapeutic levels. Barbiturates and phenothiazines, for example, both exert a depressant effect. Barbiturates, however, produce a generalized depression of the CNS, whereas phenothiazines and other major tranquilizers primarily

TABLE 2. *Classification of mood-altering drugs by site of action in the nervous system*

Generalized effects	Localized effects
CNS depressants	Affective centers
Alcohol	Antipsychotics
Barbiturates	Phenothiazines
Nonbarbiturate sedative-hypnotics	Butyrophenones
Benzodiazepines	Thioxanthenes
Anesthetics	Antidepressants
Volatile solvents	Tricyclics
Cannabinoids (low dose)	MAO inhibitors
CNS STIMULANTS	Psychotogenic
Amphetamines	Hallucinogens
Cocaine	Opioids and opioid antagonists
Caffeine	
Nicotine	

depress the limbic system, exerting a beneficial effect on psychologic functioning. Recognition of this explains why general CNS depressants carry a strong risk of associated respiratory depression, whereas this side-effect is unlikely with respect to the major tranquilizers. Autonomic effects of the phenothiazines, however, can be quite important and result in considerable hypotension.

The classification of mood-altering substances to be used in this text

TABLE 3. *Classification of mood-altering drugs affecting the cardiovascular system by function*

Alcohol
Sedative-hypnotics and minor tranquilizers
Barbiturates
Nonbarbiturate sedatives
Benzodiazepines
Major tranquilizers
Phenothiazines
Rauwolfia alkaloids
Butyrophenones
Thioxanthenes
Drugs used for affective disorders
Tricyclic antidepressants
Lithium carbonate
MAO inhibitors
Marijuana
Hallucinogenic agents
Narcotic analgesics and antagonists
Stimulants
Amphetamine
Cocaine
Methylphenidate
Caffeine
Nicotine

represents a combination of those previously described. Since the primary objective is to present to the practicing physician an organized discussion of the effects of these substances on the cardiovascular system, the basic classification is functional in accordance with current use (Table 3). A more detailed description of the pharmacology of each agent may be found in the appropriate chapters.

BIOAVAILABILITY

In evaluating the action of a drug on an organ system, it is important to determine whether the observed response is related to the drug or to other factors associated with its use. Bioavailability is the percentage of the active drug contained in a specific product that enters the circulation in an unchanged form after administration (2,3). Although in the laboratory setting the bioavailability of an active ingredient is primarily a function of its physiochemical properties, in the clinical setting bioavailability can be greatly modified by other factors, such as formulation of the drug product, individual patient characteristics, and concurrent administration of other substances.

Formulation of Drug Product

Bioavailability, secondary to formulation of the drug product, is greatest with respect to mood-altering agents purchased on the streets. Not only are the observed effects often determined by the nature of the contaminants in these substances rather than by the "pure" drug, but, in addition, there may frequently be a complete absence of the specific drug desired. The contents of a glassine bag of heroin, for example, may contain anywhere from 0 to 10% heroin as well as numerous adulterants (Chapter 12). An analysis of illict heroin seized on the West Coast showed 11 of 23 specimens to have no detectable narcotic agents. A larger series of 200 confiscated bags of heroin analyzed by the Medical Examiner's Office of the City of New York found 30 specimens to be completely free of narcotics, containing substances varying from baking powder to marijuana (4).

An analysis of street drugs by a large pharmaceutical laboratory revealed 23% of the samples identified as marijuana, 16% as stimulants, 35% as hallucinogens, and 55% as opiates to either not contain the substances requested by the purchaser or to be completely free of all mood-altering drugs (5). Of the total of 1,833 specimens analyzed, 360 (20%) did not contain the alleged drug but a combination of other agents, and 96 (5%) contained no psychoactive ingredients whatsoever.

A somewhat better estimate of bioavailability can be obtained with the commonly ingested mood-altering substances, such as coffee, tea, alcohol, and nicotine. The settings in which these substances are used, however, are far from conducive to assessing the amount of drug reaching the circulation

TABLE 4. *Cardiac medications with statistically significant differences in bioavailability*[a]

Bishydroxycoumarin
Diazoxide
Digoxin
Diphenylhydantoin
Hydrochlorthiazide
Spironolactone
Theophylline
Triamterene
Warfarin

[a] Adapted from ref. 3.

TABLE 5. *Cardiac medications exhibiting clinically important differences in bioavailability*[a]

Bishydroxycoumarin
Digoxin
Diphenylhydantoin
Theophylline preparations

[a] Adapted from ref. 3.

The caffeine concentration of coffee and tea has been shown to vary considerably, depending on potency of brew (Chapter 14). Similarly, the amount of alcohol absorbed from a cocktail is dependent on the amount of alcohol used as well as the dexterity of the specific bartender.

Complete control with respect to bioavailability is only possible at the level of pharmaceutical formulation. Yet even in such instances, variations in bioavailability can exist because of the physical state of the actual drug, the presence of an active excipient, the degree of pressure used in tablet fabrication, and the rate at which the drug enters into solution, which in turn influences its absorption (3). It is not surprising, therefore, that most studies of comparative bioavailability reveal statistically significant differences in many cardiovascular drugs (Table 4). Fortunately, the clinical relevance of these differences in most instances is rather small, because statistically significant differences in bioavailability of 10% or less would be unlikely to influence the therapeutic outcome (Table 5) (2). Although a number of drugs have been shown to have their clinical therapeutic effectiveness altered by formulation factors, there is little evidence that any important differences in therapeutic effectiveness exist with the commonly prescribed mood-altering drugs.

Effect of Aging

Exclusive of the manufacturing process, bioavailability will also vary depending on the route of administration, absorption, distribution, metabo-

TABLE 6. *Factors influencing bioavailability of mood-altering agents*[a]

Formulation of drug product
Purity
Presence of excipients
Characteristics of drug
Inactivation prior to absorption
Incomplete absorption
Biotransformation prior to reaching general circulation
Interaction with other substances in gastrointestinal tract
Patient characteristics
Age
Gastrointestinal alterations in pH motility, flora, and perfusion
Preexisting disease states
Hepatic dysfunction
Poor vascular perfusion
Genetic Factors

[a] Modified from ref. 2.

lism, biotransformation, and excretion of a particular agent (Table 6). All these factors may in turn be greatly influenced by individual variation. Bioavailability has been found to differ in the same person from one time to another or on successive days. The age of the subject may also be important. In the laboratory setting, reduced microsomal enzyme activity and impaired enzyme induction have been demonstrated in aging mice (6,7). Clinically, it is well recognized that children and infants are more sensitive to drug effects than adults (8). Conversely, elderly patients have frequently been shown to exhibit an altered response to different drugs related to alterations in absorption distribution, biotransformation, and elimination that occur with the aging process (9,10).

Age has been associated with elevated plasma levels of amobarbital (11), diazepam (12), as well as other drugs. Evidence suggests that these differences may be of clinical relevance. Greenblatt et al. (13), in a review of adverse reactions to flurazepam amoung 2,542 hospitalized patients taking this drug, found toxicity to increase with age, being 1.9% in those under age 60 and 7.1% in those over 80 ($p < 0.001$). Although the incidence of toxicity was dose related, the prominence of untoward effects in the aged was noted at all doses. The overall incidence of toxicity was 12.3% at daily doses of 30 mg or more flurazepam but was 39% in patients over age 70 receiving this dose. An increased drug effect in elderly persons taking nitrazepam was also found by Linnoila and Viukari (14).

These changes may be due to age-associated impaired enzyme activity or differences in the initial space of distribution. Even if body weight remains constant, cell mass and body fluid appear to decrease at a constant rate associated with a proportional decrease in the volume of distribution of drugs. Exogenous age-related factors may also exert a confounding influence.

TABLE 7. *Adverse mood-altering drug effects in underlying diseases frequently present in the elderly*[a]

Disease State	Drug	Effect
Asymptomatic organic brain disease	Atropine	Can precipitate confusional episodes
Cerebrovascular disease	Sedatives and tranquilizers	Can precipitate urinary incontinence and syncope
	Antidepressants	Syncope
	Chlorpromazine	Syncope
Organic dementia	Barbiturates and opiates	Confusion at times accompanied by auditory or visual hallucinations

[a] Modified from ref. 2.

Smoking and coffee consumption can significantly affect metabolic clearance rate and are usually of lesser prevalence in the elderly (15). In addition, problems with patient compliance, more specifically, difficulty in taking medications as prescribed, may be more prominent in the elderly, resulting in a greater tendency toward adverse drug reactions. Regardless of the reasons for untoward drug effects in the elderly, the frequency of underlying disease and the prescription of multiple medications in this population, most commonly involving drugs affecting the cardiovascular system and the CNS, mandates a working knowledge on the part of the physician of basic principles of pharmacokinetics and drug interactions (Table 7).

Presence of Disease

Preexisting disease states also affect bioavailability. The degree of biotransformation of a drug metabolized in the liver may be affected by the presence of hepatic disease, with subsequent decrease in hepatic function and portal blood flow. Patients with cirrhosis have been shown to have a more than twofold prolongation in half-life of diazepam (12). Similarly, disease of the cardiovascular system, resulting in a decrease in flow, may affect not only absorption but also metabolism of certain drug products.

Genetic Factors

Genetic factors may also influence bioavailability. The rate of activation of drugs metabolized in the liver, such as the acetylation of isoniazid and hydralazine, is known to be genetically determined. Since psychotropic drugs are specifically sought or prescribed solely for their mood-altering effects, it is entirely possible that the actions of these drugs with respect to mood may also be influenced by individual genetic variations. The majority of people consuming alcohol or caffeine do so in moderation, without the development of dependence. Recent evidence suggests that genetic factors may indeed play a role in the production of such dependency (16,17).

PHARMACOKINETICS AND DRUG INTERACTIONS

Assuming an acceptable level of bioequivalence among generically equivalent drugs, the actual biologic effect of a drug can be modified by its absorption, distribution, extent of binding in tissues, metabolism, and excretion (Fig. 1). These properties constitute the pharmacokinetics of drug action, as contrasted to pharmacodynamics, which describes the physiologic and biochemical effects of a particular drug. The pharmacokinetics of a drug may be influenced by similar factors affecting bioavailability and by concomitant use of other drugs. Drug interactions are especially relevant when describing the effects of mood-altering drugs on the cardiovascular system, as these medications are frequently prescribed to persons with cardiac disease or to the elderly in whom consumption of multiple medications is quite

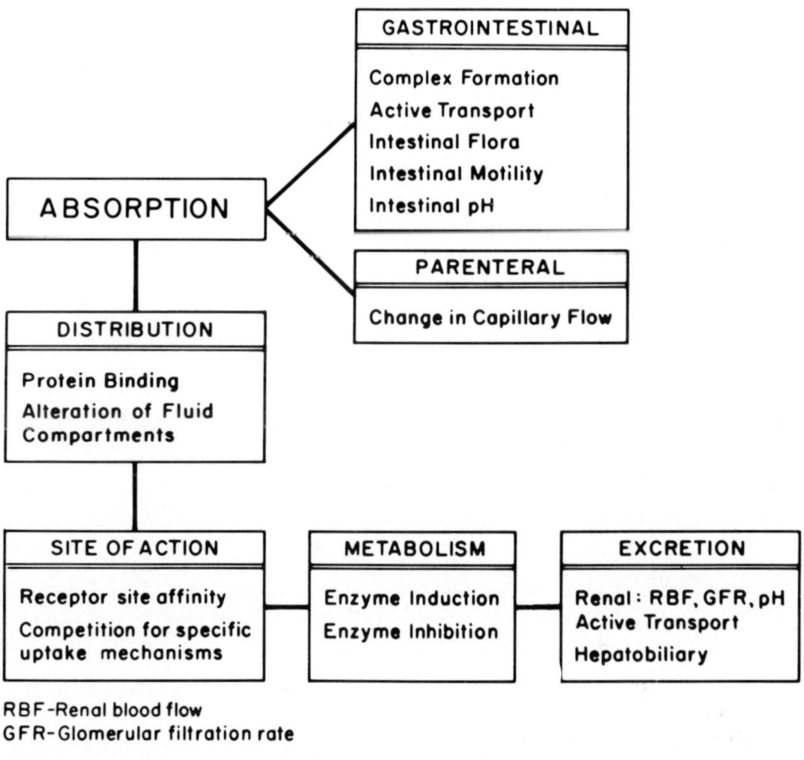

FIG. 1. Basic mechanisms of drug interactions. RBF, renal blood flow; GFR, glomular filtration rate.

prevalent (Chapter 1). Unfortunately, such medication may sometimes be dispensed without adequate consideration of the interactions that may ensue.

Although it is not the purpose of this chapter to provide a comprehensive discussion of pharmacokinetics or drug interactions, it is important to briefly review the factors that may modify the effects of a drug. Sections describing clinically relevant pharmacokinetic interactions between specific mood-altering substances and cardiac medications can be found in each of the subsequent chapters.

Absorption

Absorption of a particular drug after oral administration is dependent on many variables, including its physiochemical properties, degree of aqueous solubility, rate of dissolution, and concentration at and circulation to the absorptive site. Absorption may also be affected in several ways by simultaneous administration of a second drug. The presence of another drug may result in complexing of the two substances in the gastrointestinal tract, with a subsequent diminished absorption and corresponding lower blood level of both agents. This is commonly seen with combined use of divalent cations, such as aluminum or magnesium in antacids and the tetracyclines. When active transport of a substance is required across the intestinal wall, inhibition of the necessary enzymes may result in decreased absorption (17).

Intestinal flora normally present in the gut may also affect the bioavailability of a drug with coadministration of an antibiotic, resulting in either increased or decreased absorption, depending on the medication involved. Medications affecting gastric emptying or intestinal motility may influence absorption of other pharmacologic agents through effects on solubility and/or dissolution rate (18).

Changes in intestinal pH may result in enhanced or diminished absorption by altering the ionization of a drug. Nonionized drugs are lipid soluble and tend to be more rapidly absorbed through the lipoprotein membrane of cells lining the gastrointestinal tract than ionized agents. For example, medications poorly ionized at the pH of gastric fluid with good absorption rates have their absorption diminished by the consumption of antacids, which elevate intraluminal pH. A rise of pH can also result in delayed gastric emptying, with a subsequent alteration in the absorption rate of a second agent, the direction of change depending on whether the site of absorption is in the stomach or duodenum.

Surfactants, such as sorbitol, may facilitate absorption of another drug through increasing its solubility, allowing a greater amount to be available for passage through intestinal mucosa.

Parenteral administration of mood-altering drugs and vasoactive medications, such as epinephrine or methylcholine, results in an altered absorption from subcutaneous or intramuscular reservoirs secondary to vasoconstriction.

Distribution

Once absorption has occurred, the distribution of the drug within the body becomes important. Initial distribution is dependent on cardiac output, regional blood flow, and the specific physiochemical properties of the drug. Drugs that have a high degree of lipid solubility will rapidly transverse cell membranes. Tissue accumulation is dependent on the active transport and extent of binding of a drug and its solubility in fat. Considerable tissue accumulation will result in a prolongation of the effect of the drug.

Protein Binding

Although attachment of drugs to any of the constituents of blood may occur, most agents are variably bound to plasma protein (usually albumin), with the unbound portion responsible for activity. There are many charged sites on the albumin molecule that could theoretically function as receptors for appropriate agents. Practically, however, there are only one or two primary binding sites available for any specific agent. Koch-Weser and Sellers (19) have emphasized that when assessing the importance of percentage of drug bound to serum albumin, knowledge of the concentration of both the drug and of serum albumin is essential. Individual variation in binding affinity of drug with albumin related to age, body temperature, pH, and ionic strength also exists.

Binding of drugs to plasma albumin is nonselective. Competition of drugs for similar binding sites can therefore be quite important, even if the degree of displacement is minimal. The clinical actions of drugs highly bound to albumin are dependent on the serum concentration of free drug. As an example, when digitoxin, which is 98% bound and 2% free, is used with a second drug that displaces only 10% of bound digitoxin, a sixfold increase of free digitoxin results (2 to 12%), with probable adverse clinical effects (17,19). Such reactions are especially important when the margin between the clinical therapeutic and toxic effects of the drug is small or when hepatic or renal dysfunction exists and the ability to metabolize and clear the drug from the circulation is diminished. In most instances, this type of interaction involves highly bound acidic rather than neutral or basic drugs (Table 8). Cardiovascular agents that are highly bound to albumin include bishydroxycoumarin, clofibrate, diazoxide, digitoxin, diphenylhydantoin, chlorothiazide, furosemide, ethacrynic acid, hydralazine, quinidine, trichlormethiazide, and warfarin (19). Mood-altering drugs exhibiting a high degree of plasma protein binding include some of the barbiturates, chloralhydrate, the phenothiazines, some of the tricyclic antidepressants and their active metabolites, and diazepam. Concomitant use of agents from each group may result in clinically important drug interactions.

TABLE 8. *Drugs exhibiting a high affinity for serum albumin*

Cardiovascular drugs	Mood-altering drugs
Bishydroxycoumarin	Barbiturates[a]
Chlorothiazide	
Clofibrate	Chloral hydrate
Diazoxide	Diazepam
Digitoxin	Phenothiazines
Diphenylhydantoin	Tricyclic antidepressants[a]
Ethacrynic acid	
Furosemide	
Hydralazine	
Quinidine	
Trichlormethiazide	
Warfarin	

[a] A high degree of protein binding exists for some, but not all, agents in these groups.

Cellular Reservoirs

Distribution of drugs may also be affected through accumulation in cellular reservoirs or by storage in physical solution in fatty tissue. Redistribution of a drug to these reservoirs may considerably alter the duration of clinical effect by a more rapid removal from the primary receptor site.

Receptor Sites

The observed response to a drug can be influenced through a pharmacokinetic interaction that alters the affinity of its receptor site. An example of this can be seen in the quinidine-coumarin interaction. Quinidine enhances the affinity of receptor sites to coumarin, thereby decreasing its anticoagulant effect (20).

Fluid Compartments

Drugs that alter the fluid compartments can either enhance the effect of another drug through increasing the concentration of the latter or, as in the case of diuretics, may result in an increased excretion of substances normally passively reabsorbed by renal tubules (17). Agents that selectively affect blood flow may also alter the action of another drug, thereby increasing or decreasing the potential for toxicity.

Metabolism

Many drugs are metabolized in the liver through the microsomal ethanol-oxidizing system (MEOS). Other hepatic enzyme systems also participate in biotransformation or metabolism, as do other tissues. The hepatic MEOS is located in the endoplasmic reticulum and catalyzes glucuronide conjugation and oxidation of most drugs, especially those with a high degree of lipid solubility. Biotransformation through hydrolysis or reduction may occur in the MEOS, as well as in non-MEOS.

Activity of the MEOS can be influenced by many drugs and varies greatly among individuals, depending on genetic factors. Susceptibility to induction also exhibits a good deal of individual variability. Chronic administration of a drug may induce its own metabolism as well as that of other agents. This can be seen most prominently with the barbiturates and some nonbarbiturate hypnotics (21). This system may also be induced by drugs not normally metabolized through this pathway. An example of this is alcohol, which has a dual effect on the MEOS. Acute administration will result in an enzyme inhibition, whereas chronic ethanol intake will stimulate enzyme induction (see Chapter 4).

Interference with biotransformation of a drug by another drug is a common clinical phenomenon. Drugs may compete for sites for degradation on the endoplasmic reticulum. Enzyme induction of microsomal enzymes, on the other hand, causes an acceleration of drug metabolism, a decrease in plasma level, and a subsequent diminished therapeutic effect and diminished potential for toxicity (21). Correspondingly, interference with drug metabolism through enzyme inhibition will prolong the action of an agent or increase its therapeutic effect. Persistence of this inhibition may require the continued presence of the inhibiting drug or may persist after the drug is discontinued until a new enzyme has been synthesized.

Competition for binding sites on the albumin molecule may also enhance hepatic metabolism of a drug. Entry into the hepatocyte through simple diffusion is prevented by albumin binding. Availability of the drug for hepatic biotransformation is therefore increased with increased displacement from binding sites. This would not be true for drugs concentrated in the hepatic cell by active transport, as dissociation from albumin would occur in proportion to a decreased free-drug concentration (17).

Excretion

Drugs filtered at the glomerulus and passively reabsorbed through different concentration gradients may be affected by alterations in glomerular filtration rate, renal blood flow, and avidity of binding to serum albumin. Negligible amounts of albumin pass through the normal glomerulus. Only the free portion of the drug is readily filtered, with the rate of glomerular filtration proportional to the extent of albumin binding (19). Pharmacologic interactions may occur during excretion of drugs or their metabolites from the body. Tubular secretion may also play a prominent role in the excretory process. Displacement of one drug from its binding site by another agent may facilitate excretion of the former with an attendant diminished duration of clinical effect. Alteration of urinary pH affects drug clearance in a manner similar to that described in absorption from the intestinal tract. An agent that causes urine alkalinization results in an increased ionization of acidic drugs, with a diminished reabsorption of such agents from the urine. Conversely, basic agents in an alkaline urine will have a diminished renal clearance. Competition among agents for identical transport systems can slow tubular secretory mechanisms with subsequent lengthening of half-lives.

If hepatobiliary elimination is an important route of excretion, drugs that affect biliary action can cause impressive changes in pharmacologic activity.

REFERENCES

1. World Health Organization Expert Committee on Addiction Producing Drugs (1967): WHO Tech. Rep. Series No. 407, p. 6.
2. Koch-Weser, J. (1974): Bioavailability of drugs I. *N. Engl. J. Med.,* 291:233.
3. Koch-Weser, J. (1974): Bioavailability of drugs II. *N. Engl. J. Med.,* 291:503.
4. Stimmel, B. (editor) (1975): Getting off and coming down. In: *Heroin Dependency,* pp. 98–111. Stratton, New York.
5. The Pharm Chem Newsletter (1975): Summary of street drug results. Palo Alto, California, 1974, 4(4).
6. Kato, R., Takanata, A., and Onoda, K. I. (1970): Studies on age difference in mice for the activity of drug metabolizing enzymes of liver microsomes. *Jpn. J. Pharmacol.,* 20:572.
7. Adelman, R. C. (1971): Age dependent effects in enzyme induction—A biochemical expression of aging. *Exp. Gerontol.,* 6:75.
8. Brown, A. K., and Zuelzer, W. W. (1958): Studies on the neonatal development of the glucuronide conjugating system. *J. Clin. Invest.,* 37:332.
9. Bender, A. D. (1966): Pharmacologic aspects of aging. A survey of the effect of increasing age on drug activity in adults. *J. Am. Geriatr. Soc.,* 12:114.
10. Triggs, E. J., and Nation, R. L. (1975): Pharmacokinetics in the aged. A review. *J. Pharmacokinet. Biopharm.,* 3:387.
11. Irvine, R. E., Grove, J., Toseland, P. A., et al. (1974): The effect of age on the hydroxylation of amylobarbitone sodium in man. *Br. J. Clin. Pharmacol.,* 1:41.
12. Klotz, U., Avant, G. R., Hoyumpa, et al. (1975): The effects of age and liver disease on the disposition of diazepam in adult man. *J. Clin. Invest.,* 55:347.
13. Greenblatt, D. J., Allen, M. D., and Shader, R. I. (1977): Toxicity of high dose flurazepam in the elderly. *Clin. Pharmacol. Ther.,* 21:355.
14. Linnoila, M., and Viukari, M. (1976): Efficacy and side effects of nitrazepam and trioridazine as sleeping aids for psychogeriatric in-patients. *Br. J. Psychiatry,* 128:566.
15. Vestal, R. E., Norris, A. H., Tobin, J. D., et al. (1975): Antipyrine metabolism in man. Influence of age, alcohol, caffeine and smoking. *Clin. Pharmacol. Ther.,* 18:425.
16. Contevio, F., and Chiarelli, B. (1962): Study of the inheritance of some daily life habits. *Hereditary,* 17:347.
17. Wolff, P. H. (1972): Ethnic differences in alcohol sensitivity. *Science,* 175:449.
18. Prescott, L. (1969): Pharmacologic drug interactions. *Lancet,* 2:1239.
19. Koch-Weser, J., and Sellers, E. M. (1976): Binding of drugs to serum albumin. *N. Engl. J. Med.,* 294:311.
20. Deykin, D. (1970): Warfarin therapy. *N. Engl. J. Med.,* 283:801.
21. Kosman, M. E. (1974): Pharmacokinetic drug interactions. Sedative, hypnotic and antianxiety agents. *JAMA,* 229:1485.
22. World Health Organization Expert Committee on Drug Dependence (1973): WHO Tech. Rep. Series No. 526.
23. Davison, W. (1976): Unwanted drug effects. In: *Rrug-induced Diseases,* edited by L. Meyer and H. M. Peck. Excerpta Media, Amsterdam.

Chapter 3

Anxiety, Stress, and Cardiovascular Disease

It is apparent that mood-altering drugs, whether prescribed or self-administered, are usually taken to relieve anxiety or to produce a euphoric state. The chapters that follow describe in some detail the effects that these drugs may have on the cardiovascular system. Prior to considering the potential cardiac toxicity of these agents, it is important to assess the effects that psychologic stress, in the absence of any therapeutic interventions, might have on the heart and vasculature.

If anxiety or persistent stress can adversely effect the heart, then the use of psychotropic drugs may mitigate or even eliminate risks associated with undue anxiety. Conversely, if the anxiety is not totally relieved, an interaction may occur between the physiologic changes induced by these drugs and those seen under stress, resulting in an adverse clinical response. A knowledge of the physiologic response to stress and the corresponding effects on the cardiovascular system is therefore of considerable relevance.

Decades ago, Selye (1), in a letter to the editor of *Nature,* emphasized to the scientific community the importance of stress in producing disease. Since that time, more than 100,000 publications have evolved dealing with the role of stress in both health and disease (2). These studies firmly established that both physical and emotional stress can sufficiently upset homeostasis, adversely effecting many organ systems, including the heart and blood vessels.

STRESS IN THE LABORATORY SETTING

The response of the organism to stress is marked by a sympathetic adrenergic discharge of catecholamines accompanied by a release of ACTH and corticoids. This elevation in plasma catecholamines increases myocardial oxygen consumption and oxygen wasting, resulting in a diminished myocardial efficiency and myocardial hypoxia (3). There is a rise in plasma cholesterol levels, lipoproteins, triglycerides, and free fatty acids (FFA). The hyperlipidemia may affect deposition of triglycerides and cholesterol in vessel walls, resulting in an increased rate of atheroma formation. The elevation in circulating FFA is also associated with an enhancement of platelet stickiness, which in turn can induce intravascular platelet aggregation with subsequent atheroma and thrombus formation (2,4). It has been suggested that the elevation in FFA may also exert an irritative effect on the vessel wall associated with subendothelial hemorrhages and small mural thrombi (5).

Hypertension

In rats chronically stressed on high sodium diets, malignant hypertension with hyalinizing cardiovascular and renal disease develop (6). This effect is most marked after unilateral nephrectomy, a procedure that alone can induce such lesions. The changes observed are considered to result from an interference in the feedback mechanism between aldosterone and the renin-angiotensin system. The stress-induced increase in catecholamine secretion is also associated with a vasoactive pressor response, which can occur even in adrenalectomied animals. Such effects are transient, however, and alone they rarely lead to sustained hypertension. Epinephrine and norepinephrine can potentiate the effects of increased corticosteroid production and, therefore, may play a synergestic role in the production of hypertensive disease.

Myocardial Dysfunction

Cardiomyopathies associated with myocardial necrosis can be produced experimentally by the administration of steroids in combination with a high sodium diet or sudden exposure to stress (7,8). Davidson (9) observed that noise stress administered to cardiomyopathic rats resulted in sudden death in 2 to 6% of these animals. The administration of antidepressants to the rats in a basal state was not associated with any additional adverse effects. When these animals were subjected to standard noise stress and then given tricyclic antidepressants, a sudden increase in unexpected deaths occurred, with 79% of animals succumbing, usually secondary to the onset of ventricular fibrillation.

In control noncardiomyopathic rats given tricyclic antidepressants and then subjected to noise stress, no deaths occurred. The onset of ventricular fibrillation in the cardiomyopathic rats could be blocked most effectively by concurrent treatment with propranolol. This was associated with a decrease in mortality from 70 to 90% to 2 to 10%. Similar protective effects, although of a lesser magnitude, were also achieved with sodium pentobarbital, phenothiazines, and diazepam. These findings suggest that arrhythmia formation in experimental cardiomyopathies may be enhanced by the use of mood-altering drugs when administered in the continued presence of stress.

Electrocardiographic Alterations

The vulnerable period threshold for ventricular fibrillation has been shown to be lowered in the normal laboratory animal exposed to stress (10). This is considered to be secondary to an enhancement in sympathetic activity predisposing to ventricular fibrillation. An increase in parasympathetic tone conversely has been shown to have a protective affect against ventricular fibrillation, especially in the presence of augmented sympathetic activity (11,12). DeSilva et al. (13) found the threshold at which repetitive extra systoles (RES) occur to be reduced by 45% in dogs in an adversive compared to a nonadversive environment. Reduction in threshold was accompanied by a significantly greater elevation in heart rate and blood pressure. The administration of morphine sulfate in the adversive environment resulted in a significant elevation of RES threshold, whereas no effect on this threshold was noted subsequent to morphine administration in the nonadversive setting. Elimination of sympathetic activity with beta-adrenergic blockade is accompanied by variable changes in vulnerability to vagal stimulation although sympathectomy in dogs can elevate the ventricular fibrillation threshold protecting against ventricular fibrillation. Cholinergic blockage with atropine can interfere with the protective influence of morphine on the RES threshold in the adversive state (12), suggesting that the protective influence of increased vagal activity is predetermined by the prevailing level of sympathetic tone.

CLINICAL STUDIES

Although the adverse cardiovascular effects induced by stress in the laboratory setting are impressive, it must be remembered that these data cannot easily be extrapolated to humans. Numerous publications, however, have described the clinical effects of stress in normal individuals, as well as in those with cardiovascular disease. The discussion that follows is a summary of these findings rather than an exhaustive review. The interested reader is referred to the bibliography at the end of the chapter.

Metabolic Response to Stress

It is well known that stressful situations, whether physical or emotional, are associated with a rise in blood pressure, pulse rate, and cardiac output. These findings have been consistently demonstrated to be associated with an increased excretion of both catecholamines and 11-hydroxycorticosteroids, as well as an elevation in plasma levels of FFA, triglycerides, and cholesterol (14–16). Taggart and Carruthers (17), measuring these biochemical alterations in racing car drivers at various times within a 3-hr period following a race, found the increase of plasma catecholamines and FFA concentrations to coincide at the exact time of maximal stress. The rise in triglycerides, however, was delayed, suggesting a conversion of FFA to triglyceride.

Several investigators have suggested that the actual emotions evidenced in a stress situation may be related to the ratio of epinephrine and norepinephrine produced (18). Funkenstein et al. (19) proposed that norepinephrine release is associated mainly with anxiety and fear. Ax (20) also described subjects exhibiting fear to show physiologic responses resembling those seen with epinephrine injection, whereas persons exhibiting anger respond in a manner compatible with a combination of epinephrine-norepinephrine release (21,22). This response to catecholamine excretion has been found to be more marked in hypertensives than in normals, although the resting level of catecholamines may be essentially the same in both groups (23). An exaggerated response can also be seen in patients with other cardiac diseases (2).

Alterations in Hemostasis

Clinical alterations in hemostasis similar to those seen in the laboratory setting have also been observed in stress states. Friedman et al. (24), in reviewing the clotting time in groups of accountants subjected to various stresses, found that a marked acceleration in blood clotting time consistently occurred during severe occupational stress, returning to normal during periods of relative relaxation. Gordon et al. (25) found stressful procedures, such as cardiac catheterization in conscious patients, to be associated with a rise in platelet aggregation in response to an increase in ADP levels. Levites and Haft (26) similarly noted exercise to induce platelet aggregation.

Electrocardiographic Alterations

Repolarization Abnormalities

The elevation in circulating catecholamines induced by stress may also adversely affect the electrocardiogram (ECG). Froberg et al. (27) recorded

ECG changes in Swedish officers deprived of sleep for up to 75 hr. In these individuals, ST segment depression was common, requiring several days of rest for the patterns to return toward normal. Studies of workers exposed to industrial medium-frequency and high-frequency noise found them to exhibit bradycardias with intraventricular conduction disturbances and T-wave depressions, most frequently seen at the end of the work day (28). Taggart et al. (29,30) reviewed ECGs taken from experienced bus drivers in busy city traffic. This study involved 32 normal individuals and 24 with coronary heart disease. In both groups of patients, there were periods of increased heart rates exceeding 140/min. ST segment changes unrelated to tachycardia developed in three of 32 normal individuals and 13 of 24 coronary heart disease patients. In the coronary group, these changes were associated with T-wave changes, which in several patients were of sufficient magnitude to be of clinical concern. Similar findings were reported by Bellet et al. (14), who reviewed electrocardiographic changes after 2 hr of automobile driving in patients with coronary heart disease.

Stress has also been shown to prolong the QT interval (31). Congenital QT prolongation is known to be associated with sudden death secondary to ventricular fibrillation. There are, however, many asymptomatic persons with acquired QT prolongation. Stress situations may precipitate various arrhythmias in such persons. Even in the absence of documented prolongation of the QT interval, cases of psychogenic ventricular tachycardia have appeared in the literature (32). In most instances, the arrhythmias were paroxysmal tachycardias appearing in persons with structurally normal hearts subjected to emotional pressures. The specific type of arrhythmia reported ranged from relatively mild supraventricular tachycardias to heart block and ventricular tachycardia, sometimes ending in death. Precipitating factors have included violent arguments, strenuous exertions, or other severe emotional stresses (33,34).

Alterations in Rhythm

Psychologic stress has long been believed to produce alterations in cardiac rhythm in both healthy people and in those with preexisting cardiac disease. Fatal ventricular arrhythmias are commonly invoked as the mode of exodus in the "frightened to death" syndrome, which has appeared over the centuries in all cultures (33–35).

ECG monitoring of individuals speaking publicly has shown the appearance of more than six ventricular ectopic beats per minute in six of 23 healthy persons and considerably more ectopy in five of seven with coronary heart disease (36). Naturally occurring, unrecognized environmental stress may also induce arrhythmias in persons with preexisting coronary artery disease. Taggart et al. (29), monitoring heart rate in 24 persons with coronary heart disease when they were driving their car along a familiar route, noted multiple ventricular ectopic beats in five people (20%).

Psychologic stress induced in the laboratory setting has been demonstrated to have an effect on persons with coronary heart disease. Lown et al. (37) studied the effect of psychologic stress testing in 19 persons with advanced grades of ventricular arrhythmias. Ventricular premature beats were significantly increased in 11 (60%), with a twofold or greater increase in arrhythmias developing in seven, and paroxysms of ventricular tachycardia developing in one. These changes were reproduced by activating autonomic reflex activity in the absence of psychologic stress, suggesting that stress-induced arrhythmias are introduced through an integrated response of the central nervous system.

Arrhythmia formation in mitral valve prolapse has recently been shown to be enhanced by stress. Combs et al. (38) artificially induced a stress state in 15 persons with mitral valve prolapse and found the amplitude of the systolic click to be increased in five, with an equal number showing changes in rhythm. The arrhythmias consisted of new ventricular ectopic beats in three patients, an increase in ventricular ectopy in one, and the development of a new coronary sinus rhythm in one. Since mitral valve prolapse is now recognized as a not-uncommon finding in surveys of supposedly healthy populations, the effects of stress in precipitating arrhythmias known to be associated with this disorder may be of importance.

Coronary Heart Disease and Myocardial Infarction

One of the earliest associations of stress and cardiovascular disease can be found in the works of William Harvey (39). In 1628, he wrote of a man who died:

> . . . having receiving injury and affront from one more powerful than himself, and upon whom he could not have his revenge, was overcome with hatred and spite and passion, which he yet communicated to none, that at last he fell into a strange distemper, suffering from extreme oppression and pain of the heart and breast.

Two centuries later, the patient with coronary heart disease was described by Osler (40) as "a keen and ambitious man, the indicator of whose vengence is always set full speed ahead."

Occupational Risk Factors

More recent investigations performed in this century among large population groups have suggested that stress associated with modern industrialized society as well as specific professional roles is associated with a greater incidence of both hypertension and coronary heart disease (CHD). Russek and Russek (41), in a review of statistical surveys on 12,000 professional men in 14 occupational categories, found the incidence of coronary heart disease to be strikingly related to the relative stressfulness of occupational activity. Syme et al. (42) found that men who changed jobs more frequently had a ratio of coronary heart disease three times higher than that of occupationally stable men, suggesting that stress associated with vocational roles does have an adverse effect on the cardiovascular system.

Russek (43), in a second survey of the prevalence of coronary artery disease among physicians, found general practitioners in each field to have a prevalence rate of two to three times those of specialists. These findings were confirmed by Morris et al. (44), who noted full-time practitioners to have twice the incidence of coronary heart disease as other members of the profession.

The frequent presence of multiple confounding variables makes it difficult to assess the meaningfulness of a positive association between emotional stress and coronary heart disease. Several investigators have attempted to take these variables into account and have found the association between stress and cardiovascular disease independent of possible confounding factors. Groen et al. (45), in a study of coronary heart disease in Benedictine and Trappist monks, noted no differences between these groups in the presence or absence of CHD in any monk under the age of 65. Although both of these groups live in rural areas removed from the stresses of life, the Benedictines have a diet similar to that of other Europeans, whereas Trappists abstain from fish, meat, eggs, and butter. Mann et al. (46) have noted that although the East African Masai, a pastoral group free from the stresses of modern society, are relatively free from coronary disease, their diet includes a considerable intake of animal products and dairy fat. These findings suggest that stress, independent of diet, may be associated with an acceleration in the development of coronary artery disease. It should be emphasized, however, that considering the physiologic response to stress, it is not unreasonable to hypothesize that adverse effects of stress may be most prominent in the presence of a diet particularly rich in animal fat.

Other factors associated with anxiety include environmental toxins and consumption of alcohol, caffeine, and nicotine. These variables must also be considered in assessing the association between stress and coronary heart disease.

The Coronary-Prone Personality

Surveys of personality traits in individuals with myocardial infarction have revealed fairly uniform findings. Russek and Zohman (47), in a survey of 100 young coronary patients, noted severe emotional strain of occupational origin to be observed in 91% of the subjects as compared to 20% of the controls. Although smoking was also quite prevalent in this group, it was thought to be an indication of emotional tension rather than a causative factor in producing CHD.

Weiss et al. (48) have also noted that patients with CHD often have a history of gradually increasing tension weeks, months, or even years prior to the actual onset of coronary artery occlusion. The frequency of these associations with the development of coronary-prone personality types was recorded by Friedman and Rosenman (49), who divided men predisposed to clinical coronary disease into three basic behavioral patterns. Group A was found to be characterized by the presence of intense ambition, competitive drive, a persistent desire for recognition and advancement, continuous involvement in multiple and diverse functions, yet with a sense of time urgency propelling them to accelerate their rate of execution of such functions, and extraordinary mental and physical alertness. Group B exhibited a precisely converse behavioral pattern, whereas group C exhibited behavioral patterns essentially similar to those of men in group B, with the added element of a chronic anxiety state.

Unfortunately, this classification was based on retrospective analyses and, therefore, is subject to criticism. Indeed, in a prospective study, Mordkoff and Parsons (50) were unable to find differences in personality between individuals and subsequent development of myocardial infarction. Mai (51) similarly was unable to document this relationship and suggested that the predicted pattern may follow rather than precede a cardiac event, the findings representing a psychologic response to an infarct rather than an etiologic factor.

Although the classification of Friedman and Rosenman may be criticized, the biochemical differences noted in type A as compared to type B persons have been quite impressive. Type A persons have been found to have higher serum lipids and an increased excretion rate of catecholamines in response to puzzle solving, with the plasma norepinephrine of a type A individual rising 30% above that of a type B (52). The incidence of clinical coronary heart disease was seven times more frequent in type A than in type B persons, with a prospective study revealing 22 of 25 deaths due to coronary artery disease over 5 years in the type A group. In one study, regardless of the cause of death on autopsy, coronary atherosclerosis was found to be six times more common in the type A person (49).

Summary

Available evidence confirms an association between stress and coronary heart disease. There is no question that other variables may adversely or beneficially influence this relationship. The consumption of diets high in fat, associated with a low exercise level and the use of mood-altering agents, such as nicotine and caffeine, may well be associated with an even higher rate of coronary heart disease. On the other hand, the presence of a type A personality in the absence of other risk factors may not be marked by an outcome different from that seen in individuals exhibiting a type B or type C state. Certainly, more work is needed in this area to better define this relationship.

Hypertension

The increased secretion of catecholamines and steroids in response to stress may be associated with renal vasoconstriction and increased secretion of renin, angiotensin, and aldosterone. This is accompanied by sodium retention, which in turn sensitizes the vasculature to vasoconstriction. This process allows a relationship between stress and hypertension to be easily postulated. Indeed, several investigators have demonstrated elevated urinary levels of norepinephrine in hypertensives at rest, with higher-than-usual elevations in response to exercise. An increased response to epinephrine and norepinephrine infusions has been observed in persons with anxiety and essential hypertension as compared to normals (53–56). Hypertensive patients have also been shown to manifest a greater rise of FFA, triglycerides, phospholipids, and cortisol, as well as an increase in urinary 3-methoxy-4-hydroxymandelic acid following psychic stress as compared to normotensives (57).

Population surveys as early as 1945 demonstrated an association of stress with elevations in blood pressure. Graham (58) reported an incidence of asymptomatic hypertension in 27% of 695 men exposed to desert warfare for a 1-year period. Even when no immediate danger existed, these men showed evidence of a stress state associated with hypertension, which subsided only after relief of anxiety. Harburg et al. (56) found blood pressure levels among inner-city blacks to be significantly correlated with different patterns of life stress, with lower socioeconomic working class persons in the high-stress area having higher blood pressures after adjusting for sex, age, and weight. In the middle socioeconomic class, individuals with higher blood pressure levels were found to have higher occupational achievement goals, aspiring to much more than normotensive controls.

Similarly, the incidence of hypertension in air traffic controllers exposed to considerable stress was found to be four times greater than that in second class airmen, with those controllers working with high traffic densities revealing more evidence of hypertension than those working in low-traffic density areas (59). Morrison and Morris (60), in a survey of 302 London bus drivers and conductors, found the average systolic blood pressure in drivers charged with the stressful chore of negotiating London traffic to have substantially higher elevations in blood pressure than conductors.

Confounding Variables

Once again, however, there are multiple confounding variables that must be considered. First, none of these studies involved matched control groups to account for differences observed. Family histories were not routinely obtained to see if there was a greater prevalence of hypertension in the families of those persons enrolled in jobs of high stress. Finally, dietary factors, such as consumption of alcohol, caffeine, high salt-containing foods, and smoking, were not routinely controlled. All these factors have independently been associated with elevations of both systolic and diastolic blood pressure, in some instances accompanied by increased catecholamine excretion.

Summary

A review of the abundant literature on this subject shows conflicting findings (61–63). It does appear that elevation in blood pressure can be induced by stress; conversely, individuals can voluntarily reduce their blood pressure with appropriate conditioning techniques, such as transcendental meditation. The precise pathogenesis of sustained hypertension in response to stress, however, has not been clearly demonstrated. Unlike the typography of the coronary-prone patient, a hypertensive personality has not been well described. Patients with hypertension suffer from anxiety symptoms, as well as symptoms of depression. However, in the few controlled studies, no significant differences have been found with respect to anxiety between these individuals and their control groups. Personality differences that have been observed in hypertensives might well be the result rather than the cause of concomitant associations or reactive states.

SUMMARY

The evidence presented in the literature suggests that psychologic stress, in the absence of any confounding variables, can affect cardiovascular physiology, may be associated with or predispose to coronary heart disease, and, in persons with cardiac disease, can enhance the development of arrhythmias or other adverse clinical changes. The frequent positive association of anxiety and consumption of caffeine, a possible risk factor in coronary artery disease, and nicotine, a known risk factor, may further intensify the development of an untoward response.

Proscription of all stimulants, such as alcohol or caffeine-containing beverages, however, may serve to heighten the anxiety level in persons psychologically dependent on these substances. Medical advice concerning total abstinence of those substances not positively identified as risk factors must be individualized, based on a careful assessment of the needs and personality of each person.

The use of psychotropic agents to relieve anxiety, especially in the cardiac patient, can be quite helpful in relieving the added physiologic burden of persistence of undue anxiety. Since many of these drugs are also associated with hemodynamic changes, however, they should be prescribed only when reassurance or counseling is unsuccessful or inappropriate in providing relief.

In the following chapters, the specific effects of mood-altering drugs on the cardiovascular system are reviewed in an attempt to provide additional insight into the risks as well as the benefits associated with their use.

REFERENCES

1. Selye, H. (1936): A syndrome produced by diverse nocuous agents. *Nature,* 138:32.
2. Selye, H. (1976): *Stress in Health and Disease,* p. 762. Butterworth, Boston.
3. Page, I. H. (1959): Atherosclerosis: A commentary. *Fed. Proc.,* 18:47.
4. Haft, J. I., and Fani, K. (1973): Intravascular platelet aggregation in the heart induced by stress. *Circulation,* 47:353.
5. Raab, W., and Humphreys, R. J. (1947): Drug action upon myocardial epinephrine-sympathin concentration and heart rate. *J. Pharmacol. Exp. Ther.,* 89:64.
6. Green, D. M. (1953): Experimental hypertension. *Ann. Intern. Med.,* 39:334.
7. Selye, H. (1976): *Stress in Health and Disease,* p. 796. Butterworth, Boston.
8. Ibid, p. 796.
9. Davidson, W. J. (1977): Psychotropic drugs, stress and cardiomyopathies. In: *Stress and the Heart,* edited by D. Wheatley, pp. 63–86. Raven Press, New York.
10. Lown, B., Verrier, R., and Corbalan, R. (1973): Psychological stress and threshold for repetitive ventricular response. *Science,* 182:834.
11. Rabinowitz, S. H., Verrier, R. L., and Lown, B. (1976): The effects of vago-sympathetic stimulation on the repetitive extrasystole (RE) threshold. *Circulation,* 53:622.
12. Kolman, B. S., Verrier, R. L., and Lown B. (1975): The repetitive extrasystole as an index of vulnerability to ventricular fibrillation in the dog. *Circulation,* 52:578.
13. DeSilva, R. A., Verrier, R. L., and Lown, B. (1978): The effects of psychological stress and vagal stimulation with morphine on vulnerability to ventricular fibrillation (VF) in the conscious dog. *Am. Heart J.,* 95:198.
14. Bellet, S., Roman, L., and Kostis, J. (1969): The effects of automobile driving on catecholamine and adrenocortical excretion. *Am. J. Cardiol.* 24:365.
15. Nestel, P. J. (1969): Blood pressure and catecholamine excetion after mental stress in labile hypertension. *Lancet,* 1:692.
16. Carruthers, M. E. (1969): Aggression and atheroma. *Lancet,* 2:1170.
17. Taggart, P., and Carruthers, M. (1971): Endogenous hyperlipidemia induced by emotional stress of racing car drivers. *Lancet,* 1:363.
18. Wenke, M. (1966): In: *Advances in Lipid Research, Vol. 14,* edited by R. Paoletti and D. Kritchovsky. Academic Press, London.
19. Funkenstein, D. H., King, S. H., and Drolette, M. (1954): The direction of anger during a laboratory stress inducing session. *Psychosom. Med.,* 16:404.
20. Ax, A. F. (1953): The psychological differentiation between fears and anger in humans. *Psychosom. Med.,* 15:433.
21. Von Euler, V. S. (1964): Quantitation of stress by catecholamine analysis. *Clin. Pharmacol. Ther.,* 5:398.
22. Frankenhauser, M., and Rissler, A. (1970): Catecholamine output during relaxation and anticipation. *Percept. Mot. Skills,* 30:745.
23. Nestel, P. J. (1969): Blood pressure and catecholamine excretion after mental stress in labile hypertension. *Lancet,* 1:692.
24. Friedman, M., Rosenman, R. H., and Carroll, V. (1958): Changes in the serum cholesterol and blood clotting time in men subjected to cyclic variation of occupational stress. *Circulation,* 17:852.
25. Gordon, J. L., Bowyer, D. E., Evans, D. W., and Mitchinson, M. J. (1973): Human platelet reactivity during stressful diagnostic procedures. *J. Clin. Pathol.,* 26:958.
26. Levites, R., and Haft, J. I. (1974): Effects of exercise-induced stress on platelet aggregation. *Clin. Res.,* 22:285A (Abstr.).

27. Froberg, J., Karlsson, C. G., Levi, L., et al. (1969): Conditions of work and their influence on psychological and endocrine stress reactions. *Lab. Clin. Stress Res.,* 8:1.
28. Shatalov, N. N., Saitanov, A. O., and Glotova, K. V. (1962): On the state of the cardiovascular system under conditions of exposure to continuous noise. *Gig. Tr. Prof. Zabol.,* 6:10.
29. Taggart, P., Gibbons, D., and Sommerville, W. (1969): Some effects of motor car driving on the normal and abnormal heart. *Br. Med. J.,* 4:130.
30. Taggart, P., and Carruthers, M. (1977): Behavior patterns and emotional stress in the etiology of coronary heart disease: cardiological and biochemical correlates. In: *Stress and the Heart,* edited by D. Wheatley, p. 33. Raven Press, New York.
31. James, T. N. (1969): QT prolongation and sudden death. *Mod. Concepts Cardiovasc. Dis.,* 38:35.
32. Hai, H. (1977): Psychogenic ventricular tachycardia. *Circulation* [*Suppl. III*], 156:55.
33. Bernreiter, M. (1956): Cardiac arrhythmias in physical or emotional stress. *Mo. Med.,* 53.19.
34. Engel, G. L. (1971): Sudden and rapid death during psychological stress. Folklore or folk wisdoms *Ann. Intern. Med.,* 74:771.
35. Bernreiter, M. (1956): Cardiac arrhythmias in physical or emotional stress. *Mo. Med.,* 53:19.
36. Taggart, P., Carruthers, M., and Somerville, W. (1973): Electrocardiogram, plasma catecholamines and lipids and their modification by oxprenolol when speaking before an audience. *Lancet,* 2:341.
37. Lown, B., DeSilva, R. A., and Lenson, R. (1978): Role of psychologic stress and autonomic system changes in provocation of ventricular premature complexes. *Am. J. Cardiol.,* 41:979.
38. Combs, R., Shah, P. M., Shulman, J., et al. (1977): Effects of psychological stress on click and rhythm in mitral valve prolapse. *Circulation,* 56:111 (Abstr.).
39. Harvey, W.: *Exercitatio Anatomica De Motu Cordis Et Sanguinis In: Animabilus.* Frankfurtam-Main 1628.
40. Osler, W. (1896): Lectures on angina pectoris and allied states. *N.Y. Med. J.,* 4:224.
41. Russek, H. I., and Russek, L. G. (1961): Behavior patterns and emotional stress in the etiology of coronary heart disease: Sociological and occupational aspects. In: *Stress and the Heart,* edited by D. Wheatley, p. 15. Raven Press, New York.
42. Syme, S. L., Hyman, M. M., and Enterline, P. E. (1964): Some social and cultural factors associated with the occurrence of coronary heart disease. *J. Chronic Dis.,* 17:277.
43. Russek, H. I. (1962): Emotional stress and coronary heart disease in American physicians, dentists and lawyers. *Am. J. Med. Sci.,* 243:716.
44. Morris, J. N., Heady, J. A., and Barley, R. G. (1952): Coronary heart disease in medical practitioners. *Br. Med. J.,* 1:503.
45. Groen, J. J., Tijong, B. K., Willebrant, A. F., et al. (1959): Influence of nutrition, individuality and different forms of stress on blood cholesterol: Results of an experiment of 9 months duration in 60 normal volunteers. *Voeding,* 19.
46. Mann, G. V., Schaffer, R. D., and Rich, A. (1965): Physical fitness and immunity to heart disease in the Masai. *J. Atheroscler. Res.,* 2:1308.
47. Russek, H. I., and Zohman, B. L. (1958): Relative significance of heredity, diet and occupational stress in coronary heart disease of young adults. Based on an analysis of 100 patients between the ages of 25 and 40 years and a similar group of 100 normal control subjects. *Am. J. Med. Sci.,* 235:266.
48. Weiss, E., Dolin, B., and Rollin, H. R. (1957): Emotional factors in coronary artery occulsion. *Arch. Intern. Med.,* 99:628.
49. Friedman, M., and Rosenman, R. H. (1959): Association of specific overt behavior patterns with blood and cardiovascular findings: Blood cholesterol level, blood clotting time, incidence of arcus senilis and coronary artery disease. *JAMA,* 169:1286.

50. Mordkoff, A. M., and Parsons, O. P. (1967): The coronary personality. A critique. *Psychosom. Med.,* 29:1.
51. Mai, F. M. M. (1968): Personality and stress in coronary disease. *J. Psychosom. Med.,* 12:275.
52. Friedman, M., Byers, S. O., Diamant, J., and Rosenman, R. H. (1975): Plasma catecholamine response of coronary-prone subjects (Type A) to a specific challenge. *Metabolism,* 24:205.
53. Esler, M. D., and Nestel, P. J. (1973): High catecholamine essential hypertension: Clinical and physiological characteristics. *Aust N.Z. J. Med.,* 3:117.
54. Vlachakis, N. D., Guia, D. de, Mendlowitz, M., Antram, S., and Wolf, R. L. (1974): Hypertension and anxiety. A trial with epinephrine and norepinephrine infusion. *Mt. Sinai J. Med.,* 41:615.
55. Kimura, K. (1974): Pathophysiological significance of sympathetic activity in cardiovascular disease. *Jpn. Circ. J.,* 38:181.
56. Harburg, E., Schull, W. J., Erfurt, J. C., and Schork, M. A. (1970): A family set method for estimating heredity and stress. I. A pilot survey of blood pressure among Negroes in high and low stress areas, Detroit, 1966–1967. *J. Chronic Dis.,* 23:69.
57. Godicke W., Graff, C., Baumann, R., Naumann, E., and Ziprian H. (1971): Influence of experimentally produced mental stress on serum lipids, plasma cortisol and 3 methoxy-4 hydroxy maydelic acid excretion in essential hypertensives. *Dtsch. Gesundheitsw.,* 26:1973.
58. Graham, J. D. P. (1945): High blood pressure after battle. *Lancet,* 1:239.
59. Cobb, S., and Rose, R. M. (1973): Hypertension, peptic ulcer and diabetes in air traffic controllers. *JAMA,* 224:489.
60. Morrison, S. L., and Morris, J. N. (1959): Epidemiological observations on high blood pressure without apparent cause. *Lancet,* 2:864.
61. Cochrane, R. (1971): High blood pressure as a psychosomatic disorder. A selective review. *Br. J. Soc. Clin. Psychol.,* 10:61.
62. Gutman, M. C., and Benson, H. (1971): Interaction of environmental factors and systemic arterial blood pressure. A review. *Medicine,* 50:543.
63. Davies, M. H. (1971): Is high blood pressure a psychosomatic disorder. A critical review of the evidence. *J. Chronic Dis.,* 24:239.

Chapter 4

Alcohol 1: Acute and Chronic Effects on the Heart and Vasculature

Alcohol abuse is recognized as the nation's most serious public health problem (Chapter 1). Although precise figures concerning incidence and prevalence are difficult to obtain, a generally accepted figure is 95 million persons, consuming alcohol, with 9 million considered to be physically dependent on this drug (1). Economic costs attributable to the misuse of alcohol are equally impressive, with an estimated annual figure of $31.4 billion, only a portion of which relates to direct health care costs. Excess mortality due to alcohol abuse accounts for 7% of all male deaths in the United States (2). Hospitalizations for alcohol-related illnesses have been reported to be as high as 47% in municipal hospital settings (3,4).

Alcohol may exert an effect on the cardiovascular system in many ways. In the normal nonalcoholic subject, acute administration may result in hemodynamic changes. These changes, when occurring in persons with underlying cardiac disease, may have considerable deleterious effects. Even in the absence of clinically important hemodynamic changes, however, interactions of alcohol with cardiac medications in persons with preexisting cardiac disease can also interfere with desired therapeutic actions. Finally, contin-

TABLE 1. *Alcohol content of commonly consumed beverages*

Beverage	Approximate % alcohol by volume	Approximate amount alcohol in one drink[a]	
		Oz	grams
Beers and ales	3–8	0.36–0.96	9–18
Table wines	8–14	0.32–0.56	10–17
Dessert wines	15–20	0.45–0.60	14–18
Liqueurs	20–60	0.30–0.90	7–22
Distilled spirits	35–50	0.52–0.75	16–18

[a] Assuming a typical serving to consist of 12 oz beer, 4 oz table wine, 3 oz dessert wine, and 1.5 oz liqueurs and distilled spirits.

TABLE 2. *Alcohol content of commonly used drugs*[a]

Proprietary or common name	Alcohol content (%)
Antihistamines/decongestants	
Benadryl® elixir	14
Chlor-Trimeton® syrup	7
Dimetapp® elixir	2.3
Neosynephrine® elixir	8
Polaramine® syrup	6
Propadrine® elixir	16
Cough/cold preparations	
Nonprescription	
Coldene®	15
Dristan®	12
Nyquil®	25
Robitussin®	3.5
Robitussin-DM®	1.4
Trind®	15
Vicks 44®	10
Prescription	
Cheracol®	3
Dimetane® expectorant	3.5
Novahistine® expectorant	5
Phenergan® expectorant	7
Robitussin A-C® expectorant	3.5
Terpin hydrate elixir	42
Terpin hydrate with codeine elixir	42
Gastrointestinal drugs	
Belladonna tincture	67
Butibel® elixir	7
Donnagel®	3.8
Donnagel®-PG	5
Donnatal® elixir	23
Respiratory drugs	
Brondecon® elixir	20
Elixophyllin® elixir	20
Isuprel® Compound Elixir	19
Marax® syrup	5
Quibron® elixir	15
Miscellaneous	
Decadron® elixir	5
Feosol® elixir	5
Geritol®	12
Kaon elixir	5
Phenobarbital elixir	14
Tempra® syrup	7
Tylenol® elixir	7

[a] Adapted from ref. 149.

uous alcohol consumption may have a direct deleterious structural effect on the cardiovascular system different from those changes seen in nonalcoholic persons and in individuals with previous underlying cardiac disease.

The effects of alcohol may be related to (a) a direct action of alcohol or its metabolites, (b) induced alterations in electrolyte distribution, (c) associated nutritional deficiences, or (d) the effects of other components in alcoholic beverages. It is therefore important to consider briefly the vehicles in which alcohol is consumed as well as the general pharmacologic actions of this drug prior to reviewing its actions on the cardiovascular system.

There are currently five types of alcoholic beverages consumed: beer, table wine, dessert or cocktail wines, liqueurs or cordials, and distilled spirits (Table 1). Each type of beverage, in addition to containing ethyl alcohol, may contain other alcohols, aldehydes, ketones, esters, salts, acids, vitamins, minerals, or amino acids. Each of these ingredients may exert a separate systemic effect, although the major effects exerted on the body by consumption of these beverages are related to the action of ethanol (CH_3,CH_2,OH) or its metabolites. In the sections that follow, consistent with common usage, alcohol refers only to ethanol, unless otherwise specified.

In addition to intentional consumption of alcoholic beverages, alcohol is a common ingredient in many oral medications (Table 2). The alcohol content of these medications is variable. Elixers usually contain between 10 and 25%, whereas spirits and tinctures may be as much as 95% alcohol. Persons with chronic debilitating disorders, especially of the respiratory tract, may unwittingly consume considerable quantities of alcohol. For example, a chronic bronchitic taking 45 cc Elixophyllin® elixir four times daily would be ingesting 1.2 oz of pure alcohol. This would be equivalent to approximately 10 oz of 12% table wine, 2.4 oz of 100-proof liquor, or 30 oz of beer. In persons with coexisting cardiac or respiratory disease, a potential exists for the development of adverse clinical effects.

PHARMACOLOGY

Alcohol is readily absorbed from the intestinal tract, although the rate varies greatly, not only among individuals but also in the same person upon replicate administration (5). Absorption is facilitated in the presence of an empty intestinal tract and, conversely, is inhibited in the presence of food in the stomach. Distribution is widespread and uniform in body water, occurring within 1 hr after absorption has been completed.

Alcohol cannot be stored in the body and is secreted unchanged through the lungs and the kidneys to only a minor degree (5 to 10%) (6). In general, alcohol is metabolized at the rate of 0.19 g/kg/hr, with more rapid rates occurring in heavy drinkers. The major effects of alcohol (Table 3) occur during its metabolism. Oxidation of alcohol is accompanied by the (a) reduction of nicotinamide adenine dinucleotide (NAD); (b) activation of the micro-

TABLE 3. *Metabolic effects of alcohol*[a]

Carbohydrate metabolism
Hypoglycemia
Decreased oxidation of galactose[b]
Protein metabolism
Decreased albumin and transferrin synthesis[b]
Increased lipoprotein synthesis
Lipid metabolism
Hypertriglyceridemia
Increased liver triglycerides
Increased VHDL
Increase in NADH/NAD Ratio
Increased production lactate
Hyperuricemia
Hyperporphobilinogenemia
Decreased citric acid-cycle activity
Increase in acetaldehyde levels
Metabolic effects
Decrease in serum magnesium and phosphate
Increased catecholamine release
Decreased β-adrenergic receptor sensitivity
Increased oxygen consumption
Decreased 2–3-diphosphoglycerate in the red blood cell
Decreased vitamin activation
Hepatic effects
Decreased β-adrenergic receptor sensitivity
Increased oxygen consumption
Decreased 2–3-diphosphoglycerate in the red blood cell
Decreased vitamin activation
Hepatic effects
Fatty liver
Hepatitis
Cirrhosis

[a] Data from ref. 150.
[b] Seen with acute alcohol consumption.

somal-ethanol oxidizing system (MEOS), and (c) accumulation of acetaldehyde and acetate.

General Metabolic Effects

The greatest portion of alcohol is initially degraded into acetaldehyde and hydrogen through oxidation by alcohol dehyrogenase in the liver (Fig. 1). The hydrogen produced from this reaction combines with NAD to form NADH (7). The hepatocyte subsequently utilizes this hydrogen rather than that from existing fatty acids for energy production, synthesis of fat, and reduction of pyruvate to lactate. This last reaction reverses the normal metabolic pathway in which lactate is converted to pyruvate. The end results of

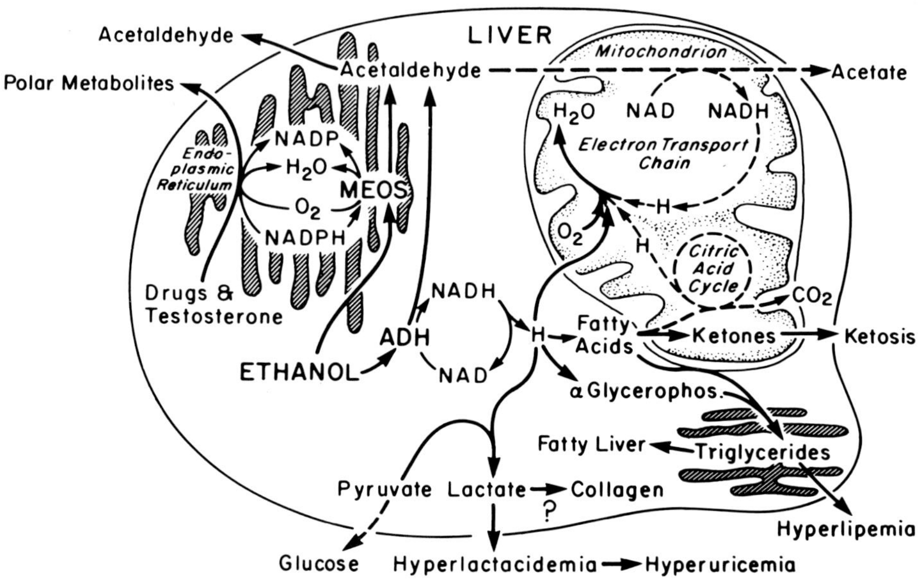

FIG. 1. Oxidation of ethanol in the hepatocyte and its link to fatty liver, hyperlipemia, hyperuricemia, hyperlactacidemia, ketosis, hypoglycemia, and drug and acetaldehyde metabolism. NAD, nicotinamide adenine dinucleotide; NADH, reduced NAD; NADP, nicotinamide adenine dinucleotide phosphate; NADPH, reduced NADP; MEOS, microsomal ethanol-oxidizing system; ADH, alcohol dehydrogenase. *Broken lines,* pathways that are depressed by ethanol. (Reprinted from ref. 151.)

these reactions are hypoglycemia, hyperlactidemia, and hyperlipemia. Acetaldehyde is then oxidized through acetaldehyde dehydrogenase to acetic acid, which is subsequently oxidized to two molecules of carbon dioxide and two molecules of water.

Alcohol also alters cellular amino acid metabolism with accumulation of certain amino acids in the liver. Acutely, inhibition of albumin synthesis occurs, as well as a decreased synthesis of other specific carrier proteins. Lipoprotein formation in the liver is stimulated, however, and may contribute to the hyperlipidemia noted.

Effects on Lipid Metabolism

Lipid abnormalities have been well documented in alcoholics. In the past, most attention has been focused on the reduced uptake of free fatty acids (FFA) and the hypertriglyceridemia produced in response to a heavy alcohol challenge or found in chronic alcoholics, primarily those with a primary type 4 hyperlipoproteinemia. Serum cholesterol levels have also been demonstrated to be increased with alcohol and, correspondingly, rapidly decline during abstinence (8–12). In most instances, these findings are based on studies dealing with chronic alcoholics or persons acutely challenged with considerable quantities of alcohol. The triglyceride response has also been demonstrated to be variable, depending on the resting level of triglyceridemia and existing dietary factors (12).

Since lipoprotein synthesis is stimulated by alcohol, changes in lipoprotein levels would be expected in the presence of continued alcohol use. Recently, the Cooperative Lipoprotein Phenotyping Study, utilizing data from five distinct populations, analyzed plasma lipids, relating this analysis to the quantity of alcohol consumed (13). Correlation between alcohol consumption and high density lipoprotein (HDL) cholesterol and triglyceride levels was noted in all populations. The elevations in HDL-cholesterol levels were graded over the range of quantity of alcohol consumed. Consumption of 5 to 6 oz of alcohol weekly was associated with a HDL-cholesterol 10% higher than that seen in a nondrinker. Triglyceride levels were also directly related to alcohol intake, although less so than HDL-cholesterol.

Changes in low density lipoprotein (LDL) cholesterol generally exhibited a negative variance with increasing alcohol consumption, although with a lesser consistency among different population groups. Correlations between alcohol intake and very low density lipoprotein (VLDL) cholesterol were not demonstrated. Analysis of the data to eliminate potentially confounding variables, such as type of alcoholic beverage consumed, drugs, or diet, did not alter these findings.

The relationship between elevated levels of HDL-cholesterol and diminished prevalence of coronary heart disease is only beginning to be defined in the literature. The relevance of the association of HDL-cholesterol and alcohol consumption with respect to coronary heart disease in alcoholics remains unclear and is discussed further in the section on coronary artery disease.

Lipid Metabolism and Disulfiram

Although withdrawal from alcohol is associated with a decline in serum cholesterol, recent work by Major and Goyer (14) suggests that the treatment of alcoholism with disulfiram (Antabuse®) may not only prevent this decline but may result in an elevation of serum cholesterol levels. The administration of 500 mg/day disulfiram was associated with a mean rise of serum cholesterol over basal values of 34 mg% in 3 weeks and a mean increase of 74 mg% in 6 weeks. This increase in serum cholesterol was not seen in subjects taking the same disulfiram dose in combination with 50 mg/day pyridoxine or in control groups. The control groups sustained a mean decrease in serum cholesterol of 33 mg% upon initiating abstinence.

The authors suggest that these changes are related to the production of carbon disulfide during the metabolism of disulfiram, which in turn results in a state of pyridoxine deficiency causing hypercholesterolemia. In addition, carbon disulfide has also been shown to stimulate the incorporation of acetate to cholesterol and accelerate the hepatic turnover rate of cholesterol (15). Regardless of the precise mechanism involved, however, these findings warrant further investigation, since carbon disulfide produced in an industrial setting has been associated with an increased risk of atherosclerosis in humans (16).

Effects on Ionic Transfer

In the experimental animal, alcohol interferes with active transport of potassium, phosphate, and sodium across cell membranes, resulting in an intracellular depletion of potassium and phosphate; it also produces an increased liberation of epinephrine (17–19). Magnesium and zinc have also been shown to be released from the heart during ethanol infusion (20). Clinically, alcoholics have often been found to be magnesium deficient. This may relate to a direct effect of alcohol on tubular resorption or may be associated with symptoms accompanying alcohol consumption which favor magnesium deficiency, such as vomiting, diarrhea, hyperhydrosis, and hyperaldosterone states in the presence of cirrhosis and ascites (21). The clinical effects of these changes with respect to myocardial function must be more clearly defined. Although deficits in magnesium can cause myocardial dilatation with mitochondrial swelling similar to experimentally induced alcoholic cardiomyopathy (22), clinically, magnesium deficiency is not a requisite for the cardiomyopathy seen in alcoholics. However, ionic shifts may account for the sinus tachycardia and T-wave alterations seen in the electrocardiograms (ECGs) of asymptomatic alcoholics without known cardiac disease (23,24).

In humans, losses of potassium, and magnesium from the left ventricle, have been noted following acute administration of 12 oz of alcohol, accompanied by a decrease in left ventricular uptake of FFA and an enhanced triglyceride uptake (25).

Alcohol can also cause a depression in phosphate concentrations in the blood. The magnitude of hypophosphatemia produced may be of clinical importance when alcohol is consumed with aluminum-containing antacids, which are also associated with a decerase in blood phosphate (26). Severe hypophosphatemia has been associated with low intracellular stores of adenosine triphosphate (ATP) and specific cellular dysfunction both *in vivo* and *in vitro* (27–29). O'Connor et al. (30) recently described the effect of hypophosphatemia on myocardial performance in humans before, during, and after repletion with intravenous potassium phosphate. Repletion of serum phosphate to a normal concentration was associated with an improved myocardial stroke work, as manifested by an increase in left ventricular stroke work per beat at a constant afterload ($p < 0.01$) and a decrease in mean pulmonary artery wedge pressure ($p < 0.02$). The relevance of these findings with respect to the hemodynamic changes observed after alcohol ingestion in alcoholics remains to be determined. Hypophosphatemia occurring in the presence of chronic alcoholism, however, may be yet another contributory factor to myocardial dysfunction.

Metabolic Effects of Acetaldehyde

As alcohol consumption persists, adaptive proliferative changes occur in the endoplasmic reticulum, resulting in the induction of the MEOS, which continues the process of alcohol metabolism (31,32). Although at low to moderate levels of alcohol ingestion the alcohol dehydrogenase system predominates, at higher levels of consumption the MEOS begins to assume a greater metabolic role. Activation of the MEOS affects the disposition of other drugs usually metabolized by this system. In addition, structural changes occur in the mitochondria, which result in a decreased functional capacity, including a diminished oxidization of acetaldehyde to acetate with subsequent acetaldehyde accumulation. Acetaldehyde accumulation is greater in chronic alcoholics than in nondrinkers or occasional drinkers and may also contribute to deleterious myocardial effects (33). At concentrations similar to that found in the blood of alcoholics, acetaldehyde has been shown to depress myocardial protein synthesis, interfere with mitochondrial function, and elevate circulating catecholamines (34–36).

Pharmacologically, acetaldehyde has a positive iontropic effect and, at the blood levels produced by moderate ethanol consumption, is not a myocardial depressant. The ability of the myocardium to respond to catecholamine release, however, may determine whether the net effect of alcohol administration is stimulatory or depressant. In the presence of normal myocardial function, catecholamine release might result in an augmentation of cardiac output, whereas the impaired heart might exhibit an inability to respond to catecholamines, with a depressant effect predominating. Continuous alcohol administration or persistent stress might ultimately serve to deplete catecholamine stores, impair adrenergic activity, and result in an inability to respond to stress.

Cardiac Metabolism and Alcohol

The mechanism by which ethanol acutely influences myocardial action has not been clearly defined. Since myocardial sarcoplasm lacks alcohol dehydrogenase, it is unlikely that similar effects relating to a shift of intracellular NAD to NADH redox potential would occur in the heart. A similar change might occur, however, through the appearance of lactate in the blood, which increases after ethanol ingestion. An increased utilization of lactate by the heart could affect the redox state, causing a shift from aerobic to anaerobic metabolism. Profound changes in metabolic pathways secondary to hypoxia and anaerobic glycolysis may explain the cardiac depressant effect of alcohol, as well as the findings of increased lipid deposits frequently seen in the myocardium of persons dying from alcoholic heart disease (37).

An increase in concentration of mitochondrial-derived enzymes, such as isocitric and malic dehydrogenases, similar to that found during hepatic metabolism of ethanol, has been found in coronary sinus blood of alcoholic subjects consuming large amounts of alcohol. This enzyme leakage suggests an alteration in intramitochondrial metabolic pathways or membrane permeability. Pathologic examinations of samples of myocardium have documented mitochondrial damage, suggesting a serious disturbance in oxidative metabolism and energy production (38). Prolonged ethanol ingestion associated with decreased myocardial mitochondrial respiration and diminished calcium binding and uptake by the sarcoplasmic reticulum can exert deleterious effects on contractility, since myocardial contractility is modulated by sarcoplasmic release and uptake of calcium (39,40).

Chronic ethanol consumption also results in a decrease in extraction and oxidation of FFA by the heart and an increased myocardial uptake of triglycerides (41).

Summary

Alcohol has multiple effects on normal homeostasis. The intensity and frequency of these effects depend on several factors, including preexisting nutritional status, presence of acute or chronic alcohol consumption, genetic factors controlling enzyme induction, simultaneous administration of other drugs, and age of the drinker. This last factor is too seldom considered in assessing the individual response to drinking. Vestal et al. (5), using alcohol infusions in 50 healthy subjects aged 21 to 81 years, found the peak alcohol concentration of blood water to be significantly correlated with age ($p < 0.01$). This was related to the smaller volume of distribution and the decreased lean body mass occurring more frequently in the elderly. These findings help to explain the differences in mood-altering effects of similar quantities of alcohol seen in the elderly as compared to younger persons and may reinforce a recommendation of moderation in drinking in older individuals.

DRUG INTERACTIONS WITH ALCOHOL

Although most ingested alcohol is metabolized by alcohol dehydrogenase, chronic use of large quantities of alcohol increases the activity of the MEOS and, providing an acute alcohol challenge is not present, can increase the rate of metabolism of many drugs (Table 4) (42).

Oral Anticoagulants

The half-life of both coumadin and diphenylhydantoin (Dilantin®) may be diminished by up to 50% in alcoholic subjects, with an attendant diminution in anticoagulant and antiarrhythmic or anticonvulsant effect (43). Acute

TABLE 4. *Selective alcohol-drug interactions*

Drug	Effect
Chloramphenicol	Disulfiram-like reaction
Coumarin derivatives	Chronic alcohol consumption: decreased anticoagulant effect; Acute alcohol consumption: enhanced anticoagulant effect
Digoxin	Increased sensitivity to digitalis toxicity
Diphenylhydantoin	Chronic alcohol consumption: decreased anticonvulsant and antiarrhythmic effect; Acute alcohol consumption: enhanced effect, potential for toxicity
Disulfiram	Flushing, tachycardia, hypotension, dyspnea
Griseofulvin	Disulfiram-like reaction
Hypoglycemics (oral)	
Chlorpropamide (Diabinase®)	Disulfiram-type reaction
Phenformin (DBI®)	Lactic acidosis
Tolbutamide	Disulfiram-type reaction
Marijuana	Enhanced euphoria
Narcotics	Enhanced CNS depression
Nitroglycerin	Enhanced hypotension
Phenothiazines	Enhanced CNS effects, elevation of blood alcohol
Quinacrine (Atabrine®)	Disulfiram-like reaction
Sedatives and hypnotics	Chronic alcohol consumption: diminished sedative effect; Acute alcohol consumption: enhanced CNS depression
Chloral hydrate	Enhanced CNS depression, flushing, headache, tachycardia
Stimulants	Variable
Tolazoline (Priscoline®)	Disulfiram-like reaction
Tricyclic antidepressants	Impairment of motor skills

consumption of an intoxicating amount of ethanol, however, will result in an inhibition of coumadin metabolism and an increase in anticoagulant effect with the potential for toxic reactions. A similar inhibition of diphenylhydantoin metabolism will also occur.

Sedatives and Tranquilizers

Alcohol belongs to the sedative-hypnotic group of agents and as such exerts a generalized depressant effect on the central nervous system (CNS). A combination of alcohol with such drugs or with other medications causing respiratory depression results in a synergistic depressant effect. Experimentally, a potentiation of the depressant effect of alcohol on the myocardium has also been observed with the use of sedative agents (44).

This effect is modified by the presence of acute or chronic consumption of these drugs. Acute alcohol intoxication inhibits pentobarbital metabolism, whereas chronic ingestion of alcohol enchances its metabolism. Chronic pentobarbital administration can more rapidly decrease blood alcohol levels (45,46). Similar interactions can occur with other drugs in this group, notably, meprobamate, benzodiazepines, chloral hydrate, and glutethimide (47).

These interactions are usually secondary to enchancement or depression of the MEOS, although other mechanisms may play a role. Hayes et al. (48) have suggested that alcohol might enhance the absorption of diazepam since administration of diazepam mixed with alcohol has been found to result in a twofold increase in mean plasma diazepam levels over that found when it is administered with water.

Chloral Hydrate

The interaction of alcohol with chloral hydrate may be of specific concern in persons with cardiovascular disease. This interaction was noted as early as 1872 by Björnstrom (43), who reported facial erythema and angina in two patients regularly receiving chloral hydrate after ingesting a half bottle of beer. The reaction could be eliminated by discontinuing the chloral hydrate therapy prior to drinking and precipitated by reinstituting this drug. More recently, Bardodêj (49) and Sellers et al. (50) noted that in patients pretreated with chloral hydrate for 5 to 7 days, tachycardia and a widened pulse pressure developed with ingestion of alcohol. An enhanced CNS effect of alcohol was also noted. This was associated in one subject by marked vasodilation accompanied by flushing, palpitations, and headache. The cause of this reaction remains to be clearly defined. It is unlikely that increasing acetaldehyde levels are responsible, as Sellers et al. (51) demonstrated that acetaldehyde concentrations actually fall with concomitant administration of these agents. Regardless of etiology, however, the combined use of alcohol and chloral hydrate in persons with cardiovascular disease should be avoided whenever possible.

Tricyclic Antidepressants

Combined use of alcohol and tricyclic antidepressants has also been shown to have deleterious effects (52). Motor skills have been shown to be impaired within the first several days of tricyclic therapy combined with alcohol ingestion (53). Ingestion of alcohol by a patient maintained on chlorpromazine can also result in an enhancement of blood alcohol levels (54) secondary to the effect of chlorpromazine on alcohol dehydrogenase.

Narcotics

The acute consumption of alcohol and the use of narcotic agents results in an increase in CNS depression. It is an impressive and sobering fact that even in deaths considered to be caused by narcotic use, up to 50% of such persons are found to have detectable levels of blood alcohol on toxicologic examination, with 25% of cases having levels exceeding 0.10 g% (55).

Stimulants

Studies of the interaction between alcohol and CNS stimulants have reported variable findings. Although it is commonly believed that caffeine can effectively antagonize the depressant effect of alcohol, no evidence exists to substantiate this belief.

Marijuana

Alcohol use with marijuana is considered by marijuana smokers to result in an enhancement of the euphoria. Although little pharmacologic work has been published documenting this relationship, considering the actions of both agents, a synergestic effect would be expected.

Digitalis

Digitalis was once clinically recommended for the treatment of acute alcoholism (56). The intracellular and extracellular shifts in potassium and magnesium induced by alcohol in reality, however, can heighten sensitivity to digitalis. Neumann and Walter (57) demonstrated a lowering of the LD_{50} in glycoside-maintained cats receiving acute infusions of ethanol. This experimentally induced alteration in sensitivity to digitalis may explain the increased incidence of arrhythmias noted in elderly alcoholic patients (58).

Vasodilators

Consumption of alcohol in the presence of vasodilator therapy may also result in adverse effects. Hypotension has been reported with the combination of alcohol and nitroglycerin. Depending on individual sensitivity, this reaction may be of clinical importance (59).

Other Constituents of Alcoholic Beverages

Adverse drug interactions with alcoholic beverages may also be related to the presence of associated congeners rather than ethanol. Consumption of alcohol in combination with tyramine, found in chianti wines, may result in acute hypertensive reactions in patients taking monoamine oxidase (MAO) inhibitors (60). Cobalt, when added to beer as a foam stabilizer, has been responsible for the development of cardiomyopathy (see below). Alcohol can enhance absorption of iron from the intestine. When alcohol is combined with iron, as in some French wines that are mixed in iron-containing vessels (as the Bantu do during brewing of beer) or consumed along with iron supplements, deposition of iron in the tissues can occur with resultant deleterious effects (61).

Disulfiram

Disulfiram (Antabuse®) is used frequently in the treatment of alcoholism. When taken with ethanol, an accumulation of acetaldehyde occurs. This is accompanied by symptoms of flushing, tachycardia, dyspnea, and hypotension. With severe reactions, respiratory depression, syncope, shock, arrhythmias, congestive heart failure, and myocardial infarction may occur. Use of disulfiram in elderly patients or in persons with preexisting heart disease, therefore, is not recommended. Other drugs also having a disulfiram-like effect include tolbutamide, chlorpropamide, griseofulvin, and quinacrine.

HEMODYNAMIC EFFECTS

An association of alcohol and heart disease was first recorded as early as 1873 by Walsh (62), who described a form of cirrhosis of the heart in persons dying of chronic alcoholism. It is only in the recent past, however, that attention has been directed to the effects of acute or relatively short-term ingestion of alcohol on the cardiovascular system.

Animal Studies

Regan et al. (63) studied hemodynamic parameters and histologic myocardial abnormalities in dogs maintained in a constant nutritional state, with alcohol constituting 36% of their caloric intake. After an 18-month period, these animals did not differ from controls with respect to body weight, serum proteins, vitamins, or electrolytes. Hemodynamic measurements revealed comparable values for heart rate, aortic pressure, and ejection fraction before and after angiotensin infusion. Stroke output postangiotensin was significantly higher in control animals, whereas a significantly greater rise in end-diastolic pressure was noted in the alcohol-fed animals, indicating a reduced ventricular compliance. These findings were associated with a significant prolongation of QRS duration and conduction time from His bundle to onset of ventricular depolarization (64). Histologic sections of the myocardium revealed an interstitial accumulation of glycoprotein-like material and a dilatation of the intercalated disks.

Leidtke and DeMuth (65) studied the effects of alcohol after experimental, nonpenetrating chest trauma in dogs. In such a setting, significant decreases in cardiac index and arterial pressure occurred, indicating a loss in peripheral compensatory mechanism as compared to changes seen in control animals. The ethanol-treated animals had a 92% mortality, as compared to 11% in the control group. The majority of the deaths were attributed to electrical-mechanical dissociation.

Similar adverse findings were reported by Beard et al. (66) in studying the cardiovascular response to hemorrhage in dogs after exposure to ethanol. After daily intubation with alcohol for a 4-week period, survival from a sublethal hemorrhage was markedly decreased. Once again, fatal arrhythmias were the most common mode of exodus.

The relevance of these findings with respect to mortality in humans following trauma, which not infrequently is associated with alcohol ingestion, remains to be determined.

Healthy, Nonalcoholic Persons

The earliest studies of the actions of alcohol on the normal human heart were performed in 1930 by Grollman (67), who demonstrated that small amounts of alcohol could produce a transient rise in heart rate, cardiac output, and blood pressure in nondrinkers. Subsequently, conflicting reports have appeared concerning the acute effects of ethanol ingestion in nondrinkers. This variability may be related in part to the dose of alcohol administered, mode and duration of administration, type of hemodynamic variable measured, time of measurement, and effects of the presence of alcohol prior to testing on the baseline hemodynamic state.

Riff et al. (68) administered 6 oz of 90-proof bourbon whiskey to volunteers who had a history of consuming no more than two bottles of beer or 3 oz of whiskey per day. Measurements of heart rate, arterial pressure, and cardiac output were recorded in the resting state and postexercise, before and after alcohol consumption. In the resting state, no difference in hemodynamic parameters was noted between control and experimental groups. Following ingestion of alcohol, peak blood alcohol levels were noted within 30 min in all subjects. Heart rate and cardiac index increased significantly, reaching a maximum 30 min postingestion. There was little or no change reported in stroke volume or arterial pressure. Left ventricular contractility was similarly unimpaired. The calculated peripheral resistance decreased. No effect of alcohol was seen on the hemodynamic response to exercise. This rate-dependent increase in cardiac output with alcohol ingestion was also found by Juchems and Klobe (69). That these findings could be reproduced even with small amounts of alcohol was confirmed by Gould et al. (70), who administered a cocktail consisting of 2 oz of 86.8-proof Canadian whiskey to normal volunteers with a resulting increase in cardiac index. An increase in stroke volume in these persons, however, was found to be responsible for the rise in output.

Systolic Time Intervals

These studies suggest that in the normal subject, acute consumption of alcohol is not associated with any adverse hemodynamic effects. The use of stroke volume and cardiac output to assess myocardial performance, however, does not provide as sensitive measurements as systolic time intervals (STI). Subsequent studies of left ventricular function in normal volunteers utilizing STI, as well as controlling for the duration of administration of alcohol and the time of measurement, demonstrated acute hemodynamic responses to alcohol ingestion. Ingestion of 4- to 6-oz cocktails was associated with a transient impairment of left ventricular contractility, as manifested by increases in preejection period (PEP), isometric contraction time, PEP/left ventricular ejection time (LVET) ratio, and heart rate ($p < 0.01$). A significant fall in systolic blood pressure, with decreases in LVET and QS2, was noted ($p < 0.01$ and 0.05, respectively) (71–73). Maximum changes were seen within 60 min of ingestion. Although statistically significant, the magnitude of these changes in STI is small. These observations, seen in a relatively small number of subjects, may represent diurnal changes. Diurnal variations in STI, however, are marked by a decrease in all parameters measured, whereas decreased intervals in these studies were seen only with LVET and QS2 (74).

Echocardiography

A myocardial depressant effect of acute alcohol ingestion in nonalcoholics has also been demonstrated by echocardiography (75). Ingestion of 0.79 cc alcohol/kg in less than 30 min and 1.59 cc/kg in under 60 min (approximately 4 and 6 oz, respectively) resulted in a significant decrease in fractional change in the minor axis of the left ventricle at both 30 and 60 min postalcohol ingestion. These changes reverted to normal within 1 hr, although persistence of elevated blood alcohol levels was noted throughout the 3-hr study period. A lack of correlation between hemodynamic effect and blood alcohol has been noted by several investigators (76,77). Although the reasons for this lack are unclear, it may be related to the presence of compensatory responses initiated in the autonomic nervous system. Alterations in cardiovascular reflexes resulting from single doses of alcohol of 0.3 or 0.6/kg have been noted by Zsotér and Sellers (78). Response pre- and postalcohol ingestion to the Valsalva maneuver, deep breathing, hyperventilation, and head up tilt was tested in 20 subjects. Alcohol was found to modify all reflexes but not to a clinically or physiologically important extent.

Alcoholics Without Evidence of Cardiac Disease

The studies described above suggest that acute ingestion of nonintoxicating amounts of ethanol in normal subjects results in subtle myocardial depression unrelated to the effects of alimentation or increase in afterload. These changes appear to be short lived, and a return to normal values occurs within hours (73). Interestingly, the magnitude of such changes has been shown to be correlated with past drinking history. Timmis et al. (79) studied the acute effects of 50% alcohol (100-proof vodka) in persons classified as having light (1 oz/day), average (1 to 2 oz/day), or heavy (2 oz/day or more) consumption of alcohol. Progressive increases of STI were seen based on drinking classification. The degree of myocardial impairment in some of the heavy drinkers on control measurements was severe enough to preclude detection of further cardiac depression subsequent to acute exposure and tended to be proportionate to the quantity of alcohol consumed. In one patient in this group, complete abstinence from alcohol resulted in a return of values to control levels within 2 months, with acute ingestion of alcohol resulting in the expected prolongation of STI.

The hemodynamic effects of acute alcohol administration in persons with a history of chronic alcoholism but without impaired myocardial function in a baseline state are somewhat different. After 12 oz of scotch, Regan and his co-workers (80) noted an increase in left ventricular end-diastolic pressure (LVEDP) and a decrease in stroke output, which reverted toward control levels within 4 hr. With angiotensin infusion, stroke volume could not be increased in response to increasing LVEDP as seen in nonalcoholic subjects. This response appeared to be dose related in that similar findings could not be reproduced with lesser concentrations of alcohol.

Zambrano et al. (81), in a study of 60 unselected ambulatory alcoholics in the absence of acute ethanol administration, noted a significantly higher heart rate as compared to normal subjects. LVET, when corrected for heart rate, was depressed, with the PEP/LVET ratio increased secondary to a low ejection time, suggesting the presence of persistent cardiac malfunction even in the absence of symptoms. Cardiac reactivity to stress has also been found to be impaired in alcoholics as compared to nonalcoholics. Noxious auditory stimuli were associated with a diminished response of increasing heart rate in alcoholics in both the presence and absence of alcohol (82). It is possible that this altered response to stress with acute alcohol consumption may be associated with an even greater augmentation in catecholamine secretion with associated deleterious effects.

Nonalcoholic Persons with Preexisting Cardiac Disease

Hemodynamic studies of the effects of alcohol in coronary patients have not been forthcoming until recent years. After alcohol consumption, equivalent to three to four whiskeys, patients with coronary artery disease have been noted to exhibit a progressive decrease in arterial pressure, cardiac output, left ventricular work, and tension time index, both at rest and during light exercise. No change was seen in cardiac rate or peripheral resistance. These changes were accompanied by ECG alterations consisting of T-wave flattening and ST segment depression (70,76,83).

Kentala et al. (84) studied the effect of alcohol on cardiac rhythm in

10 persons with a past history of acute myocardial infarction. The subjects were tested in a baseline state and 30 min after consumption of 0.5 g/kg alcohol, with each subject serving as his/her own control. The heart rate-blood pressure product was increased significantly by alcohol at a submaximal workload ($p < 0.01$). In five of the 10 patients, Holter monitoring revealed changes in cardiac rate subsequent to alcohol ingestion, consisting of an increased rate of atrial ectopy, appearance of ventricular ectopic beats, and/or multiple sinus arrests. Clinically, these changes were unassociated with any symptoms.

A more sophisticated study of the effects of alcohol on cardiac conduction in cardiac patients was conducted by Gould et al. (83), who recorded ECGs with and without atrial pacing before and after administration of 2 oz of 86.8-proof Canadian whiskey administered orally in less than 10 min. ECGs were taken at 5, 10, and 15 min subsequent to drinking. No significant changes were noted in P-A or A-H intervals subsequent to alcohol ingestion. At rapid atrial pacing rates, however, alcohol significantly lengthened the HQ and HS intervals. Second degree heart block occurred at lower pacing rates after alcohol than in the control state. The postsuppression, sinoatrial node recovery time was increased in the majority of patients after alcohol ($p < 0.05$).

In a rather unusual study, Klein and Harmjanz (85) infused a 7.5% solution of alcohol in patients with myocardial and valvular disease who underwent diagnostic cardiac catherization. Before and after the infusion, multiple endomyocardial biopsies were performed and examined by electron microscopy. Subsequent to ethanol infusion, all patients showed alterations of myocardial cell organelles, most prominently of the mitochondria, as well as changes in the sarcoplasm reticulum. The mean alcohol concentration in blood of the subjects at biopsy was 0.38 g%, which approximates a concentration obtained after the consumption of two or three beers or a glass of whiskey. These findings must be interpreted with a great deal of caution, however, as conclusions from electron microscopy must be drawn from examination of multiple specimens preferably performed by individuals without previous knowledge about the history of the specimens studied.

Coronary Blood Flow

The effect of alcohol on coronary blood flow is controversial. Alcohol has been used in the treatment of angina pectoris for more than two centuries with apparent success (86,87). Its use has been predicted on its proposed vasodilatory effect on the coronary vasculature associated with an increase in coronary flow. However, conflicting findings have been reported.

Mendoza et al. (88), measuring coronary flow with 81 Rb subsequent to intravenous infusions of alcohol in anesthetized dogs and humans, found a dose-related response. At blood alcohol concentrations of 50 mg%, there was a consistent but nonsignificant increase in coronary flow. At blood alcohol levels of 200 mg%, coronary flow increased by 60% and coronary vascular resistance declined. Ganz (89) found alcohol to decrease coronary resistance with a corresponding increase in coronary flow. Although left ventricular work decreased, myocardial oxygen consumption increased, paralleling the increase in coronary flow and oxygen contact on the coronary sinus. More recent studies have revealed little or no change in coronary flow with the administration of alcohol (90,91). In addition, exercise-induced electrocardiographic changes characteristic of ischemia have not been able to be prevented by alcohol ingestion (90–92). The absence of a salutary clinical effect of alcohol on either angina- or ischemic-induced changes in the ECG in the presence of an enhancement of coronary flow may be partially explained by the absence in most studies of techniques to determine inhomogeneous perfusion (93). A decrease in coronary vascular resistance in normal vessels may result in a diversion of blood flow from cardiac muscle fed by sclerotic vessels now dependent on arterial collaterals for their blood supply.

One study has found a beneficial effect of alcohol in patients with peripheral vascular disease. Turnipseed et al. (94) reported intravenous infusions of alcohol to produce increased blood flow in ischemic limbs at blood concentrations sufficiently low so as to diminish the possibility of intoxication or myocardial depressant effect. Further investigation in this area is warranted.

Summary

In summary, the hemodynamic changes reported following oral doses of ethanol are dependent on dose, rate of administration, presence of prior alcohol consumption or cardiac disease, time of measurement, and specific variables measured (Table 5). Acute ingestion of small amounts of alcohol in the normal nonalcoholic subject is associated with definite but clinically minimal hemodynamic changes. Larger amounts produce a transient myocardial depression. In persons with a history of alcoholism, the administration of even small amounts of alcohol may be accompanied by myocardial depression. These hemodynamic changes return to normal with abstinence. In persons with heavy, chronic ethanol consumption and some of myocardial impairment, continued ingestion of alcohol may allow a progression to symptoms characteristic of alcoholic cardiomyopathy.

Alcohol has an unequivocal hemodynamic depressant effect in patients with cardiac disease, which results in a decrease in left ventricular function. Electrocardiographic changes can include an increased ectopy as well as a depression in cardiac conduction. The magnitude of these changes varies with individual susceptibility. It should also be emphasized, however, that the clinical relevance of these findings is still unclear. Alcohol should not

TABLE 5. *Hemodynamic effects of ingestion of alcohol*

Group	Dose distilled spirits (oz)	Heart rate	Cardiac output	Stroke volume	Blood pressure	Peripheral vascular resistance	Left ventricular contractility				
							PEP	ICT	LVET	PEP/LVET	QS^2
Normals	2–6	NC/↑	↑	NC/↑	NC	↓	↑	↑	↓	↑	↓
Alcoholics	12	↑	↓	↓	NM	NM	↑/NC	NM	↓	↑	NM
Cardiac patients	4	NC	↓	↓	↓	NC	↑	↑	↓	↑	NM

↑, Increase; ↓, decrease; NC, no change; NM, not measured; PEP, preejection period; ICT, isovolumic contract time; LVET, left ventricular ejection time; QS^2, interval between Q-wave of ECG and second heart sound.

be routinely proscribed in patients with cardiac disease, as minimal or judicious use of alcohol may in fact have a beneficial psychologic effect. Injudicious use of alcohol or administration of alcohol to persons particularly susceptible to its hemodynamic effects is unwarranted. For this reason, individual evaluation is mandatory prior to formulating recommendations for altering drinking patterns in cardiac patients.

ELECTROCARDIOGRAPHIC ALTERATIONS

Animal Studies

Effects of chronic consumption of alcohol on the conduction system have been studied in laboratory animals by Ettinger et al. (64). Dogs received 36% of their caloric intake as ethanol for periods ranging from 7 to 33 months. In animals maintained on ethanol for more than 1 year, QRS widening, manifested by prolongation of H-Q intervals on His bundle tracings, was noted. At autopsy, light microscopy revealed an accumulation of mucopolysaccharide-like material in the interstitium. It is of interest that several of these animals died suddenly and unexpectedly, perhaps secondary to altered conduction with resultant ventricular arrhythmias (95). Cardiac conduction abnormalities were seen in animals with 1 year or more of ethanol ingestion. H-Q and QRS prolongation were noted in proportion to the intensity and severity of alcoholism and irrespective of cardiac enlargement. Structural changes in the myocardium were also noted, consisting of disruption of intercalated disks and interstitial deposits of Alcian-Blue staining material. These changes may be responsible for the reduced fibrillation threshold, although a tendency toward arrhythmias in laboratory animals chronically fed alcohol has been noted (96–98). The clinical implications of these findings remain to be determined.

Clinical Findings

Feinstein et al. (99), in a small study of four normal subjects, monitored electroencephalogram (EEG) and ECG during sleep under control conditions after administration of 8 oz of alcohol. The rate of premature atrial and ventricular contractions in all three subjects was found to be unchanged, although the duration of sleep increased, and EEG-recorded evidence of arousal diminished was noted. Friedman et al. (100) similarly did not note any electrocardiographic changes in 10 normal volunteers when blood alcohol levels previously associated with myocardial depression were produced. However, although arrhythmias associated with alcohol ingestion in normal men in a baseline state might not be apparent, under stressful situations associated with increased catecholamine release, such changes might have important clinical implications.

Electrocardiographic changes in 1,000 ambulatory alcoholics without any known past or present history or symptoms of previous coronary disease or nutritional disturbances have been recognized (101). These alterations consist of T-wave changes, sinus tachycardia, and conduction defects. A relationship appeared to exist between the interval between the last drink and the changes noted. Seventy percent of persons who had been drinking the day the ECG was taken had abnormal findings, with T-wave changes in 21% and a sinus tachycardia in 50%. This is contrasted to a 5% incidence of electrocardiographic alterations noted in 5% of persons who had not taken a drink for 2 days prior to their ECG. These changes were reproducible by intravenous infusion of ethanol at 1 ml/kg hr in three of nine volunteers.

These findings have been confirmed by other investigators (102,103), who have reported an incidence of abnormal ECG findings in asymptomatic patients varying from 16 to 57%. High fidelity ECG recordings have been noted by Wu et al. (104) to detect additional abnormalities not readily observable on conventional recordings. In a study of 36 alcoholics without evidence of clinical heart disease or hypertrophy, the PRc, QRS, and QTc intervals were prolonged and the septal Q frequently absent. Singer and Lundberg (105) reported ventricular dysrhythmias in a patient resulting in grand mal seizures and syncope after consumption of an alcoholic beverage.

The clinical relevance of these changes in alcoholics without known cardiac disease remains to be defined. However, it is of interest that Kramer et al. (106), in a study of sudden death in Baltimore, reported an impressive incidence of sudden, unexplained death in young male alcoholics. These persons all had fatty liver at autopsy. These findings were corroborated by Sundby (107), who noted an increased incidence of sudden death in a group of alcoholics being treated in an ambulatory care setting. Since ventricular fibrillation is not an uncommon antecedent in instances of sudden death, it is possible that the arrhythmogenic effect of acute alcohol ingestion might have in some way contributed to these individuals' demise.

Withdrawal

Abstinence, when associated with the withdrawal phenomenon, can result in electrocardiographic changes. Abbasakoor et al. (108), studying the withdrawal effects of alcohol on the ECG in 36 alcoholics without known cardiac disease, found only three patients not to exhibit ECG changes. Sinus tachycardia was most frequently observed (86%), with nonspecific T-wave changes (56%) also quite prominent. Ventricular arrhythmias occurred in 14 (39%) patients, with unifocal premature ventricular contractions (PVC) noted in 12 and multifocal PVC or ventricular tachycardia in two (6%). Supraventricular arrhythmias occurred in 3 (9%) patients. Similar findings have been confirmed by other investigators (109,110).

The etiology of the electrocardiographic changes is unclear. The appearance of arrhythmias is not correlated with blood alcohol level. The percentage of abnormal tracings, however, does vary inversely between the consumption of the last drink and time of ECG measurements. Since catecholamine excretion is increased during and after alcohol consumption, the relative excess of epinephrine and norepinephrine may result in a propensity toward arrhythmias. Other factors, such as hypokalemia or excessive smoking, frequently seen as a response to anxiety during withdrawal, may also be contributing factors. Vetter et al. (110) reported the incidence of arrhythmias to be 45% in hypokalemic patients, as compared to 11% in persons with normal serum potassium.

Although the electrocardiographic changes during withdrawal may be of no clinical relevance in healthy subjects, in persons with cardiac disease or in the presence of alcoholic cardiomyopathy, the changes may be far from innocuous and may be a cause of the sudden death that has been known to occur in alcoholics.

ALCOHOL CONSUMPTION AND CORONARY HEART DISEASE

The relationship of alcohol consumption to the production of coronary heart disease has not been clearly defined, although either a negative or a positive association might be hypothesized. Alcohol use is known to be associated with an increase in serum triglyceride, a known coronary risk factor. In persons with preexisting atheromatosis disease, the ability of alcohol to induce tachycardia and decrease left ventricular compliance may result in increased myocardial oxygen consumption. When the vasodilatory capacity of the coronary vasculature is limited by atheromatous disease, angina or myocardial infarction can occur. Indeed, myocardial infarction has been documented in chronic alcoholics without preexisting coronary artery disease. Regan et al. (111) have reported acute myocardial infarction in 12 persons with chronic alcoholism, 10 of whom had no evidence of obstructive coronary artery disease on angiography or postmortem examination. Autopsies revealed the presence of a glycoprotein-like material interstitially, as well as interstitial concentric periarterial fibrosis. These lesions might have led to ischemia and infarction due to restriction of coronary vasodilation during periods when increased coronary blood flow was required. Lipid deposits in the myocardium of persons succumbing to alcoholic cardiomyopathy have also been demonstrated (37,39) (see Chapter 5).

Knowledge of the actions of alcohol with respect to lipid metabolism might also permit the hypothesis of a negative association between alcohol consumption and coronary artery disease. Alcohol-induced elevation in HDL may have a protective effect. The presence of alcoholic liver disease, with a relative rise in estrogen levels, may also serve to exert a protective influence.

Epidemiologic Studies

Pathologic studies based on postmortem examinations have revealed a negative association between chronic alcoholism and/or hepatic cirrhosis and atherosclerosis of the coronary vasculature (112–114). Unfortunately, these studies were not controlled for potentially confounding variables, such as hypertension, age, diabetes, or gout. When such variables have been considered, a negative association has not been demonstrated (115–117). However, autopsy studies in persons with alcoholic cardiomyopathy have consistently revealed the large coronary vasculature to be relatively free of atherosclerosis (118–119).

Unfortunately, historic data obtained from autopsy cases are usually based on retrospective chart reviews. Even when controlled for confounding variables, it is frequently difficult to obtain an adequate pattern of alcohol consumption. Prospective studies, although difficult to design, are more valuable. Barboriak et al. (120) questioned 900 nondiabetic male patients undergoing coronary arteriography about their alcohol intake. On the basis of this survey, all patients were divided into abstainers and light, moderate, and very heavy drinkers. The extent of coronary artery disease on catheterization was scored and related to alcohol intake, correcting for age, hypertension, and smoking history. The coronary artery occlusion scores of abstainers and occasional drinkers were significantly higher than for those patients with high alcohol consumption ($p < 0.01$). This negative association was present for all but the youngest age groups and was not related to the existence of hypertension and/or smoking.

These data are suggestive of a negative association between alcohol ingestion and coronary artery disease. However, this study was performed in symptomatic persons appearing for cardiac catheterization. A better method of clarifying the relationship of alcohol to coronary heart disease is to study the drinking habits in large population groups followed prospectively to determine the development of coronary heart disease. Initial epidemiologic surveys either were unable to reveal a statistically significant association or demonstrated a positive association (121–123). More recent investigations, however, report a negative association of coronary heart disease with increasing alcohol consumption.

Klatsky et al. (124), in a review of multiphasic health screening examinations that controlled for confounding variables and provided data on alcohol consumption an average of 17 months before the occurrence of a first myocardial infarction, found an appreciably higher proportion of abstainers among cases at risk. Stason et al. (125), reviewing the data of the Boston Collaborative Drug Surveillance Program, found evidence of a lower rate of nonfatal myocardial infarction in subjects consuming six or more drinks per day. However, patients dying prior to or soon after hospital admission were excluded from the study, as were individuals with the diagnosis of alcoholism or cirrhosis.

Yano et al. (126), in a 6-year study of 7,705 men living in Hawaii, found a strong negative association between moderate alcohol consumption (up to 16 cc/day) and the risk of nonfatal myocardial infarction and death from coronary heart disease. This association remained significant in multivariate analysis correcting for other risk factors. The relationship persisted when individuals who had stopped drinking before the baseline examination because of latent coronary heart disease or coronary-prone health conditions were excluded from this study. An analysis of these data revealed a significant difference to exist between current drinkers and both exdrinkers and lifetime abstainers ($p < 0.01$). Surprisingly, the incidence of acute coronary insufficiency was greater in those patients with the largest alcohol consumption than in those with smaller consumption or nondrinkers; however, the trend was not statistically significant.

A review of autopsy cases in the Honolulu heart study revealed alcohol consumption at the time of the baseline examination to be distinctly lower in those individuals dying from myocardial infarction than in those dying from other causes. No relationship was noted between the severity of coronary arteriosclerosis and alcohol consumption independent of the evidence of myocardial infarction.

Summary

Although heavy use of alcohol is clearly toxic to cardiac muscle, and even moderate use may be associated with evidence of deterioration of left ventricular function, especially in patients with cardiac disease, pathologic and epidemiologic data do not preclude a beneficial effect on the coronary vasculature by occasional or even moderate use of alcohol. This beneficial effect is unrelated to the coexistence of hepatic dysfunction as the levels of drinking in most of the epidemiologic studies were rather modest, with persons with cirrhosis being eliminated from the study group. The mechanisms responsible for this negative association remain to be more clearly defined. The effects of alcohol with respect to lipid metabolism, however, may play a prominent role.

ALCOHOL CONSUMPTION AND HYPERTENSION

The association between alcohol use and hypertension has been considered for more than six decades since the initial observation by Lian in 1915 (127). Many of the data presented can be divided into retrospective analysis based on mortality rates and epidemiologic surveys in which multivariate risk analyses are performed to delineate the various factors associated with coronary artery disease.

Since alcoholism is considered the leading cause of cirrhosis of the liver, observations of the relationship of mortality from hypertension with mortality from cirrhosis have been suggestive of a relationship between alcoholism and hypertension. Mathews (128), in a review of mortality tables for England and Wales from 1949 to 1953, found that death from hypertension and stroke was highest in those groups, with the highest death rates for cirrhosis. In hypertensive persons, the observed number of cirrhotic deaths was 873 versus an expected number of 519 ($p < 0.001$). These findings suggest that the socioeconomic groups that have the highest death rates from cirrhosis of the liver also have the highest death rates from hypertension and stroke.

The prevalence of hepatic dysfunction, as determined by serum concentrations of alanine and asparate aminotransferase, in ambulatory hypertensives has recently been noted to be increased when compared to normotensives. Enzyme elevations were higher in male hypertensives than in normotensives, with a tendency for higher concentrations of enzymes in those persons with greater alcohol intakes (129).

Epidemiologic Surveys

Although these findings in isolation cannot lend credence to a causal relationship between alcohol use and hypertension, prospective epidemiologic surveys have also noted a similar association (130). D'Alonzo and Pell (102), in a review of 922 problem drinkers and a selected matched control group, found the prevalence of hypertension, as defined by a systolic blood pressure of 160 mm Hg or more and a diastolic blood pressure of 95 mm Hg or more, to be 2.3 times as high in the drinking population. Tachycardia was also threefold more frequent among the known drinkers. These findings were independent of body weight or the presence of coronary artery disease. It should be emphasized that although the differences between drinkers and nondrinkers were significant, most drinkers presented with neither hypertension (60%) nor tachycardia (82%).

Similar findings occurred in the Los Angeles Heart Study (131), which showed that 432 men drinking at least three times weekly had statistically significant higher systolic blood pressures than nondrinkers or persons consuming less than this amount. In the Framingham Heart Study (132), heavy alcohol use (2,957 mm alcohol per month) was also associated with higher mean systolic blood pressures. In both surveys, however, although the findings were statistically meaningful, the magnitude of the changes recorded (1.6 and 7 mm Hg, respectively) cannot be considered to be of practical importance. In addition, the effects of confounding variables, such as cigarette smoking and consumption of caffeine-containing beverages, were not taken into account.

Confounding Variables

Smoking

Confounding variables, especially cigarette smoking, must be considered in evaluating the relationship between alcohol consumption and hypertension. People consuming large amounts of alcohol tend to smoke an equally impressive number of cigarettes and, not infrequently, are heavy coffee drinkers (133,134). The increased cardiovascular risk associated with cigarette smoking is well known. It is therefore imperative that all studies of causal relationships between alcohol and cardiovascular disease consider this variable. Klatksy et al. (135,136), in a survey of 83,974 men and women, classified respondents as to the degree of alcohol consumption and prevalence of hypertension. Their data were also crossclassified for several confounding variables. The prevalence of hypertension in subjects taking six or more drinks a day when compared to nondrinkers doubled in whites and was approximately 50% greater in blacks. Prevalence rates in heavy drinkers as compared to controls were as follows: black men, 15 versus 10%; black women, 24 versus 14%; white men, 11 versus 5%; and white women, 11 versus 6%. The mean magnitude of these changes varied with the different demographic groups, ranging from 5 to 10.8 mm Hg for systolic blood pressure to 10 to 4.5 mm Hg in diastolic blood pressure. In general, increases of blood pressure paralleled increases in alcohol consumption. The association between blood pressure and drinking was found to be independent of cigarette smoking, coffee use, past history of drinking, educational status, and body weight as determined by adiposity levels.

A similar association was also found by Dyer et al. (137) in an analysis of data from epidemiologic surveys of two large midwestern utility companies (1,465 and 1,899 persons, respectively). In both of these cohorts, analysis of covariance showed the persistence of an increased risk for hypertension in heavy drinkers after removal of confounding variables, such as cigarette smoking, coffee consumption, and weight.

Genetic Factors

Several other factors may also exert a confounding influence on the association between alcohol use and hypertension. Familial studies have suggested that hypertension tends to occur with greater frequency in families (138). Similarly, identical twins are much more likely to exhibit similar blood pressures than nonidentical twins or siblings (139). Genetic factors predisposing to both hypertension and excessive alcohol use have been postulated. The possibility of both of these traits within individuals may allow for both hypertension and alcoholism without assessing a causal relationship. Myrhed (140) and Hrubec et al. (141) studied both monozygotic and dizygotic twin pairs. A relationship between chronic alcohol use and hypertension was confirmed but found to exist independent of genetic factors.

Lifestyle

Differing dietary habits between alcoholics and nonalcoholics could also affect the association between alcohol use and hypertension. Although dietary habits were reviewed in several of the studies, inquiry was not made as to whether specific dietary patterns were more common among drinkers, e.g., if there was heavy salting of foods or use of condiments. This may represent an additional confounding variable. The effect of lifestyle has also been inadequately studied. As discussed earlier (Chapter 2), many investigators have demonstrated the association of stress with a sustained hypertensive vascular response (142–144). It is reasonable to assume that regular drinkers resort to alcohol to relieve the anxieties of daily living; and these anxieties, independent of the alcohol, may account for the minimal elevations of blood pressures found.

Measurement Techniques

Finally, the temporal relationship between alcohol consumption and measurement of blood pressure can be of importance. The heavy drinker might have abstained for a day or more prior to the routine examination. In such instances, the blood pressure could have been measured during a subclinical alcohol withdrawal state, known to be associated with excessive activity of the sympathetic nervous system. Conversely, if alcohol was acutely consumed prior to the physical examination, a transient elevation in blood pressure and heart rate might occur. Although such changes in heart rate and blood pressure are less in the chronic alcoholic as compared to the nondrinker, the magnitude of changes reported in most studies is not great and could be accounted for by either acute consumption of alcohol or presence of withdrawal phenomena.

Summary

Recent evidence suggests a relationship between the quantity of alcohol consumed and the elevation of both systolic and diastolic blood pressures, independent of many confounding variables associated with an increased risk of hypertension. Although the magnitude of changes reported is statistically significant, these changes are of a degree that does not permit a direct cause and effect relationship to be definitively concluded. Further prospective studies designed to account for the confounding variables mentioned above are needed. In addition, extension of basic metabolic research concerning the effect of acute and chronic alcohol consumption on cathecholamine metabolism and the renin-angiotensin system would be of considerable value in further defining this association.

ALCOHOL CONSUMPTION AND DEATH DUE TO CARDIOVASCULAR DISEASES

The evidence presented above suggests that although excessive alcohol consumption is associated with an increased prevalence of hypertension, a positive association of alcohol use with angina and/or myocardial infarction either does not exist or, in fact, a negative association may be more common. As might be expected from these data, the relationship between alcohol use and mortality due to cardiovascular disease remains unclear. It is generally accepted, however, that alcoholics have a higher death rate from all causes than the nondrinking population. Depending on the specific population surveyed, a highly consistent relationship between alcohol consumption and mortality has been noted, with the risk of death in alcoholics to be two to three times that of nondrinkers. Several studies have revealed this excess mortality to be beyond that which would be expected after controlling for age, hypertension, heart rate, serum cholesterol, relative weight, or smoking (145–148). Data regarding mortality due to cardiovascular disease and alcohol consumption have shown far less uniform findings. Of the 11 surveys reported in Table 6, five noted an increased risk of death due to cardiovascu-

TABLE 6. *Cardiovascular mortality in heavy consumers of alcohol*

Study	Increased risk of death over nondrinking population	
	All causes	Cardiac disease
Schmidt and DeLint (145)	2.03	1.74
State of California (146)	2.36	Minimal
Pell and D'Alonzo (102)	3.22	2.28
Dahlgren (147)	None	None
CP Gas Company (130,137)	2.56	4.41–5.21[a]
Western Electric (130,137)	2.46	1.66–1.74[a]
Framingham (125,132)	NSM	None
Klatsky et al. (124)	NSM	None
Los Angeles Heart Survey (131)	NSM	None
Wilhelmsen et al. (148)	NSM	1.95
Yano et al. (126)	NSM	None

[a] Includes cardiovascular-renal diseases, coronary heart disease, and sudden deaths.

NSM, not specifically measured.

lar diseases associated with alcohol intake, and six reported the absence of such an association. In fact, in two of the studies a significant negative association was noted between alcohol consumption and mortality due to myocardial infarction. In contrast, a review of the data by Dyer et al. (130) (137) showed the risk of death due to cardiovascular diseases, including sudden death and coronary heart disease, to be as much as five times that of the nondrinking population.

There are several reasons for these discordant findings. First, the definition of heavy drinking varies widely. An increase in mortality may become significant only at extreme levels of alcohol consumption. Studies reporting the absence of an association might have insufficiently isolated the heavy drinkers. However, the study by Yano et al. (126), which reports cardiovascular effects over a wide range of alcohol consumption, was unable to document any significant relationship with respect to mortality and cardiovascular disease.

A second problem relates to the diagnosis of the actual cause of death. In most instances, the cause of death is obtained from the death certificate in absence of an autopsy. Since heavy alcohol consumption might be associated with coronary-like clinical symptoms and sudden death due to causes other than coronary artery disease, absence of autopsy findings may result in an erroneous assignment of causes of death to cardiovascular diseases. The presence of primary cardiomyopathy is also known to be associated with an increased mortality. Individuals with this specific disorder should be separated from prospective surveys. Failure to do so can result in an unusually high mortality due to cardiac disease in alcoholic populations.

SUMMARY

In summary, ample evidence exists that both acute and chronic administration of alcohol results in hemodynamic changes in the alcoholic and the nonalcoholic. Alcohol, even in the presence of an adequate diet in the laboratory setting, has been shown to be cardiotoxic. Epidemiologic studies have documented an association between alcohol use and hypertension, as well as an increased risk of death from all causes. Evidence suggests, however, that the prevalence of atherosclerosis, angina, and myocardial infarction in chronic alcoholics is less than that in nonalcoholics. A positive association between alcohol consumption and high density cholesterol also has been documented. The net effect on the cardiovascular system with respect to moderate or minimal consumption of alcohol has not been adequately resolved. Although the physician should not condone excessive consumption of alcohol, neither should minimal drinking in individuals with cardiovascular disease be vigorously proscribed unless adverse effects on the particular individual can be demonstrated or a coexisting physical condition preclude such use.

REFERENCES

1. Second Special Report to the U.S. Congress on alcohol and health from the Secretary of Health, Education and Welfare, June 1974. DHEW Publ. No. ADM 75–212, U.S. Government Printing Office, Washington, D.C. 1975.
2. Berry, R. E., and Boland, J. P. (1975): *The Economic Cost of Alcohol Abuse.* New York Free Press, New York.
3. McCusker, J., Cherubin, C. E., and Zimberg, S. (1971): Prevalence of alcoholism in general municipal hospital population. *N.Y. State J. Med.,* 71:751.
4. Barchha, R., Stewart, M. A., and Guaze, S. B. (1968): The prevalence of alcoholism among general hospital ward patients. *Am. J. Psychiatry,* 125:681.
5. Vestal, R. E., McGuire, E. A., Tobin, J. D., et al. (1977): Aging and ethanol metabolism. *Clin. Pharmacol. Ther.,* 21:343.
6. Wallgreen, M., and Berry, H. (1970): *Actions of Alcohol, Vol. 1,* pp. 17–73. American Elsevier, New York.
7. Isselbacher, K. J. (1977): Metabolic and hepatic effects of alcohol. *N. Engl. J. Med.,* 296:612.
8. Lieber, C. S. (1973): Liver adaptation and injury in alcoholism. *N. Engl. J. Med.,* 288:356.
9. Ostrander, L. D., Lamphiear, D. E., Block, W. D., et al. (1974): Relationship of serum lipid concentrations to alcohol consumption. *Arch. Intern. Med.,* 134:451.
10. Barboriak, J. J. (1974): Hyperlipemia in alcoholics. *O. J. Stud. Alcohol,* 35:15.
11. Stahelin, H., Wissen, C., and Sommer, P. (1974): Alcoholic hyperlipidemia. *Int. J. Vitam. Nutr. Res.,* 44:507.
12. Ginsberg, H., Olefsky, J., Farquhar, J., et al. (1974): Moderate ethanol ingestion and plasma triglyceride levels: A study in normal and hypertriglyceridemic persons. *Ann. Intern. Med.,* 80:143.
13. Casteilli, W. P., Gordon, T., Hjortland, M. C., et al. (1977): Alcohol blood lipids: The cooperative lipoprotein phenotyping study. *Lancet,* 2:153.
14. Major, L. F., and Goyer, P. F. (1978): Effects of disulfiram and pyridoxine on serum cholesterol. *Ann. Intern. Med.,* 88:53.
15. Vasak, V., and Kopecky, J. (1967): On the role of pyridoxamine in the metabolism of the toxic action of carbon disulfide. In: *Toxicology of Carbon Disulfide,* edited by H. Brieger, p. 35. Excerpta Medica, Amsterdam.
16. Tiller, J. R., Schilling, R. S., and Morris, J. N. (1968): Occupational toxic factors in mortality from coronary heart disease. *Br. Med. J.,* 4:407.
17. Israel-Jacard, Y., and Kalant, H. (1966): Effect of ethanol on electrolyte transport and electrogenesis in animal tissues. *J. Cell. Comp. Physiol.,* 65:127.
18. Klingman, G. I., and Goodall, M. M. C. (1957): Urinary epinephrine and levarterenol excretion during acute sublethal alcohol intoxication in dogs. *J. Pharmacol. Exp. Ther.,* 121:313.
19. Perman, E. S. (1961): Effect of hydration on the urinary excretion of adrenalin and noradrenalin on the blood sugar of rats. *Acta Physiol. Scand.,* 51:68.
20. Wendt, V. E., Wu, C., Balcon, R., et al. (1965): Hemodynamic and metabolic effects of chronic alcoholism in man. *Am. J. Cardiol.,* 15:175.
21. Wacker, W. E. C., and Parisi, A. F. (1968): Magnesium metabolism. *N. Engl. J. Med.,* 278:772.
22. Susin, M., and Henderson, P. B. (1967): Fine structural changes induced in rat myocardium by sodium L thyroxine and by magnesium deficiency. *Arch. Pathol.,* 83:86.
23. Van Ark, C. R., Ballantyne, F., III, and Reynolds, E. W., Jr. (1973): Electrolytes and the electrocardiogram. *Cardiovasc. Clin.,* 5:270.
24. Burch, G. E., and Giles, T. D. (1977): The importance of magnesium deficiency in cardiovascular disease. *Am. Heart J.,* 94:649.
25. Regan, T. J., Levinson, G. E., Oldewurtel, H. A., et al. (1969): Ventricular function in noncardiacs with alcohol fatty liver: Role of ethanol in the production of cardiomyopathy. *J. Clin. Invest.,* 48:407.
26. Becker, C. L., Roe, R. L., and Scott, R. A. (1974): *Curriculum on Pharmacology, Neurology and Toxicology,* p. 69. New York Medical Press, New York.

27. Williams, H. E., and Fitzgerald, F. T. (1975): Hypophosphatemia. *West. J. Med.,* 122:482.
28. Lotz, M., Zisman, E., and Bartter, F. C. (1968): Evidence for a phosphate depletion syndrome in man. *N. Engl. J. Med.,* 278:409.
29. Klock, J. C., Williams, H. E., and Mentzer, W. C. (1974): Hemolytic anemia and somatic cell dysfunction in severe hypophosphatemia. *Arch. Intern. Med.,* 134: 360.
30. O'Connor, L. R., Wheeler, W. S., and Bethune, J. E. (1977): Effect of hypophosphatemia on myocardial performance in man. *N. Engl. J. Med.,* 297:901.
31. Lieber, C. S. (1973): Liver adaptation to injury in alcoholism. *N. Engl. J. Med.,* 288:356.
32. Teschke, R., Hasumura Y., and Lieber, C. S. (1974): Hepatic microsomal ethanol oxidizing system solubalization, isolation and characterization. *Arch. Biochem. Biophys.,* 163:404.
33. Korsten, M., Matsuzaki, S., Feinman, L., et al. (1975): High blood acetyldehyde levels after ethanol administration: Difference between alcoholic and nonalcoholic subjects. *N. Engl. J. Med.,* 292:386.
34. Davis, V. E., Brown, H., Hoff, J. A., et al. (1967): The alteration of serotonin metabolism to 5 hydroxytryptophol by ethanol ingestion in man. *J. Lab. Clin. Med.,* 69:132.
35. Davis, V. E., Brown, H., Hoff, J. A., et al. (1967): Ethanol induced norepinephrine metabolism in man. *J. Lab. Clin. Med.,* 69:787.
36. Schreiber, S. S., Oratz, M., Rothschild, M. A., et al. (1974): Alcoholic cardiomyopathy II: The inhibition of cardiac microsomal protein synthesis by acetyladehyde. *J. Mol. Cell. Cardiol.,* 6:207.
37. Wendt, V. E., Ajloni Bruce, T. A., et al. (1966): Acute effects of alcohol on the human myocardium. *Am. J. Cardiol.,* 17:804.
38. Pachinger, O. M., Tillmanns, H., Fauvel, J. M., et al. (1973): The effect of prolonged administration of ethanol on cardiac metabolism and performance in the dog. *J. Clin. Invest.,* 52:2690.
39. Ferraus, V. J., Hibbs, R. G., Weilbaecher, D. G., et al. (1965): Alcoholic cardiomyopathy: A histochemical study. *Am. Heart J.,* 69:748.
40. Bing, R. J., Tillmanns, H., Fauvel, J., et al. (1974): Effect of prolonged administration of alcohol on calcium transport in heart muscle of the dog. *Circ. Res.,* 35:33.
41. Marciniak, M., Grudbjarnason, S., and Bruce, T. A. (1968): The effect of chronic alcohol administration on enzyme profile and glyceride content of heart muscle, brain and liver. *Proc. Soc. Exp. Biol. Med.,* 128:1021.
42. Kater, R. M. H., Zieve, P., Tobon, F., et al. (1969): An accelerated metabolism of drugs in alcoholics. *Gastroenterology,* 56:412.
43. Björnstrom, F. (1872): On the effect of alcoholic beverages and simultaneous use of chloral hydrate. *Ups. Lakare Foren. Fordandl.,* 8:114.
44. Newman, W. H., and Valicenti, J. E. (1971): Ventricular function following acute alcohol administration. *Am. Heart J.,* 81:61.
45. Misra, P. A., Léfèvre, A., Ishii, H., et al. (1971): Increase of ethanol, meprobamate and phenobarbital metabolism after chronic ethanol administration in man and rats. *Am. J. Med.,* 51:346.
46. Rubin, E., Gang, H., Misra, P., et al. (1970): Inhibition of drug metabolism in acute ethanol intoxication: A hepatic microsomal mechanism. *Am. J. Med.,* 47:801.
47. Mould, G. P. (1972): Interaction of glutethimide and phenobarbitone with ethanol in man. *J. Pharm. Pharmacol.,* 24:894.
48. Hayes, S. L., Pablo, G., Radomski, T., et al. (1977): Ethanol and oral diazepam absorption. *N. Engl. J. Med.,* 296:186.
49. Bardodêj, Z. (1975): Intolerance alkoholu pochloralhydratu. *Cesk. Farm.,* 14: 478.
50. Sellers, E. M., Carr, G., Bernstein, J. G., et al. (1972): Interaction of chloralhydrate and ethanol in man II. Hemodynamics and performance. *Clin. Pharmacol. Ther.,* 13:50.

51. Sellers, E. M., Lang, M., Koch-Weser, J., et al. (1972): Interaction of chloral-hydrate and ethanol in man I. Metabolism. *Clin. Pharmacol. Ther.,* 13:37.
52. Lockett, M. F., and Milner, G. (1965): Combining the antidepressant drugs. *Br. Med. J.,* 1:921.
53. Milner, G., and Landaver, A. A. (1973): The effects of doxepin alone and together with alcohol in relation to driving safety. *Med. J. Aust.,* 1:837.
54. Milner, G., and Landaver, A. A. (1971): Alcohol, thioridazine and chlorpromazine effects on skills relating to driving behavior. *Br. J. Psychiatry,* 118:351.
55. Cherubin, C., McCusker, J., and Baden, M. (1972): The epidemiology of death in narcotic addicts. *Am. J. Epidemiol.,* 96:11.
56. Loomis, H. P. (1900): The treatment of acute alcoholism by large doses of digitalis. *JAMA,* 35:377.
57. Neumann, W., and Walter, R. (1942): Beein Flussung der auswertung von digitalisstoffen durch alkohol. *Arch. Exp. Pathol. Pharmakol. (Berlin),* 199:412.
58. Kissen, B. (1974): *Interactions of Ethyl Alcohol and Other Drugs in the Biology of Alcoholism, Vol. 3,* edited by B. Kissen and H. Begleiter, p. 145. Plenum Press, New York.
59. Shafer, N. (1965): Hypotension due to nitroglycerin combined with alcohol. *N. Engl. J. Med.,* 273:1169.
60. Tacker, M., Creavin, P. J., and McIsaac, W. M. (1970): Alterations in tyramine metabolism by alcohol. *Biochem. Pharmacol.,* 19:604.
61. Powell, L. W. (1975): The role of alcoholism in hepatic iron storage disease. *Ann. N.Y. Acad. Sci.,* 252:124.
62. Walshe, W. H. (1873): *Diseases of the Heart and Great Vessels,* p. 359. Smith, Elder & Company, London.
63. Regan, T. J., Khan, M. I., Ettinger, P. O., et al. (1974): Myocardial function and lipid metabolism in the chronic alcoholic animal. *J. Clin. Invest.,* 57:740.
64. Ettinger, P. O., Lyons, M. M., Oldewurtel, T. A., et al. (1976): Cardiac conduction abnormalities produced by chronic alcoholism. *Am. Heart J.,* 91:66.
65. Liedtke, A. J., and DeMuth, W. E. (1975): Effects of alcohol on cardiovascular performance after experimental nonpenetrating chest tissue. *Am. J. Cardiol.,* 35:243.
66. Beard, J. D., Knott, D. H., Simpson, J. R., et al. (1973): Cardiovascular response to hemorrhage in dogs after alcohol. *Q. J. Stud. Alcohol,* 34:1304.
67. Grollman, A. (1930): The action of alcohol, caffeine and tobacco on the cardiac output (and its related function of normal man). *J. Pharmacol. Exp. Ther.,* 39:313.
68. Riff, D. P., Jain, A. C., and Doyle, J. T. (1969): Acute hemodynamic effects of ethanol on normal human volunteers. *Am. Heart J.,* 78:592.
69. Juchems, R., and Klobe, R. (1969): Hemodynamic effects of ethyl alcohol in man. *Am. Heart J.,* 78:133.
70. Gould, L., Zahir, M., Demartino, A., et al. (1971): Cardiac effects of a cocktail. *JAMA,* 218:1799.
71. Gould, L., Reddy, R., Groswann, K., et al. (1973): Cardiac effects of two cocktails in normal man. *Chest,* 63:943.
72. Timmis, G. C., Ramos, R. G., Gordon, S., et al. (1974): Ethanol induced changes of myocardial performance in normal adults. *Cardiology,* 59:184.
73. Ahmed, S. S., Levinson, G. E., and Regan, T. J. (1973): Depression of myocardial contractility with low doses of ethanol in normal man. *Circulation,* 43: 378.
74. Weissler, A. M., Kamen, A. C., Bornstein, R. S., et al. (1965): The effect of deslanoside on the duration of the phases of ventricular systole in man. *Am. J. Cardiol.,* 15:153.
75. Delgado, C. E., Fortuin, N. J., and Ross, R. S. (1975): Acute effects of low doses of alcohol on left ventricular function by echocardiography. *Circulation,* 51:535.
76. Conway, N. (1968): Hemodynamic effects of ethyl alcohol in patients in coronary heart disease. *Br. Heart J.,* 30:638.

77. Wong, M. (1963): Depression of cardiac performance by ethanol unmasked during autonomic blockage. *Am. Heart J.,* 86:508.
78. Zsotér, T. T., and Sellers, E. (1977): Effect of alcohol on cardiovascular reflexes. *J. Stud. Alcohol,* 38:1.
79. Timmis, G. C., Ramos, R. C., Gordon, S., et al. (1975): The basis for differences in ethanol induced myocardial depression in normal subjects. *Circulation,* 51:1144.
80. Regan, T. J., Levinson, G. E., Olbewurtel, H. A., et al. (1969): Ventricular function in noncardiacs with alcoholic fatty liver: The role of alcohol in the production of cardiomyopathy. *J. Clin. Invest.,* 48:397.
81. Zambrano, S. S., Mazzotta, J. F., and Sherman, B. S. (1974): Cardiac dysfunction in unselected alcoholic patients: Noninvasive screening by systolic time intervals. *Am. Heart J.,* 87:318.
82. Lehrer, P. M., and Taylor, H. A. (1974): Effects of alcohol on cardiac reactivity in alcoholics and nonalcoholics. *Q. J. Stud. Alcohol,* 35:1044.
83. Gould, L., Reddy, C. U. R., Patel, N., et al. (1974): Effects of whiskey on heart consumption in cardiac patients. *Q. J. Stud. Alcohol,* 35:26.
84. Kentala, E., Luurila, O., and Salaspuro, M. (1976): Effects of alcohol ingestion on cardiac rhythm in patients with ischemic heart disease. *Ann. Clin. Res.,* 8:408.
85. Klein, H., and Harmjanz, D. (1975): Effect of ethanol infusion on the ultrastructure of human myocardium. *Med. J.,* 51:325.
86. Heberden, W. (1786): Some account of disorders of the heart. *Tr. R. Coll. Physicians,* 2:59.
87. Cecil and Loeb (1976): *Textbook of Medicine, 12th Edition,* edited by P. B. Beeson and W. McDermott. W. B. Saunders & Company, Philadelphia.
88. Mendoza, L. C., Hellberg, K., and Rickart, A. (1971): The effect of intravenous ethyl alcohol on the coronary circulation and myocardial contractility of the human and canine heart. *J. Clin. Pharmacol.,* 11:165.
89. Ganz, U. (1963): The acute effect of alcohol on the circulation and on the oxygen metabolism of the heart. *Am. Heart J.,* 60:494.
90. Gould, L. (1970): Cardiac effects of alcohol. *Am. Heart J.,* 79:422.
91. Conway, N. C. (1968): Hemodynamic effects of ethyl alcohol in coronary heart disease. *Am. Heart J.,* 76:581.
92. Russek, H. I., Naegele, C. F., and Regan, F. D. (1950): Alcohol in the treatment of angina pectoris. *JAMA,* 143:355.
93. Bing, R. J., and Hellberg, K. (1972): Coronary blood flow in relation to angina pectoris. *Circulation,* 46:1146.
94. Turnipseed, W., Vasko, J. S., and Evans, W. E. (1976): Hemodynamic effects of intravenous alcohol on patients with ischemic limb disease. *J. Surg. Res.,* 20:477.
95. Ettinger, P. O., Regan, T. J., Khan, M. I., et al. (1973): Relation of alcoholic cardiac conduction abnormalities to duration of alcoholism. *Am. J. Cardiol.,* 31: 130 (Abstr.).
96. Regan, T. J., Koroxenidis, H., Moschos, C. B., et al. (1966): The acute metabolic hemodynamic responses of the left ventricule to ethanol. *J. Clin. Invest.,* 45:270.
97. Maines, J. E., and Aldinger, E. E. (1967): Myocardial depression accompanying chronic consumption of alcohol. *Am. Heart J.,* 73:55.
98. de la Cruz, C. L., Jr., Haider, B., Ettinger, P. O., et al. (1976): Effects of ethanol on ventricular electrical stability in the chronic alcoholic animal. *Clin. Res.,* 24:419A.
99. Feinstein, R., Gooden, B. A., and Wolf, W. (1975): The effect of alcohol and barbiturate on the frequency of atrial and ventricular premature beats during sleep. *Pavlov. J. Biol. Sci.,* 10:102.
100. Friedman, H. S., Korsten, M. A., Alcorta, C., et al. (1974): Acute effect of alcohol on the resting electrocardiogram in man. *Clin Res,* 22:680A.
101. Sereny, G. (1971): Effects of alcohol on the electrocardiogram. *Circulation,* 44: 558.

102. D'Alonzo, C. A., and Pell, S. (1968): Cardiovascular disease among problem drinkers. *J. Occup. Med.,* 10:344.
103. Pader, E. (1973): Clinical heart disease and electrographic abnormalities in alcoholics. *Q. J. Stud. Alcohol* 34:774.
104. Wu, C. F., Sudhakar, M., and Jafer, G. (1976): Preclinical cardiomyopathy in chronic alcoholics: A sex difference. *Am. Heart J.,* 91:281.
105. Singer, K., and Lundberg, W. B. (1972): Ventricular arrhythmias associated with the ingestion of alcohol. *Ann. Intern. Med.,* 77:247.
106. Kramer, K., Kuller, L., and Fisher, R. (1968): The increasing mortality attributed to cirrhosis and fatty liver in Baltimore (1957–1966). *Ann. Intern. Med.,* 69:273.
107. Sundby, P. (1969): *Alcoholism and Mortality.* Oslo, Norway. Universitets fordaget 1967 National Institute for Alcohol Research and Rutgers University Center of Alcohol Studies, New Brunswick, New Jersey.
108. Abbasakoor, A., Beanlands, D. S., and MacLeod, S. M. (1976): Electrocardiographic changes during ethanol withdrawal. *Ann. N.Y. Acad. Sci.,* 272–273:364.
109. Sereny, G. (1971): Effects of alcohol on the electrocardiogram. *Circulation,* 44: 558.
110. Vetter, W. R., Cohn, L. H., and Reichgott, M. (1967): Hypokalemia and electrocardiographic abnormalities during acute alcohol withdrawal. *Arch. Intern. Med.,* 120:536.
111. Regan, T. J., Wu, C. F., and Wusse, A. B. (1975): Acute myocardial infarction in toxic cardiomyopathy without coronary obstruction. *Circulation,* 51:453.
112. Howell, W. L., and Manion, W. C. (1960): The low incidence of myocardial infarction in patients with portal cirrhosis of the liver: A review of 639 cases of cirrhosis of the liver from 17,731 autopsies. *Am. Heart J.,* 60:341.
113. Creed, O. L., Vaird, W. F., and Fisher, E. R. (1955): Severity of aortic atherosclerosis in certain diseases; necropsy study. *Am. J. Med. Sci.,* 230:385.
114. Hirst, A. D., Hadley, G. G., and Gore, I. (1965): Effect of chronic alcoholism and cirrhosis of the liver on atherosclerosis. *Am. J. Med. Sci.,* 249:143.
115. Wilens, S. L. (1947): Relationship of chronic alcoholism to atherosclerosis. *JAMA,* 135:1136.
116. Parrish, H. M., and Eberly, A. J., Jr. (1961): Negative association of coronary atherosclerosis with liver cirrhosis and chronic alcoholism—a statistical fallacy. *J. Indiana State Med. Assoc.,* 54:341.
117. Rissanen, V. (1974): Coronary and aortic atherosclerosis in chronic alcoholics. *Z. Rechtsmed.,* 75:83.
118. Pintar, K., Wolansky, B. M., and Buggay, Z. R. (1965): Alcoholic cardiomyopathy. *Can. Med. Assoc. J.,* 93:103.
119. Factor, S. (1976): Intramyocardial small vessel disease in chronic alcoholism. *Am. Heart J.,* 92:561.
120. Barboriak, J. J., Rimm, A. A., Anderson, A. J., et al. (1977): Coronary artery occlusion and alcohol intake. *Br. Heart J.,* 39:289.
121. Doyle, J. T., Heslin, A. S., Hilleboe, H. E., et al. (1957): A prospective study of degenerative vascular disease in Albany: Report of 3 years experience I. Ischemic heart disease. *Am. J. Public Health* [*Suppl.*], 47:25.
122. Morris, J. N., Kagan, A., Pattison, D. C., et al. (1968): Incidence and prediction of ischemic heart disease in London busmen. *Lancet,* 2:555.
123. Shurtleff, D. (1970): Some characteristics related to the incidence of cardiovascular disease and health, Framingham Study, 16 year follow-up. In: *The Framingham Study: An Epidemiological Examination of Cardiovascular Disease,* edited by W. B. Kannel and T. Gordon, Sect. 26. U.S. Government Printing Office, Washington, D.C.
124. Klatsky, A. L., Friedman, G. D., and Siegelaub, A. B. (1974): Alcohol consumption before myocardial infarction. *Ann. Intern. Med.,* 81:294.
125. Stason, W. B., Neff, R. K., Miettinen, O. S., et al. (1976): Alcohol consumption and nonfatal myocardial infarction. *Am. J. Epidemiol.,* 104:603.

126. Yano, K., Rhoads, G. G., and Kagan, A. (1977): Coffee, alcohol and risk of coronary heart disease among Japanese men living in Hawaii. *N. Engl. J. Med.,* 297:405.
127. Lian, N. C. (1915): L'alcoolisme, cause d'hypertension arterielle. *Bull. Acad. Med. (Paris),* 74:525.
128. Mathews, J. D. (1976): Alcohol use, hypertension and coronary heart disease. *Clin. Sci. Mol. Med.,* 51:6615.
129. Beevers, D. G. (1977): Alcohol and hypertension. *Lancet,* 2:114.
130. Dyer, A., Stamler, J., Paul, O., et al. (1976): Alcohol, cardiovascular risk factors and mortality in two Chicago epidemiologic studies. *CVD Epidemiol. Newslett.,* 20:34.
131. Clark, V. A., Chapman, J. M., and Coulson, A. H. (1967): Effects of various factors on systolic and diastolic blood pressures in the Los Angeles Heart Study. *J. Chronic Dis.,* 20:571.
132. Kannel, W. B., and Sorlie, P. (1974): Hypertension in Framingham. In: *Epidemiology and Control of Hypertension,* edited by O. Paul, pp. 553–592. Stratton Intercontinental, New York.
133. Ayers, J., Ruff, C. F., and Templer, D. (1976): Alcoholism, cigarette smoking, coffee drinking and extroversion. *J. Stud. Alcohol,* 37:983.
134. Walton, R. G. (1972): Smoking and alcoholism: A brief report. *Am. J. Psychiatry,* 128:1455.
135. Klatsky, A. L., Friedman, G. D., Siegelaub, A. B., et al. (1977): Alcohol consumption and blood pressure. *N. Engl. J. Med.,* 296:1194.
136. Klatsky, A. L., Friedman, G. D., Siegelaub, A. B., et al. (1977): Alcohol consumption among white, black or oriental men and women. Kaiser Permanente multiphasic health examination data. *Am. J. Epidemiol.,* 105:311.
137. Dyer, A. R., Stamler, J., and Paul, O. (1977): Alcohol consumption: Cardiovascular risk factors and mortality in two Chicago epidemiological studies. *Circulation,* 56:1067.
138. Schweitzer, M., Gearing, F., and Perra, G. (1967): Family studies of primary hypertension. Their contribution to the understanding of genetic factors. In: *The Epidemiology of Hypertension,* edited by J. Stamler, R. Stamler, and T. Pullman, p. 28. Grune & Stratton, New York.
139. McIlhany, M. L., Shaffer, J. W., and Hines, E. A. (1975): The heritability of blood pressure: An investigation of twins using the cold pressor test. *Johns Hopkins Med. J.,* 136:57.
140. Myrhed, M. (1974): Alcohol consumption in relation to factors associated with ischemic heart disease. *Acta Med. Scand.* [Suppl.], 1:967.
141. Hrubec, Z., Cederlof, R., and Friberg, L. (1976): Background of angina pectoris: Social and environmental factors in relation to smoking. *Am. J. Epidemiol.,* 103:16.
142. Esler, M., Julius, S., Zweifler, A., et al. (1977): Mild high renin essential hypertension: A neurogenic human hypertension. *N. Engl. J. Med.,* 296:405.
143. Henry, J. P., Stephens, P. M., and Santiseban, G. A. (1975): A model of psychosocial hypertension showing reversibility and progression of cardiovascular complications. *Circ. Res.,* 36:156.
144. Gutmann, M. C., and Benson, H. (1971): Interaction of environmental factors in systemic arterial pressure: A review. *Medicine (Baltimore),* 50:544.
145. Schmidt, W., and DeLint, J. (1972): Causes of death in alcoholics. *Q. J. Stud. Alcohol,* 33:171.
146. California State Department of Public Health Alcoholic Rehabilitation Division: Follow-up studies of treated alcoholics. Publ. No. 6, Alcoholism, Berkeley, California, 1961.
147. Dahlgren, K. G. (1951): On death rates and causes of death in alcohol addicts. *Acta Psychiatr. Neurol. Scand.,* 26:297.
148. Wilhelmsen, L., Wedel, H., and Tibblin, G. (1973): Multivariate analysis of risk factors for coronary heart disease. *Circulation,* 48:950.

149. Lipman, A. (1977): Alcohol content of commonly used drugs. *Mod. Med.*, 30:43.
150. Isselbacher, K. (1977): Metabolic and hepatic effects of alcohol. *N. Engl. J. Med.*, 296:612.
151. Lieber, C. (1978): Pathogenesis and early diagnosis of alcoholic liver injury. *N. Engl. J. Med.*, 298:890.

Chapter 5

Alcohol 2: Alcohol-Related Cardiomyopathies

An association between alcohol and myocardial disease was recognized as early as 1855 by Wood (1). The pathologic changes occurring in the myocardium were first described by Walshe in 1873 (2), who noted a localized form of cirrhosis occurring in the myocardial wall in the absence of impairment of the coronary circulation. Ten years later in Munich, Bollinger (3) described cardiac dilation and hypertrophy secondary to excessive consumption of beer. This syndrome, termed the "Munich beer heart," was attributed to the toxic effects of habitual beer consumption. The ability of alcohol to diminish cardiac contractility and cause cardiac hypertrophy was reaffirmed by Aufrecht in 1895 (4). Alcoholic heart disease, as a specific term, appeared in the literature in 1902 in a monograph by MacKenzie (5). Since that time, numerous articles have appeared in the literature confirming a positive relationship between alcohol and myocardial disease.

Clinical evidence of heart disease ascribed to alcohol is estimated to be

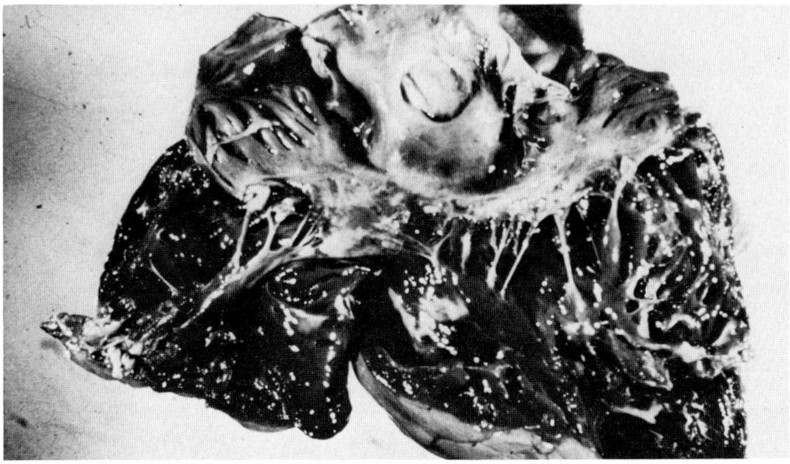

FIG. 1. Alcoholic cardiomyopathy. Endocardial fibrosis with dilatation of the right ventricle. (Courtesy of Dr. Steven Geller.)

present in up to 3% of cardiac patients in large institutions (6). All these disorders may be placed in the category of primary myocardial disease or cardiomyopathy. Pathophysiologically, primary cardiomyopathy consists of left ventricular or biventricular involvement (Figs. 1 and 2) accompanied by the following varieties alone or in combination: hypertrophic, hyperkinetic, obstructive, congestive, and restrictive (7).

The development of alcohol-related cardiomyopathy may be gradual. To define preclinical cardiac malfunction in chronic alcoholism, Spodick et al. (8) performed noninvasive polygraph recordings in ambulatory patients with a history of chronic alcoholism without clinical evidence of heart disease, patients with alcoholic cardiomyopathy, and a control group. Compared to the controls, the chronic alcoholics with or without cardiomyopathy had significantly elevated heart rates, abnormal left ventricular ejection times, and abnormal preejection periods, indicating the existence of depressed myocardial functioning. The dysfunction seen in the chronic alcoholics differed only in degree from that observed in persons with alcoholic cardiomyopathy and may represent the early stage of alcoholic cardiomyopathy without cardiomegaly. Regardless of the label, however, it is apparent that functional cardiac impairment, consisting of an elevation in left ventricular end-diastolic pressure and evidence of depressed myocardial contractility, can exist prior to the development of overt symptoms of cardiomyopathy.

Clinically, the earliest signs of involvement are seen in the hypertrophic and the hyperkinetic forms. When both are present, the development of obstructive cardiomyopathy with a true left ventricular aortic systolic gradient and obstruction of the right ventricular outflow track may occur. The appearance of heart failure in the absence of ventricular outflow obstruction or

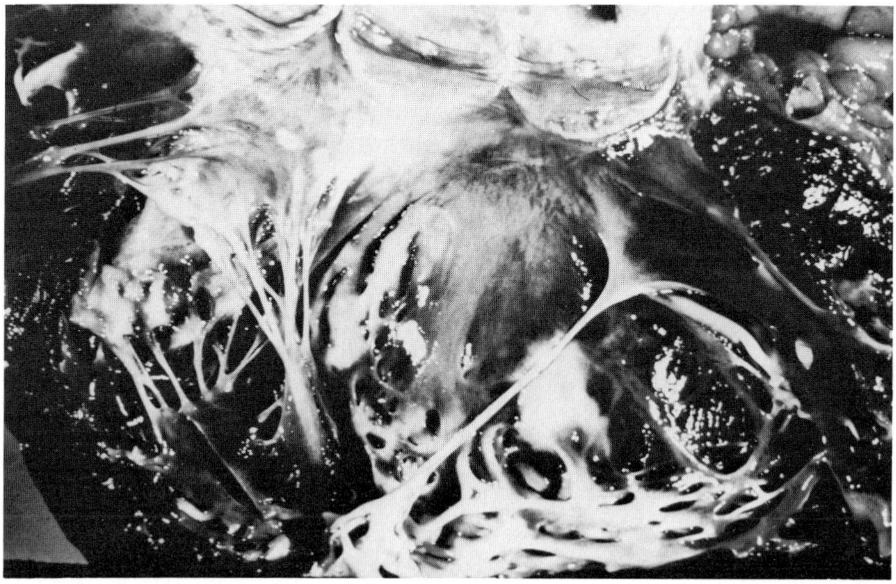

FIG. 2. Close-up view of heart in Fig. 1 showing marked endocardial fibrosis. (Courtesy of Dr. Steven Geller.)

other evidence of cardiac disease characterizes congestive cardiomyopathy. Impairment of ventricular contraction, associated with inadequate distension in end diastole, in the absence of constrictive pericarditis, suggests the presence of a restrictive cardiomyopathy.

In considering the relationship of alcohol to myocardial disease, one must distinguish between the effects of the (a) alcohol per se, (b) constituents of commercial alcoholic beverages, and (c) nutritional deficiencies associated with chronic alcoholism. Three main types of myocardial disease have been related to consumption of alcohol: (a) beriberi heart disease, (b) heavy metal cardiomyopathy in beer drinkers, and (c) cardiomyopathy secondary to the direct toxic effects of alcohol on the myocardium.

BERIBERI HEART DISEASE

Although beriberi has been recognized for centuries, cardiac involvement had not been reported until 1929 when Aalsmeer and Wenckebach (9) described a clinical syndrome in Orientals secondary to vitamin deficiency, consisting of a wide pulse pressure, bounding arterial pulse, rapid circulation time, and peripheral arterial murmurs associated with signs of right-sided congestive heart failure. This syndrome was termed Oriental beriberi. Sudden collapse (Shoshin beriberi) was also reported. Subsequently, a similar disorder, Occidental beriberi, was described in both Europe and the United States by Weiss and Wilkins (10). Almost all of those afflicted individuals in

Western countries consumed considerable quantities of alcohol, associated with a dietary deficiency of thiamin (11). Additional clinical evidence of thiamin deficiency, such as pellagra or peripheral neuritis, was also frequent, although cardiac failure was considered more likely in those without involvement of the nervous system, as the ability to work tended to place an even greater burden on the heart. The thiamin deficiency was initially thought to be related to the associated hepatic dysfunction not uncommon in chronic alcoholics. Leevy et al. (3), however, later demonstrated the absence of any difference in nutritional status between alcoholics with or without liver disease, suggesting either low dietary intake or altered intestinal absorption of thiamin as etiologic factors. Deficiencies of other vitamins were common. Other evidence of malnutrition was infrequent because of the high carbohydrate content of alcoholic beverages.

The importance of thiamin deficiency as an etiologic factor in alcoholic beriberi heart disease was considerable in the early 1900s, with approximately 100 cases of thiamin deficiency reported in one hospital in a single year (13). During the ensuing decades, nutritional deficiencies in alcoholics have become decidedly less frequent. In 1953, Figueroa et al. (14) screened 16,000 inmates for nutritional deficiencies. Few cases of overt nutritional disease were seen in the alcoholics. A more recent study of alcoholics (15) has revealed a relatively low incidence of nutritional deficiency, with only 15% presenting with low thiamin levels as determined by both dietary history and analysis of vitamin metabolites. Deficiency of riboflavin, niacin, and protein occurred in less than 10%. The improved nutritional status of many modern day consumers of alcohol makes the existence of this disorder quite infrequent in Western countries. In alcoholics presenting with cardiomyopathy who do show evidence of malnutrition, however, the existence of a thiamin deficiency must be carefully considered, especially in those individuals presenting in heart failure with a normal or elevated cardiac output.

Clinical Findings

Beriberi heart disease, as initially described, was characterized as a high output state associated with tachycardia, increased stroke and cardiac index, low peripheral vascular resistance, a narrow arteriovenous oxygen difference, and an increase in blood volume and right ventricular end-diastolic pressure. The decrease in peripheral vascular resistance was believed to be due to either opening of arteriovenous communications or paralysis of resistance vessels. The clinical picture seen in the West, however, frequently differs. Right-sided failure is commonly associated with signs and symptoms of left ventricular insufficiency rather than seen as an isolated finding, and a high output hyperkinetic state exists in only a minority of patients. Roentgenographic findings include generalized cardiac enlargement with or without pulmonary congestion. Electrocardiographic changes are nonspecific, consisting of T-wave flattening or inversion, with either a decrease in amplitude

TABLE 1. *Comparison of electrocardiographic alterations in cardiomyopathy associated with excessive alcohol consumption*

ECG Alteration	Beriberi	Cobalt	Alcoholic
Sinus tachycardias	+	+	+/−
Frequent arrhythmias	−	−	+
Conduction abnormalities	−	−	+
Abnormal progression R-wave right precordial leads	−	+	+
Left ventricular hypertrophy	+	−	+
Frequent T-wave anomalies	+/−	−	+
P-wave abnormalities	−	+	+

of the QRS or an increase in QRS amplitude, suggestive of left ventricular hypertrophy (Table 1). Laboratory findings include an increase in blood pyruvate and lactate with a decrease in blood transketolase (16).

Although the diagnosis of beriberi heart disease may be quite evident in alcoholics presenting with a classic hyperkinetic syndrome and predominant right-sided congestive heart failure, in the absence of these findings the presence of thiamin deficiency may not be apparent. This diagnosis should be considered in the presence of (a) chronic alcoholism, (b) thiamin deficiency for at least 3 months documented by either serum thiamin levels or coexisting clinical signs, such as polyneuritis or pellagra; (c) the absence of other etiologic factors relating to cardiomyopathy, and (d) a favorable clinical result subsequent to administration of thiamin. The clinical course and prognosis of this disorder is extremely variable, depending on the degree and duration of thiamin deficiency. Treatment consists of general supportive measures, digoxin, and diuretics, with parenteral administration of thiamin. The initial dose can be up to 100 mg thiamin i.m., with subsequent divided oral doses of 25 mg/day for 10 to 14 days. Since individual oral doses of more than 25 mg/day are largely unabsorbed, once the initial deficiency is corrected, maintenance dosage should not exceed 25 mg/day. Other water-soluble vitamins should be administered if coexisting deficiencies exist. If the cardiomyopathy is of short duration and thiamin is given early, an almost complete regression can occur. Heart size may diminish toward normal, with all electrocardiographic changes resolving. Unfortunately, a complete resolution infrequently occurs and mortality may be considerable, approximating 30% in severely afflicted cases. Autopsy findings consist of dilation and, occasionally, hypertrophy of the heart, with hydropic degeneration and interstitial and intracellular edema of the myocardial fibers. Myocardial fiber necrosis is rare.

Pathophysiology

Thiamine deficiency results in a diminished level of thiamine pyrophosphate, a cofactor in the decarboxylation of pyruvate to acetylcoenzyme A and alpha ketoglutarate to succinyl coenzyme A, interrupting the Krebs cycle at two separate sites. As a result, cardiac oxidative metabolism is impaired at a time when this tissue's energy needs are considerably increased due to the presence of a high output state, resulting in an alteration of ventricular performance with myocardial failure. The myocardial failure may be accentuated by the loss of peripheral vascular resistance resulting from widespread arteriovenous shunting. This peripheral effect is also considered to be secondary to thiamine deficiency as systemic vascular resistance has been shown to rise within 90 min following intravenous administration of thiamine and to return to normal within two weeks of thiamine therapy (16).

HEAVY METAL CARDIOMYOPATHY

In 1900, in the city of Manchester, England, an epidemic of heart failure and "beer" poisoning was noted in 2,000 residents (17). A Royal Commission formed to investigate this matter concluded that the syndrome was caused by the contamination of beer by arsenic. This conclusion was reached despite the fact that: (a) the persons so stricken had an unusual amount of heart failure compared to the average nonalcoholic case of arsenic intoxication; (b) the occurrence of this disorder in heavy beer drinkers was by no means uniform, as many were symptom free; and (c) the amount of arsenic found in the daily beer consumption of afflicted individuals was quite variable and rather low. It was pointed out at that time by commission members that 10 times the concentration of arsenic was prescribed to epileptics for long periods of time without side-effects. Nonetheless, after a careful epidemiologic review, the conclusion of the commission was that arsenic was indeed the etiologic agent and that "the alcoholic vehicle in the form of beer accentuated the toxic effects of arsenic." Fortunately, with improvement in the production of beer in the breweries, no other cases of cardiomyopathy in beer drinkers were reported for the next six decades.

In the 1960s, the increased use of synthetic detergents in washing glassware resulted in a thin film of detergent remaining after the cleansing process. This film prevented the appearance of foam or a "head" at the top of a glass when beer was served. This perceived dissatisfaction of beer drinkers led beer manufacturers to seek a means of restoring the head to make their product more esthetically pleasing. The use of cobalt chloride stabilized the foam.

Subsequent to preliminary animal experiments, breweries were authorized to add 1 to 1.5 ppm (1 to 1.5 mg/liter) of cobalt to beer. In the fall and winter of 1965–1966, 48 persons, all habitual consumers of large amounts of beer, were admitted to hospitals in Quebec City with an unusual type of cardiomyopathy of rapid onset. Within a short period of time, similar clinical pictures associated with heavy beer consumption were described in Omaha, Minneapolis, and Belgium (18–22). Comprehensive epidemiologic studies in Quebec, Omaha, and Belgium documented that those persons so afflicted were heavy consumers of beer containing considerable amounts of cobalt sulfate. In the series from Quebec, the brand of beer in question had approximately 10 times more cobalt sulfate than a beer of the same name manufactured in a nearby city (17).

Clinical Findings

The clinical picture of cobalt beer cardiomyopathy was quite different than that seen with previously recognized forms of primary alcoholic cardiomyopathy or beriberi heart disease (23–25). These patients presented with a relatively acute onset of left ventricular and then right ventricular failure, with symptoms appearing from 1 day to 3 months before medical advice was sought. Duration of symptoms varied greatly from less than 1 week to 1½ years. Dyspnea was the most frequent symptom, with abdominal pain also appearing frequently. Clinical signs seen in the majority of patients consisted of tachycardia, gallop rhythms, tachypnea, pulmonary rales, jugular venus distention, hepatomegaly, and peripheral edema (19,20,25).

Hemodynamics

Hemodynamic studies reported by several investigators revealed a low output state and heart failure (23,25). Elevations of right atrial pressures, pulmonary capillary wedge pressures, and left ventricular end-diastolic pressure were common. Cardiac output was decreased in the baseline state without post exercise elevation in output normally observed. Morin (24) demonstrated on follow-up study of three patients that once the acute process subsides, the cardiac response to exercise reverts to normal, even in the presence of continued consumption of alcohol.

Electrocardiographic, Roentgenographic, and Laboratory Examinations

Electrocardiographic alterations were frequent, with a sinus tachycardia of more than 90/min described in 96% of patients (18–23). Diminished amplitude of the QRS complex in the limb leads was noted in 81%, with signs suggestive of anterior infarction in 30%. P-wave abnormalities, consisting of P pulmonale or P mitrale, were seen in one-third of cases (21,23). These findings differed from those normally seen in pure alcoholic cardiomyopathy (Table 1). Arrhythmias and conduction abnormalities were quite infrequent, and there was little evidence of left ventricular hypertrophy or marked abnormalities in T-wave configuration.

Roentgenographic findings consisted of generalized cardiomegaly, pulmonary congestion, pulmonary edema, and, not infrequently, pericardial effusion (23,26). In persons in serious congestive heart failure, polycythemia, lactic acidosis, and shock, accompanied by high levels of serum glutamic oxaloacetic transaminase, creatine phosphokinase, lactic dehydrogenase, hyperbilirubinemia, hypoprothrombinemia, and increases in both circulating pyruvate and lactate were frequent.

Therapy

Therapy of heavy metal cardiomyopathy is directed to correct the heart failure and restore acid base balance to normal. Heart failure is often associated with hyperventilation and hypocapnia and, when accompanied by acidosis and lactic acidemia, can be quite refractory to cardiotonic agents and diuretics. Correction of the intracellular and extracellular acidosis, when present, is of prime importance. Although the specific therapeutic regimen for restoring pH toward normal may vary, Alexander (23) has suggested the use of tromethamine (THAM) to correct intracellular acidosis and sodium bicarbonate for the extracellular acidosis. Administration of morphine can diminish hyperventilation, lower lactate levels, and provide symptomatic relief of pulmonary edema, if present. Pericardiocentesis can be lifesaving in the presence of hemodynamically significant effusions. Digoxin, diuretics, oxygen, and potassium replacement (after correction of acidosis) are all effective in increasing cardiac output and reducing congestive failure. The use of chelating agents, such as EDTA, to remove cobalt from myocardial tissue has been suggested but has been used infrequently and has not been shown to be effective.

Prognosis

The prognosis of persons with heavy metal cardiomyopathy is not good (Table 2) (17,21,23,27–29). Despite intensive treatment for acidosis and heart failure, 55 of 166 patients (33%) reported in the literature succumbed during the initial hospitalization, with an additional 5% dying at a later time. Mortality rates varied considerably with the individual series (0 to 47%), as did the time of death. In Quebec, 15 of the 20 deaths (75%) occurred within the first 48 hr. In Omaha, only eight of 30 deaths (27%) occurred within the first 72 hr. In Minneapolis, early mortality was only 18%, but late deaths raised the total mortality to 43%.

Electrocardiographic alterations persisted for more than 4 months in approximately 27% of survivors. The prevalence of residual disability varied with the individual series. In Quebec, 10 of 18 survivors (55%) located for 1-year follow-up reported exertional dyspnea. Objective evidence of residual cardiac damage was not found, even though approximately two-thirds of these patients continued to drink considerable amounts of beer. Twelve of the 28 patients followed in Minneapolis had residual clinical disability. In Omaha, 20 of 34 survivors (58%) were found to have a normal heart size,

TABLE 2. *Prognosis in persons with cobalt beer cardiopathy*[a]

Prognosis	No.	%
Patients in series	166	—
Mortality	64	39
Acute	55	33
Late	9	6
Follow-up: total patients	68	—
Residual cardiac disability	18	26[b]
Persistent ECG changes	30	44[b]

[a] From refs. 17–19, 22, 23, 28.
[b] Percentage of 68 patients available for follow-up studies.

minimal electrocardiographic changes, and good exercise tolerance several months after treatment.

Pathology

The pathologic findings showed the frequent presence of pericardial effusions described in 82% of autopsies. Pleural effusions were infrequent; when present, they were usually small. The heart was uniformly enlarged, dilated rather than hypertrophied, with the coronary arteries free of atheromata. Mural thrombi were noted in 12 cases (26%), with thromboembolism being found in 10 (21%). On light microscopy, the pathology varied from minimal changes to marked interstitial edema, focal fibrosis, vacuolization of myocardial fibers, and accumulation of large amounts of glycogen. Electron microscopy showed extensive intracellular changes involving myofibers and mitochondria, with glycogen and lipid deposits consistently observed (23,30).

Etiology

The precise mechanism by which cobalt produces these changes remains to be defined. Although the myocardial toxicity of cobalt administered in large doses has been well documented experimentally, the amount of cobalt contained in beer should not have resulted in the degree of cardiomyopathy observed. Cobalt, when used as an antianemic agent, frequently in the form of Roncovite®, is prescribed in a much higher dosage than that ingested in persons in whom cardiomyopathy developed (daily intake of 60 mg versus approximately 8 mg) (23). Roncovite, however, also contains ferrous sulfate, which shares a common absorptive pathway with cobalt and may therefore diminish its absorption. If Roncovite is ingested during or after meals, cobalt absorption may also be decreased.

Conversely, modifying factors associated with beer drinking can enchance cobalt absorption. In the presence of iron deficiency, which may occur in chronic alcoholics, absorption of cobalt from the intestinal tract is greatly increased (31).

Other nutritional factors, such as inadequate protein intake and thiamin, magnesium, and zinc deficiencies, may play a role in sensitizing the heart to cobalt toxicity. The increased calcium concentration in water used in brewing beer may also predispose to cardiac disease. Finally, the actual effect of alcohol might serve to sensitize the heart to cobalt toxicity. Although investigators have been unable to document an increase in myocardial toxicity in animals simultaneously fed alcohol and cobalt, when rats were maintained on only beer for 36 days prior to receiving cobalt, a condition not dissimilar to that existing in the clinical setting was noted, with cobalt cardiotoxicity being enhanced (32,33).

Clinically, the toxicity of cobalt in humans was previously confined to the hematologic system and the thyroid gland; experimentally, however, cobalt is known to have multiple effects on enzyme systems (34–37). More specifically, cobalt reacts with SH groups of dihydrolipoic acid, a cofactor required in the decarboxylation of pyruvate to acetyl coenzyme A and alpha-ketoglutarate to succinyl coenzyme A (38). This effect is similar to that seen with thiamin deficiency. These enzymatic changes interfere with the Krebs cycle and oxidative metabolism. Increased triglyceride and glycogen synthesis occur, resulting in glycogen and lipid deposits. Cobalt may also diminish calcium concentration in mitochondial cytoplasm, which leads to electromechanical disturbances and competes with other metals for absorption in the gastrointestinal tract. This latter action may produce a deficiency of iron, zinc, and other trace metals. The erythropoietic effect of cobalt may be related to impaired release of oxygen from 2–3–DPG. This may be due to depletion or inactivation of 2–3–DPG or formation of a cobalt-hemoglobin complex shifting the oxygen dissociation curve to the left.

In summary, although the actual pathophysiology of cobalt cardiomyopathy is unclear, the comprehensiveness of these epidemiologic studies indicates cobalt as the responsible factor. Fortunately, in 1966, soon after the recognition of this entity in both America and Canada, the use of cobalt as an additive in beer was prohibited.

ALCOHOLIC CARDIOMYOPATHY

Primary myocardial disease in chronic alcoholism, unassociated with thiamin deficiency, is mainly congestive rather than hypertrophic or restrictive, affecting persons in all socioeconomic strata. The biochemical etiology has not been well defined; however, experimental evidence suggests a direct toxic effect of alcohol independent of nutritional status. Ettinger et al. (39) have demonstrated conduction abnormalities in dogs maintained on adequate nutrition but receiving 40% of caloric intake from alcohol for up to 3 years. Evidence has also been presented documenting a deleterious effect of alcohol ingestion over a much shorter period. Burch et al. (40) found structural abnormalities in the myocardium of mice nutritionally maintained but fed alcohol daily for periods as short as 7 to 10 weeks.

As discussed earlier, secondary metabolic effects associated with alcohol ingestion may also contribute to the pathologic changes. Depletion of potassium and magnesium and alteration in calcium binding may be to a sufficient degree to result in direct cellular damage. Virus-like particles have also been found in long-standing alcoholic cardiomyopathy (41), with an increase in viral antibody titers also documented (42). A definitive role of viruses in producing the cardiomyopathy, however, has not been demonstrated. Finally, a chronic state of alcohol-induced catecholamine excess, associated with intermittent periods of withdrawal, may exert a deleterious effect on the myocardium, which, when combined with one or more other factors, results in the pathologic changes observed.

Diagnosis

Diagnosis of alcoholic cardiomyopathy may be elusive because of the difficulty in obtaining an accurate history of alcoholism. The diagnosis is usually made on the basis of congestive heart failure appearing in persons younger than 50 years of age in the absence of any known etiologic factors and in the presence of chronic alcoholism. Since other evidence of alcoholism, such as hepatic disease and peripheral neuritis, may often be absent, careful questioning is necessary to eliminate other forms of primary myocardial disease (43, 44). It must be remembered that not only is an alcoholic frequently hesitant to admit his/her condition, but, in addition, even with a positive history, there is no clearcut relationship between the quantity, frequency, and duration of alcohol consumed and the development of cardiomyopathy. If one would assume that the development of cardiomyopathy is similar in evolution to that of cirrhosis, then this pathology may not be found even after decades of drinking (45).

Clinical Findings

Symptoms may develop insidiously, and medical attention may not be sought until the onset of arrhythmias or frank congestive failure. Gunnar et al. (46) have divided the physical manifestations into three main groups, representing progressive stages in the disease. In the first stage, the heart is of normal size, with palpitation or an intercurrent illness being the prominent symptom. Even at this time, however, a persistent sinus tachycardia and an S4 gallop are frequently present. Atrial arrhythmias or ventricular premature beats may occur. In stage two, the heart is enlarged, primarily because of left ventricular hypertrophy in the absence of hypertension. An S3 gallop may be present, and orthopnea and dyspnea on effort may exist. The third stage consists of cardiac dilatation, a diffuse apical impulse, and, frequently, signs of valvular insufficiency. A narrow pulse pressure, prolonged circulation time, and pulmonary rales are prominent, with multifocal ectopic ventricular beats and ventricular tachycardia not infrequent. In the presence of these arrhythmias, syncope may be the presenting symptom. Elevated diastolic pressures, with or without systolic elevation of blood pressure, may be seen secondary to severe congestive failure.

Electrocardiographic Changes

Electrocardiographic changes can be seen in all stages of alcoholic cardiomyopathy (Tables 1 and 3). These changes may consist of abnormal P-waves, slurred or notched QRSs, often with pseudoinfarction patterns, ST segment depression, prolonged QT intervals, and markedly deformed T-waves. These T-wave changes, when cloven, bifid, dimpled, or spinous configurations, have been considered by Evans (47) to be diagnostic. Others have also noted prominent T-waves in alcoholics in the absence of clinical myocardial disease. These alterations are now considered nonspecific (48). Arrhythmias, such as atrial fibrillation, premature unifocal or multifocal ventricular contractions, paroxysmal atrial tachycardias, and paroxysmal ventricular tachycardias, may occur. Other disorders of the conduction system are common. Sudden death in this group may occur and is probably the result of ventricular fibrillation (49,50).

TABLE 3. *Electrocardiographic abnormalities reported in alcoholic cardiomyopathy*

P-Wave
Left atrial hypertrophy
Intraartrial conduction defect
Notched P-waves
QRS
Slurred on notching of QRS
Pseudoinfarction pattern with absent QI; embryonic Q precordial leads
Left ventricular hypertrophy pattern
Decreased amplitude R-waves
Repolarization alterations
ST segment depression
Prolongation QT interval
Cloven, bifid, dimpled, or spinous T-waves

Radiologic Findings

Radiologic features include cardiomegaly, the magnitude of which depends on the extent and duration of congestive failure. The left side of the heart is usually affected more than the right. Left ventricular wall movement is diminished on fluoroscopy, and an increase in left ventricular volume is noted on angiography.

Therapy

With the onset of clinical manifestations, treatment should be directed to the presenting problems. Bed rest, with careful digitalization and diuretic therapy, is warranted. These patients are particularly sensitive to digitalis. Accompanying electrolyte disturbances, at times associated with aggressive diuresis, may intensify or provoke digitalis-toxic arrhythmias. Arrhythmias other than sinus tachycardia should be treated with appropriate medications. Nutritional deficiencies, if present, should be corrected.

The importance of anticoagulant therapy, especially in those persons with paroxysmal or persistent arrhythmias, deserves emphasis. Thromboembolism originating from endocardial thrombi have been reported in as many as 80% of persons with this disease (43,44). Anticoagulation in persons consuming considerable quantities of alcohol, however, is also hazardous. For this reason, abstinence becomes one of the first goals in therapy. Unfortunately, although abstinence may aid in recovery early in the disease process, once structural damage has occurred, there is no compelling evidence that abstinence per se will result in a reversal or halt in the progression of cardiac failure.

Bed rest has been emphasized by several investigators as an important adjunct to therapy, with a positive relationship being noted between a decrease in heart size and duration of restriction of activity (44,51,52). These changes have been quite impressive, even in the presence of considerable cardiac enlargement. Although the beneficial effects of bed rest are real, it is extremely difficult practically to accomplish this goal with most patients.

Prognosis

Demakis et al. (53) have studied the prognosis in 57 persons with stage 3 alcoholic cardiomyopathy during an average of 40.5 months. During the follow-up period, the disease was stable in 12 (21%), improved in 15 (26%), and deteriorated in 30 (53%), with 24 (42%) dying on the average of 30 months after initial diagnosis. A more favorable course was associated with a shorter duration of symptoms prior to initiation of therapy and with abstinence from alcohol. The average duration of symptoms in those patients showing clinical improvement was 4.2 months versus 11 to 17 months in those showing no improvement or a deterioration in their condition (p) $<$ 0.05). Of those improving clinically, 73% had become abstinent, as compared to 13 to 25% in the other groups ($p = 0.03$ to 0.001). A complete return to normal heart size was noted in 17% of persons, unrelated to bed rest. Similar findings have been reported by other investigators (47,52,54). McDonald et al. (52) found that heart size returned to normal in 20 of 42 patients (44%) but continued to remain normal in only 9 individuals (21%) once mobilization was initiated. Unfortunately, in most series the mortality of patients with alcoholic cardiomyopathy is considerable, reaching 40 to 45% within a relatively short period.

Pathologic Findings

On autopsy, the pericardium is usually uninvolved. There is ventricular hypertrophy and dilatation of all chambers, with left ventricular predominance (Figs. 1 and 2). Frequently, thrombi can be found. Pathologic alterations, as defined by light microscopy, are minimal, consisting of fibrosis, lipid deposition, and interstitial edema (42). On electron microscopy, dilatation of the sarcoplasmic reticulum, associated with mitochondrial degeneration, myocardial oxidative enzyme depletion, and changes in contractile proteins, occurs (55,56). The mitochondrial changes and the appearance of lysosome-like granules and lipofusium staining deposits are all similar to the pathologic changes reported in alcoholic liver injury.

The coronary arteries are usually normal, with the degree of generalized arteriosclerosis somewhat less than expected for age (57–59). The existence of small vessel disease in the myocardium was first described by Pintar et al. in 1965 (59). Others have also reported vascular abnormalities, consisting of edema, perivascular fibrosis, and vascular sclerosis in 36 to 48% of young alcoholic persons dying secondary to alcoholic liver disease or chronic alcoholism. Several investigators, however, have found little or no changes other than dilation in the small intramyocardial vessels (60,61).

REFERENCES

1. Wood, G. B. (1855): *A Treatise on the Practice of Medicine,* 2:168. Lippincott, Philadelphia.
2. Walshe, W. H. (1873): *Diseases of the Heart and Great Vessels,* Fourth Edition. Smith, Elder and Co., London.
3. Bollinger, O. (1884): Uber die Häufigkeit and Ursachen der idiopathischen Herzhypertrophie in München. *Dtsch. Med. Wochenschr.,* 10:180.
4. Aufrecht, D. (1895): Die alkoholische Myocarditis mit nachfolgender Lebererkankung und zeitweiliger Albuminurie. *Dtsch. Arch. Klin. Med.,* 54:615.
5. MacKenzie, J. (1902): *The Study of the Pulse.* Y. T. Pentland, Edinburgh.
6. Asokan, S. F., Frank, M. J., and Witham, A. C. (1972): Cardiomyopathy without cardiomegaly in alcoholics. *Am. Heart J.,* 81:13.
7. Perloff, J. K. (1971): The cardiomyopathies—current perspectives. *Circulation,* 44: 942.
8. Spodick, D. H., Pigott, V. M., and Chirife, R. (1972): Perclinical cardiac malfunction in chronic alcoholism. *N. Engl. J. Med.,* 287:677.
9. Aalsmeer, W. C., and Wenckebach, K. F. (1929): Herz and kreislauf bei der beriberikrau heit wien. *Arch. Intern. Med.,* 16:93.
10. Weiss, S., and Wilkins, R. W. (1937): The nature of the cardiovascular disturbances in nutritional disease states (beriberi). *Ann. Intern. Med.,* 11:104.

11. Blankenhorn, M. A., Vilter, C. F., Scheinker, I. M., et al. (1946): Occidental beriberi heart disease. *JAMA,* 131:717.
12. Leevy, C. M., Baker, H., Ten-Hove, O., et al. (1965): B complex vitamins in liver disease in the alcoholic. *Am. J. Clin. Nutr.,* 16:339.
13. Burch, G. E., and DePasquale, N. P. (1969): Alcoholic cardiomyopathy. *Am. J. Cardiol.,* 23:723.
14. Figueroa, W. G., Sargent, F., Imperiale, L., et al. (1953): Lack of avitaminosis among alcoholics. Its relation to fortification of cereal products and the general nutrition of the population. *J. Clin. Nutr.,* 1:179.
15. Neville, J. N., Eagles, J. A., Sampson, G., and Olson, R. E. (1968): The nutritional status of alcoholics. *Am. J. Clin. Nutr.,* 21:1329.
16. Alexander, C. S. (1971): Nutritional heart disease. *Cardiovasc. Clin.,* 4:221.
17. Morin, Y., and Daniel, P. (1967): Quebec beer-drinkers' cardiomyopathy. Etiological considerations. *Can. Med. Assoc. J.,* 97:926.
18. Sullivan, J. F., Egan, J. D., and George, R. P. (1969): A distinctive myocardiopathy occurring in Omaha, Nebraska: Clinical aspects. *Ann. N. Y. Acad. Sci.,* 156:526.
19. McDermott, P. H., Delaney, R. L., Egan, J. D., et al. (1966): Myocardosis and cardiac failure in men. *JAMA,* 198:253.
20. Morin, Y. L., Foley, A. R., Martineau, G., et al. (1967): Quebec beer-drinkers' cardiomyopathy: forty-eight cases. *Can. Med. Assoc. J.,* 97:881.
21. Têtu, A., and Samson, M. (1967): Quebec beer-drinkers' cardiomyopathy: Electrocardiographic study. *Can. Med. Assoc. J.,* 97:893.
22. Kesteloot, H., Terryn, R., Bosmans, P., and Joossens, J. V. (1966): Alcoholic perimyocardiopathy. *Acta Cardiol. (Brux.),* 21:34.
23. Alexander, C. S. (1972): Cobalt beer cardiomyopathy. A clinical and pathological study. *Am. J. Med.,* 53:395.
24. Morin, Y. (1967): Quebec beer-drinkers' cardiomyopathy: Hemodynamic alterations. *Can. Med. Assoc. J.,* 97:901.
25. Morin, Y., Têtu, A., and Mercier, G. (1969): Quebec beer-drinkers' cardiomyopathy. Clinical and hemodynamic aspects. *Ann. N. Y. Acad. Sci.,* 156:566.
26. Lapointe, A. (1967): Quebec beer-drinkers' cardiomyopathy: Radiologic aspects. *Can. Med. Assoc. J.,* 97:905.
27. Sullivan, J., Parker, M., and Carson, S. B. (1968): Tissue cobalt content in "beer drinkers' myocardiopathy." *J. Lab. Clin. Med.,* 71:893.
28. Kestelott, H., Roelandt, J., Willems, J., Claes, J. H., and Joossens, J. V. (1968): An inquiry into the role of cobalt in the heart disease of chronic beer drinkers. *Circulation,* 37:854.
29. Mercier, G., and Patry, G. (1967): Quebec beer-drinkers' cardiomyopathy. Clinical signs and symptoms. *Can. Med. Assoc. J.,* 97:884.
30. Bonenfant, J. L., Auger, C., Miller, G., Chenard, J., and Roy, P. E. (1969): Quebec beer-drinkers' myocardosis. Pathological aspects. *Ann. N. Y. Acad. Sci.,* 156:577.
31. Olatunbosun, D., Corbett, W. E. N., Ludwig, J., and Valberg, L. S. (1970): Alteration of cobalt absorption in portal cirrhosis and idiopathic hemochromatosis. *J. Lab. Clin. Med.,* 75:754.
32. Mohiuddin, S. M., Taskar, P. K., Rheault, M., Roy, R. E., Chenard, J., and Morin, Y. (1970): Experimental cobalt cardiomyopathy. *Am. Heart J.,* 80:532.
33. Wiberg, G. S., Munro, I. C., Meranger, J. C., Morrison, A. B., Grice, H. C., and Heggtveit, H. A. (1969): Factors affecting the cardiotoxic potential of cobalt. *Clin. Toxicol.,* 2:257.
34. Davis, J. E., and Fields, J. P. (1955): Cobalt polycythemia in humans. *Fed. Proc.* 14:331 (abstr.).
35. Schirrmacher, U. O. E. (1967): Case of cobalt poisoning. *Br. Med. J.,* 1:544.
36. Kriss, J. P., Carnes, W. H., and Gross, R. T. (1955): Hypothyroidism and thyroid hyperplasia in patients treated with cobalt. *JAMA,* 157:117.
37. Webb, M. (1962): The biological action of cobalt and other metals. III. Chelation of cations by dihydrolipoic acid. *Biochim. Biophys. Acta,* 65:47.
38. DeMoraes, S., and Mariano, M. (1967): Biochemical aspects of cobalt intoxication. *Med. Pharmacol. Exp.,* 16:441.

39. Ettinger, P. O., Lyons, M., Oloewurtel, H. A., et al. (1976): Cardiac conduction abnormalities produced by chronic alcoholism. *Am. Heart J.,* 91:66.
40. Burch, G. E., Colcolough, H. L., Harb, J. M., and Tsue, C. Y. (1971): The effect of ingestion of ethyl alcohol, wine and beer on the myocardium of mice. *Am. J. Cardiol.,* 27:522.
41. Hibbs, R., Ferrans, V., Black, W., et al. (1965): Virus like particles in the heart of a patient with cardiomyopathy. *Am. Heart J.,* 69:766.
42. Brigden, W. (1971): Alcoholic cardiomyopathy. *Cardiovasc. Clin.,* 4:187.
43. Ferrans, V. J., Rios, J., Gooch, A. S., et al. (1966): Alcoholic cardiomyopathy. *Am. J. Med. Sci.,* 252:123.
44. Burch, G. E., and Giles, T. D. (1971): Alcoholic cardiomyopathy. Concepts of the disease and its treatment. *Am. J. Med.,* 50:141.
45. Galambos, J. T. (1974): Alcoholic hepatitis. In: *The Liver and its Diseases,* edited F. Schaffner et al. Intercontinental Medical Book, New York.
46. Gunnar, R. M., Sutton, G. C., Pietras, R. J., et al: Alcoholic cardiomyopathy. *DM,* 1:30.
47. Evans, W. (1959): The electrocardiogram of alcoholic cardiomyopathy. *Br. Heart J.,* 21:445.
48. Horan, L. G., Flowers, N. C., Thomas, J. R., et al. (1974): The spatial vector cardiogram in ideopathic cardiomyopathy. *Prog. Cardiovasc. Dis.,* 7:115.
49. Kramer, K., Kuller, L., and Fisher, R. (1968): The increasing mortality attributed to cirrhosis and fatty liver in Baltimore (1957–1966). *Ann. Intern. Med.,* 69:273.
50. Sundby, P. (1967): *Alcoholism and Mortality.* Rutgers Center of Alcohol Studies, New Brunswick, New Jersey.
51. Burch, G. E., Walsh, J. J., and Black, W. C. (1963): Value of prolonged bed rest in management of cardiomegaly. *JAMA,* 183:81.
52. McDonald, C. D., Burch, G. E., and Walsh, J. J. (1971): Alcoholic cardiomyopathy managed with prolonged bed rest. *Ann. Intern. Med.,* 74:681.
53. DeMakis, J. G., Rahimtoola, S. H., Sutton, G. C., et al. (1974): The natural course of cardiomyopathy. *Ann. Intern. Med.,* 80:293.
54. Hamby, R. F., Catangay, P., Apiado, O., et al. (1970): Primary myocardial disease: Clinical, hemodynamic and angiocardiographic correlates in 50 patients. *Am. J. Cardiol.,* 25:625.
55. Alexander, C. S. (1967): Electron microscopic observation in alcoholic heart disease. *Br. Heart J.,* 29:200.
56. Ferraus, V., Hibbs, R., Weilbaecher, D., et al. (1965): Alcoholic cardiomyopathy. A histochemical study. *Am. Heart J.,* 69:748.
57. Massumi, R. A., Rios, J. C., and Gooch, A. S. (1965): Primary myocardial disease: Report of 50 cases and reviews of the subject. *Circulation,* 31:19.
58. Schenk, E. A., and Cohen, J. (1970): The heart in chronic alcoholism. Clinical and pathologic findings. *Pathol. Microbiol.* 35:96.
59. Pintar, K., Wolansky, B. M., and Buggay, Z. R. (1965): Alcoholic cardiomyopathy. *Can. Med. Assoc. J.,* 93:103.
60. Sackett, D. L., Lepid, R. W., Gibson, I. D., et al. (1968): Relationship between aortic atherosclerosis and the use of cigarettes and alcohol. An autopsy study. *N. Engl. J. Med.,* 279:1413.
61. Burch, G. E., and Giles, T. D. (1977): The small coronary arteries in alcoholic cardiomyopathy. *Am. Heart J.,* 94:471.

Chapter 6

Barbiturates, Other Sedatives, and Minor Tranquilizers

The use of sedatives, hypnotics, and minor tranquilizers, as discussed in Chapter 1, is quite widespread. Although patterns of prescribing practices vary with availability and physician familiarity of a particular agent, these drugs have been and continue to be prescribed most frequently by a wide variety of physician specialties.

In general, barbiturate hypnotic use has been consistently decreasing since the introduction of the benzodiazepines into clinical medicine in the early 1960s. The growth of the benzodiazepines since that time has been phenomenal. In 1967, psychotropic drugs represented 17% of the 1 billion prescriptions written by physicians, with chlordiazepoxide and diazepam accounting for almost one-third (1). By 1972, more than 70 million prescriptions were written for these two agents alone at a cost to the public of approximately $200 million. The use of flurazepam, a hypnotic benzodiazepine introduced in the United States in 1970, had progressed to account for 6.76 million prescriptions in 1976 (2). It is important to reemphasize (Chapter 1) that these medications are prescribed (a) usually without a specific diagnosis of a psychiatric disorder being made, (b) usually by physicians other than psychiatrists, and (c) for a considerable number of persons with cardiovascular diseases.

Abuse or misuse of these agents is not inconsiderable. The suicide rate in the United States has been slowly rising, with a 1976 survey showing that barbiturates account for almost 51% of suicides in four large metropolitan cities. Despite this finding, however, the frequency of barbiturate overdose is decreasing (1,2). In a recent nationwide survey of 1,265 facilities, including emergency rooms, crisis centers, and medical examiners' offices, diazepam was found to be the first or second drug of abuse noted in all drug abuse contacts (3). Unfortunately, in up to 60% of cases, diazepam was initially obtained with a physician's prescription.

These agents may be classified into three main groups: (a) barbiturates, (b) benzodiazepines, and (c) other nonbarbiturates. Practically, it is most convenient to use a classification that follows the pattern of usage, dividing these drugs into hypnotics, sedatives, and anxiolytics or tranquilizing agents.

HYPNOTICS AND SEDATIVES

The agents in the hypnotic-sedative category comprise a large group of chemically unrelated substances that should properly include alcohol, capable of inducing sedation and sleep with small doses and varying degrees of amnesia or anesthesia with larger quantities (Table 1). Prolonged and uninterrupted use of these agents can result in both physical and psychologic dependence.

Pharmacology

Chloral hydrate, first synthesized by Liebig in 1832, is the oldest of the hypnotic and sedative agents. In 1864, von Baeyer synthesized barbituric acid, the parent compound of the barbiturate drugs. Subsequent to the introduction of the first hypnotic barbiturate barbital (Veronal®) by Fisher and von Mering in 1903, barbiturates have become the commonly accepted prototype and, until recently, have been the most frequently utilized (4). Bar-

TABLE 1. *Classification of sedative and hypnotic drugs*

Generic name	Trade name
Antihistamines	
Hydroxyzine hydrochloride	Atarax, Vistaril injectable, Cartrax[6], Marax[b]
Hydroxyzine pamoate	Vistaril oral
Barbiturates	
Benzodiazepines	
Flurazepam hydrochloride	Dalmane[a]
Chloral derivatives	
Chloral hydrate	Aquachoral, Noctec, Somnos
Chloral betaine	Beta Chlor
Triclofos sodium	Triclos
Ethchlorvynol	Placidyl
Bromides	Sedamyl
Carbamates	
Meprobamate	Miltown
Mebutamate	Capla
Ethinamate	Valmid
Tybamate	Solacen, Tybatran
Paraldehyde	
Piperidinedione derivatives	
Gluthethimide	Doriden
Methyprylon	Nodular
Quinazalones	
Methaqualone	Quaalude, Sopor
Methaqualone hydrochloride	Parest, Somnfac
Scopolamine and/or methapyrline	Sleepeze, Mr. Sleep, Sominex, Nytol

[a] Other benzodiazepines used primarily as minor tranquilizers are listed in Table 3.

[b] Also contains pentaerythritol tetranitrite; also contains ephedrine sulfate and theophylline.

biturates may be classified by duration of action and plasma half-life into long-acting, short- to intermediate-acting, and ultrashort-acting drugs (Table 2) although some overlap with respect to duration of action does exist.

After oral administration, absorption depends on lipid solubility of the particular agent as well as on the dissolution of the drug in the intestinal lumen. The short-acting, lipid-soluble barbiturates in the form of sodium salts are absorbed more rapidly than long-acting barbiturates, which have a lesser affinity for lipids and are administered in a free acid form. The slow absorption rate of the long-acting barbiturates makes these agents less likely to be used for "highs" by those specifically seeking a mood-altering experience.

Distribution is widespread, depending on the plasma half-life. The half-lives of the barbiturates used as hypnotics and sedatives, such as pentobarbital, phenobarbital, and secobarbital, are relatively long, varying from 14 to 96 hr, depending on the specific agent. Some nonbarbiturates such as methyprylon and ethchlorvynol have considerably shorter half-lives of 4 to 6 hr (5). Metabolism of all these agents, with the exception of the benzodiaze-

TABLE 2. *Classification of barbiturates*

Drug	Trade name	Action	Half-life (hr)
Phenobarbital[a]	Luminal, Eskabarb	Long	24–96
Mephobarbital	NF	—	—
Metharbital	NF	—	—
Amobarbital[a]	Amytal	Short/intermediate	14–42
Butabarbital sodium	Butisol Sodium, Butazem	—	—
Pentobarbital[a]	Nembutal, Nebralin	—	21–42
Secobarbital[a]	Seconal	—	20–28
Talbutal	—	—	—
Hexobarbital	—	Ultrashort	3–8
Methohexital	Brevital	—	3–6
Thiamylal	NF	—	—
Thiopental	Pentothal	—	3–8

[a] Sodium salt also exists.

pines and chloral hydrate, results in the formation of inactive metabolites. Biotransformation of the barbiturates occurs mainly in the liver through (a) oxidation of radicals at position C5, (b) N-dealkylation, (c) desulfuration (thiobarbiturates), and (d) destruction of the barbituric acid ring. Non-metabolized barbiturates are excreted unchanged in the urine over a period of several days. Barbital metabolism differs from that of the other barbiturates, with urinary excretion representing the major route of elimination.

Cardiovascular Effects

Experimentally, some of the short-acting barbiturates can cause cardiac arrhythmias as well as decrease myocardial contractility when administered in sufficiently high doses. This may be related to an alteration of intracellular distribution of calcium in the myocardial fibrils (6). Clinically, parenteral administration of the ultrashort-acting barbiturates may result in a slight diminution of myocardial contractility accompanied by an increase in vascular tone (7). Depression of the medullary vasomotor center usually occurs with relatively little effect on the baroreceptors and autonomic nervous system. This results in a slight decrease in cardiac output with increased peripheral resistance and a maintenance of arterial pressure, unless high doses are injected. Vascular flow and volume in the extremities are increased, and there is a decrease in cerebral blood flow with a fall in cerebrospinal fluid pressure.

In appropriate oral doses, the use of barbiturates and other sedatives is associated with minimal cardiovascular effects. Similarly, when administered as preanesthetic medication to healthy persons, minimal clinical effects are seen, although a mild decrease in arterial pressure may occur. In the presence of a hypovolemic state, however, hypotension may occur with these agents. In addition, the use of thiopental in persons maintained on positive pressure respiration may result in untoward effects due to its ability to impair the cardiovascular adjustments accompanying mechanical inflation of the lung (4).

The use of hydroxyzine hydrochloride has been associated with electrocardiographic alterations similar to those seen with the phenothiazines and tricyclic antidepressants (8). Changes in T-wave morphology and/or prolongation of the QT interval were noted in 9 of 25 patients after administration of 300 mg/day hydroxyzine. These alterations may be of clinical importance when hydroxyzine is used in combination with atropine or other agents affecting repolarization.

Overdose Reactions

In usual sedative doses, barbiturates and other hypnotics or sedatives have little cardiovascular effects. When taken in toxic doses, however, these agents may produce hypotension and negative chronotropic effects. Epidemiologic data suggest that the risk of an overdose and attendant adverse sequellae is greatest for the barbiturates and least for the benzodiazepines, although misuse of agents in this latter group is most prevalent.

Hemodynamic Effects

Thorstrand (9), in a review of 50 cases of hypnotic overdose, found patients in deep coma associated with hypothermia to have a low cardiac output and a somewhat lowered blood pressure, suggestive of a reflex increase in systemic vascular resistance. Myocardial function, as evidenced by elevation in ventricular filling pressure, was increased. Electrocardiographic changes were minimal, although the QT interval was slightly prolonged in 25%.

Various hypotheses have been formulated to account for the hemodynamic changes observed. The hypovolemia in severe cases of barbiturate overdose has been attributed to a redistribution of blood to the splanchnic bed, a reduction in plasma volume, or inadequate tone of capacitance vessels. None of these hypotheses has been adequately demonstrated. Reduced myocardial force and impaired regulation of resistance vessels may also play a role. In severe overdoses, especially in older patients, the decrease in blood pressure may be accompanied by shock and subsequent hypoxia (10).

Treatment

The general principles involved in the treatment of a central nervous system (CNS) depressant overdose are the same regardless of the agent involved. These consist of (a) maintenance of an open airway, (b) artificial respiration if needed, (c) artificial circulation with closed chest massage if peripheral pulses are absent, and (d) institution of an intravenous infusion to maintain adequate hydration. Dehydration and shock, associated with reduced intravascular volume or vascular collapse, are not infrequent. Adequate hydration and careful monitoring of intake and output are essential until consciousness is resumed.

Analeptics or stimulants have been shown to be relatively ineffective in depressant overdose and, in addition, may be associated with adverse effects. Their use should therefore be proscribed. Gastric lavage in a comatose patient should not be performed if the patient is seen 6 hr after ingestion; if seen earlier, it should be deferred until cardiovascular stability has been obtained and airway patency is insured with an inflated endotracheal tube. Dialysis may be warranted, depending on the severity of the intoxication as well as the dializability of the drug. Schreiner and Teehan (11) have provided guidelines for dialysis in drug overdose.

Although clinically it is very difficult to initially identify the specific depressant drug responsible, in general the nonbarbiturate sedatives are associated with a greater degree of cardiovascular instability, including arrhythmias and hypotension. Electrocardiographic monitoring in all overdose cases is essential. Toxic reactions to several nonbarbiturate sedatives do, however, present with some distinctive features.

Glutethimide

Glutethimide (Doriden®) in large doses results in coma usually of long duration and varying intensity. Symptoms consist of hypotension, papilledema, apnea, and pulmonary edema, which may be quite severe. Management is extremely difficult and is complicated by a poor correlation between the concentration of glutethimide in plasma and the patient's clinical course. This lack of correlation has recently been related to the formation of an active metabolite 4-hydroxy-2-ethyl-2-phenylglutarimide (4-HG) (12). In addition to supportive measures, aqueous and lipid hemodialysis and hemoperfusion have been shown to be helpful in treatment of this disorder (13).

Methaqualone

Recent abuse of methaqualone has also been associated with recognition of toxic cardiovascular effects, consisting of tachycardia, acute cardiac failure, and increased vascular permeability (14).

Meprobamate

Meprobamate poisoning may also be accompanied by severe hypotension, usually adequately managed by plasma expanders and mild vasoconstricting agents. If the hypotension results from myocardial failure rather than a primary effect of meprobamate on the arterial musculature, however, the accompanying elevation in pulmonary wedge and right atrial pressures would make fluid loading hazardous. Individual assessment of each patient is mandatory to determine which factors are predominant in producing the hypotensive state. Therapy can then be directed more appropriately to the primary cause (15–17).

Overdose With Multiple Drugs

It should be emphasized that synergistic effects resulting from ingestion of multiple agents in the hypnotic-sedative category may be especially hazardous, with hypotension frequently seen. Alcohol is the drug most frequently used in combination with other hypnotics. Specific interactions between alcohol and barbiturates are common. A chloral hydrate-alcohol interaction has also been noted. Angina, tachycardia, widened pulse pressure, and marked vasodilation have been found to develop in patients maintained on chloral hydrate after consuming small amounts of alcohol (18,19). Whether these effects are secondary to a central mechanism, to a direct cardiac effect, or to action on the peripheral vascular system is unclear at present.

Summary

In summary, most patients admitted with overdose of CNS depressants can recover with supportive therapy. When the agent consumed is excreted mainly by the kidneys, forced diuresis may be helpful. Complications that develop are usually related to lack of attention given to the cardiovascular effects of the drug or to inattention in maintenance of adequate respiration. The prognosis is good, providing therapy is instituted early enough to preclude the presence of any permanent cerebral damage secondary to anoxia.

BENZODIAZEPINES

Since the synthesis of chlordiazepoxide, many other benzodiazepine derivatives have appeared on the market (Table 3), although chlordiazepoxide and diazepam are still considered to be the main prototypes.

Pharmacology

After oral administration of diazepam, peak blood levels are noted within several hours, with a half-life of 1 to 2 days. Metabolism results in the formation of a lactam and a demethylated derivative, with small amounts of free and conjugated compounds being excreted in the urine. Diazepam is rather rapidly absorbed, with peak blood levels noted in 1½ hr. Excretion is biphasic, with a rapid phase within 2 to 3 hr, followed by a slow decay over

TABLE 3. *Benzodiazepine derivatives commonly prescribed*

Generic name	Trade name
Chlordiazepoxide hydrochloride USP	Librium
Chlordiazepoxide NF	Libritabs
Chlorazepate	Tranxene
Diazepam	Valium
Oxazepam	Serax
Flurazepam	Dalmane
Flunitrazepam	
Lorazepam	Ativan
Nitrazepam	Verstran
Prazepam	
Ketazolam	
Alprazolam	
Medazepam	
Temazepam	

the next several days, during which time the drugs are biotransformed and excreted. The half-life varies from 20 to 50 hr (4).

The terminal plasma half-life of diazepam in normal individuals increases linearly with advancing age. Klotz et al. (20) have shown the half-life at age 20 to be 20 hr, increasing to 90 hr at age 80. This increase is thought to be due primarily to an increase in initial volume of distribution rather than decreased metabolism. Diazepam clearance from the plasma and plasma binding are not age dependent. Accumulation of diazepam in the plasma will probably not be of great clinical importance in the elderly with respect to possibility of an overdose reaction. This finding, however, cannot be applied to all benzodiazepine derivatives.

Metabolic clearance of chlordiazepoxide is impaired in healthy, elderly persons, with clinical toxicity to diazepam and chlordiazepoxide associated with increasing age and daily drug dosage (21,22). The use of high-dose flurazepam in the elderly has also been associated with increased untoward reactions (1.9% in those under age 60 versus 7.1% in those over 80) (21). It is reasonable to begin by prescribing the lowest possible effective dose of the appropriate benzodiazepine for the elderly patient.

The presence of hepatic disease is associated with a prolongation in half-life of diazepam of approximately twofold; in addition, it is accompanied by a twofold decrease in total plasma clearance. This reduction in clearance of diazepam is of clinical importance in the use of this agent in persons with liver disease, especially if administered with other drugs that compete with diazepam for common metabolic pathways (20). Seventy percent of the oral dose is excreted in the urine, and 9 to 10 percent in the feces. Urinary excretion is in the form of conjugated metabolites, primarily glucuronides with oxazepam conjugates predominating.

The metabolites of chlordiazepoxide and diazepam are pharmacologically active as compared to inactivity of the metabolites of nitrazepam and oxazepam. This has clinical relevance since the latter two agents may be used as hypnotics with relatively little sedation persisting after a day. Chlordiazepoxide and diazepam, although capable of producing sleep in sufficient dosage, retain a sedative effect for more than 24 hr, with cumulative effects occurring on repeated administration.

Hemodynamics

Animal Studies

The benzodiazepines can influence cardiac function through centrally mediated effects on the nervous system, secondary to depression of the hypothalamic area, as well as through stimulation of the postganglionic adrenergic and cholinergic vasodilating mechanisms. In isolated canine heart preparations, Abel et al. (23) have noted an increase in myocardial contractility, significant coronary artery vasodilatation, and increase in coronary artery blood flow. When intravenous diazepam was administered, however, no coronary dilatation was observed.

Diazepam has also been shown to elevate the threshold for shock-induced ventricular tachycardia in dogs and to potentiate the antiarrhythmic effects of lidocaine. Liebeswar (24) has demonstrated the ability of pharmacologic doses of flurazepam to prolong the duration of the action potential and to decrease its amplitude and rate of rise. In the intact animal, however, little hemodynamic alterations have been noted with the use of these agents.

Persons Without Cardiac Disease

In human volunteers without evidence of cardiac disease, hemodynamic effects of the benzodiazepines have been reported to be minimal. Although venous tone and venomotor reflexes are impaired by diazepam, these effects are insufficient to alter arterial pressure in doses of chlordiazepoxide of up to 1.5 mg/kg or diazepam up to 0.2 mg/kg (25). Somewhat larger dosages may be associated with statistically significant although clinically unimportant decreases in systolic and diastolic blood pressure (26,27).

Recent use of parenteral drugs in the benzodiazepine groups as preinduction medication for endoscopies has provided additional information concerning their hemodynamic effects. Rao et al. (28), using 20 to 120 mg diazepam (Valium®) i.v. preendoscopy in both normal persons and individuals with chronic obstructive lung disease, found increases in heart rate and peripheral vascular resistance. This was associated with a decrease in both systolic and diastolic blood pressure and a corresponding decrease in cardiac output of 20% 15 min postinjection. Minimal differences were noted in the patients with chronic lung disease and in those with normal pulmonary function. The changes reported, however, may be related to the large doses of diazepam administered, as other investigators, utilizing amounts of less than 15 mg, have not reported any clinically significant alterations in hemodynamic parameters (27–30).

Studies involving the effect of diazepam on coronary blood flow in subjects with normal coronary arteriograms have revealed several hemodynamic changes. Coté et al. (31) noted a decrease in aortic pressure, with a depression of cardiac index and a consistent fall in left ventricular end-diastolic pressure (LVEDP), accompanied by a decreased tension time index and myocardial oxygen consumption (MVO_2) subsequent to intravenous injection of 5 to 8.5 mg diazepam. Neither coronary blood flow nor coronary vascular resistance was affected.

Persons With Cardiac Disease

Benzodiazepines may be used in cardiac patients as induction agents for cardioversions, for the treatment of anxiety in patients with valvular or coronary artery disease, or as specific therapy in hypertension.

Hemodynamic effects in persons with valvular heart disease have been rarely reported. D'Amelio et al. (32) have found intravenous diazepam to produce a statistically significant decrease in both pulmonary and systemic arterial pressure as well as a decrease in heart rate in persons with mitral valve disease undergoing routine diagnostic catheterization. All these patients had normal LVEDP at time of study. Clinically, little difficulty arose with the drug's use.

Cardioversion

The pharmacologic properties of diazepam make it an ideal drug to use for cardioversion; it not only eliminates the risks associated with general anesthesia but usually produces amnesia without causing a major depression of the cardiovascular system. Greenblatt and Shader (33), in a review of more than 450 patients receiving intravenous diazepam prior to cardioversion, reported adverse hemodynamic effects to be extremely infrequent, with pain and occasional phlebitis associated with injection rate being the only consistent problems. The dose of diazepam required to produce somnolence and amnesia, however, may vary considerably. Elderly patients in congestive heart failure generally require small doses. Persons with a history of chronic alcohol consumption may require large doses. With larger doses, decreases in both diastolic and systolic blood pressure can occur (34,35).

Ventricular arrhythmias have also been reported with the intravenous use of diazepam for cardioversion (36–38), although this relationship cannot be consistently confirmed. No agent used for induction, however, is free of all side-effects. Existing evidence supports the effectiveness of diazepam and warrants continued use of this drug in cardioversion.

Coronary Heart Disease

Several studies have appeared in the literature describing the effects of diazepam on coronary blood flow in persons with coronary heart disease undergoing diagnostic coronary angiography. Ikram and co-workers (39) have found intravenous diazepam in a dose of 0.1 mg/kg body weight to markedly increase myocardial blood flow as measured by Xenon clearance in subjects with normal coronary arteries and in those with radiologically confirmed coronary artery disease. The increases measured varied from 22% over control levels in normal subjects to a 73% average increase in persons with coronary artery disease.

Unfortunately, a specific increase in coronary blood flow has not been confirmed by other investigators. Coté et al. (40), in a study utilizing 5 to 8.5 mg diazepam i.v. prior to coronary angiography in patients with coronary artery disease, noted clinically insignificant hypoventilation and a consistently significant fall in aortic pressure and LVEDP, as well as a decreased index and MVO_2 without effect on coronary blood flow, coronary vascular resistance, or heart rate. Although a fall in aortic pressure was observed, in none of the patients did a clinical hypotensive reaction develop. A subsequent study in patients with hemodynamic evidence of left ventricular failure at time of catheterization revealed similar findings, with a decrease in LVEDP being prominent (40).

These authors hypothesized that such effects could result in a diminished intraventricular cavity volume, myocardial wall tension, and left ventricular MVO_2. In an attempt to confirm this hypothesis, diazepam was administered to patients given propranolol and atropine intravenously to induce partial autonomic blockade. Although myocardial blood flow and contractility and cardiac output remained unchanged, systolic pressure and LVEDP decreased significantly. These findings suggest the ability of diazepam to exert a direct dilatory effect on peripheral vascular smooth muscle with subsequent beneficial effects on cardiac function (41). Other investigators (42,43) have reported either insignificant changes or small decrements in coronary blood flow subsequent to administration of diazepam in persons with coronary artery disease. These data suggest that diazepam may be quite beneficial in patients with coronary artery disease through (a) peripheral vasodilation, (b) lowering of aortic blood pressure and MVO_2, (c) lowering of basal metabolism accompanying its sedative action, and (d) its recognized effectiveness in diminishing anxiety and depression commonly encountered in the coronary patient.

Unfortunately, most of the reports in the literature advocating the superiority of the benzodiazepines in the cardiac patient represent uncontrolled studies. Two well-designed drug trials have recently reported the superiority of these drugs over barbiturates. Benson (44) found diazepam to be more effective than phenobarbital in regard to alleviating apprehension, depression, restlessness, and preoccupation with illness in patients with acute myocardial infarction. Hackett and Cassem (45), in a comparison of chlordiazepoxide and amobarbital in myocardial infarction patients treated in a coronary care unit, found analgesia to be required less often and in smaller doses in those patients receiving chlordiazepoxide than in those receiving barbiturates. These findings suggest that diazepam may be the sedative of choice in patients with coronary artery disease and angina. It should be emphasized, however, that the benzodiazepines by no means represent a pharmacologic panacea for the coronary patient. The elderly have been shown to be more susceptible to the sedative effects of these agents (46,47), and withdrawal associated with chronic use, although rare, has been reported (48,49).

Hypertension

Although prescription of benzodiazepines to hypertensive patients is quite common, there is little evidence supporting the efficacy of these agents in reducing blood pressure (50). Whitehead et al. (51) surveyed the effectiveness of benzodiazepines in reducing blood pressure in 32 patients compared to a matched control group attending the same hypertension clinic. Although the incidence of psychologic complaints on the initial visit were higher in the benzodiazepine group (34 versus 0%), 66% of patients received this drug in the absence of any psychologic indications. This group did experience a greater decrease in diastolic blood pressure (average 6.69 mm Hg) than the controls ($p < 0.01$). Unfortunately, this was a retrospective survey. At present, there is little objective evidence that the benzodiazepines exert a specific antihypertensive effect other than the relief of anxiety.

DRUG INTERACTIONS

Many of the hypnotics, sedatives, and minor tranquilizers are known to influence the hepatic endoplasmic reticulum, with barbiturates having the most prominent effects (Table 4). In general, the direction of the enzymatic response is both frequency and dose related. Chronic administration of barbiturates and other sedatives results in enzymatic induction, whereas acute administration of large doses may cause an inhibition of enzymatic activity. Concomitant administration of these agents with other drugs whose metabolism is dependent on the hepatic endoplasmic reticulum can result in drug interactions, many of clinical importance.

Interactions With Other Mood-Altering Drugs

The potentially hazardous effects of drinking alcohol and consuming sedative drugs are reviewed in Chapter 4. When they are taken simultaneously, synergistic respiratory depressant activity is likely to occur. Similarly, CNS

TABLE 4. *Selected drug interactions of barbiturates and benzodiazepines*

Drug	Clinical effect	
	Barbiturates	Benzodiazepines
Alcohol	Synergistic respiratory depressant activity with acute administration	Synergistic respiratory depressant activity with acute administration
Diphenylhydantoin	Increase in plasma levels	Increase in plasma levels
Digitoxin	Decrease in plasma half-life	No reported clinical effect
Oral anticoagulants	Decrease in anticoagulant effect[a]	Minimal clinical effect
Phenothiazines	Decrease in plasma levels	No reported clinical effect
Tricyclic antidepressants	Decrease in antidepressant effect	Increase in anticholinergic symptoms

[a] Potential for serious bleeding when barbiturate therapy discontinued.

depression will be enhanced if any of the individual drugs in this group are taken simultaneously.

The use of barbiturates with therapeutic doses of the tricyclic antidepressants has been associated with a decrease in antidepressant effect believed to be related to an induction of the hepatic enzyme system responsible for tricyclic metabolism (52,53). The use of barbiturates in tricyclic overdose has been associated with a potentiation of adverse effects and is therefore contraindicated (54). Additive depressant effects and an increase in anticholinergic symptoms have also been reported with continued use of chlordiazepoxide and the tricyclics. Unlike barbiturates-tricyclic interactions, however, serious adverse effects are rare (53,55,56). For this reason, if convulsions present as a manifestation of tricyclic antidepressant overdose, a benzodiazepine, such as diazepam, is the preferred agent for treatment (53,57).

Plasma levels of phenothiazines have been shown to decrease and urinary phenothiazine excretion increase in patients simultaneously given barbiturates (58). This effect is secondary to the induction of hepatic enzymes responsible for phenothiazine metabolism. The clinical significance of this interaction remains to be defined.

Interactions With Cardiac Medications

Oral Anticoagulants

Hypnotic-sedative drugs can interact with several medications routinely prescribed to persons with cardiovascular disease. Clinically, the most important interactions involve the oral anticoagulants.

Barbiturates

Of all the sedatives, the barbiturates have the most prominent effect on metabolism of the coumarin derivatives. Concurrent barbiturate administration may necessitate the doubling of the anticoagulant dosage to maintain the desired prothrombin time. This interaction occurs with all barbiturates, although phenobarbital exerts the most potent effect. Antlitz et al. (59) studied the effect of butabarbital (120 mg/day for 2 weeks) in 12 patients stabilized on either warfarin or phenprocoumon (Liquamar®). The average dose of each anticoagulant had to be increased significantly by 63 and 42%, respectively, after the barbiturate was administered. This increase was necessary within 1 week after initiation of barbiturate therapy, with the effect persisting for at least 6 weeks subsequent to discontinuing the drug.

Gross and Dickhaus (60), in a study of eight patients stabilized on dicumarol subsequent to administering phenobarbital (90 mg/day), noted the dicumarol requirements to increase by an average of approximately 33%. Despite the increase in dicumarol dosage, the prothrombin time in these patients indicated a diminishing anticoagulant effect. Downward adjustment of anticoagulant dosage was necessary approximately 1 month after the phenobarbital was discontinued.

MacDonald et al. (61) administered single doses of warfarin to 10 healthy volunteers followed by 120 mg phenobarbital daily for 3 weeks. On the nineteenth day of barbiturate therapy, the subjects were given another single dose of warfarin. The serum warfarin level, serum half-life, and prothrombin time were all significantly lower in the barbiturate-treated subjects than in controls. A barbiturate-free period of 1 week was necessary to restore the previous anticoagulant response.

Evidence suggests that the barbiturate-warfarin interactions may be dose related, although most of the studies contain too small a number of patients to permit definitive conclusions. Interactions with the oral anticoagulants vary with the specific barbiturate administered. Dicumarol absorption from the intestine is inhibited by heptabarbital administration, whereas it is little affected by the other barbiturates (62). In most studies, phenobarbital appears to be a slightly more potent enzyme inducer of anticoagulant metabolism.

The main importance of this interaction is the propensity for hemorrhage when the sedative is discontinued rather than the initial difficulty in establishing adequate levels of anticoagulants. Microsomal enzyme activities usually return to normal within 2 or 3 weeks after cessation of barbiturate therapy. If an adjustment in warfarin dosage is not made, the potential for serious hemorrhage exists. MacDonald and Robinson (61) found that patients on oral anticoagulants for myocardial infarction who were also given barbiturates exhibited poor anticoagulation control and lower prothrombin times than other patients. In a review of 67 bleeding episodes in these patients, the prior coadministration of enzyme-inducing agents was found to be a factor in 14 patients (21%), two of whom died.

Chloral Hydrate

Chloral hydrate interacts with warfarin in a somewhat complex manner. During early therapy with both agents, trichloroacetic acid, a major metabolite of chloral hydrate, accumulates in the plasma and, having a higher infinity for plasma albumin, displaces warfarin. This results in an increase in unbound plasma warfarin and enhancement of anticoagulant action (63,64). With time, however, hepatic enzyme induction occurs with an increased rate of warfarin metabolism and inhibition of anticoagulation. Although these interactions have been pharmacologically documented, recent studies suggest that their clinical importance may be minimal (65,66).

Benzodiazepines

Interactions between the oral anticoagulants and the benzodiazepines are minimal and of little clinical importance (67,68). Although more carefully designed studies are needed, to date these agents are indicated in persons maintained on anticoagulant therapy.

Digitalis

A lowering of plasma digitoxin levels and a diminished digitoxin half-life have been reported in persons maintained on digitoxin and given phenobarbital (69). Concomitant use of these two drugs is also associated with an acceleration of conversion of digitoxin to digoxin (70). Although the interaction does not uniformly occur, concomitant use of digitoxin and phenobarbital should be avoided when possible; underdigitalization, with its attendant adverse effects, may be of sufficient magnitude to be clinically important.

Antiarrhythmics

Induction of the hepatic microsomal system by barbiturates can affect the metabolism of quinidine, diphenylhydantoin, and lidocaine. Data et al. (71) have found the serum half-life of quinidine to diminish by an average of 50% with concomitant use of these agents. Similarly, an increase in diphenylhydantoin blood levels to toxic concentrations has also been reported (72), although clinical importance of this interaction may show individual variation (73,74). Several reports have also appeared in the literature describing an increase in diphenylhydantoin levels with concomitant administration of benzodiazepines. Although this interaction may also be of clinical importance, the paucity of published data warrants further investigation (75). Lidocaine metabolism can also be affected in a similar manner. The clinical relevance of this interaction has not been clearly defined (76,77).

Antihypertensives

Interaction at a metabolic level has been reported with barbiturate administration and the simultaneous use of alpha-methyldopa (78) and monoamine oxidase inhibitors (79), but the clinical importance of these reactions has not been demonstrated.

Summary

The use of hypnotics and sedatives may act on the hepatic microsomal system to affect the metabolism of other drugs usually detoxified through this pathway. The magnitude of this effect varies with the individual drug, the barbiturates being the most influential and the benzodiazepines the least. If a sedative or tranquilizing agent is warranted in the presence of consumption of other drugs metabolized by the liver, one of the benzodiazepines would be the agent of choice. Even with these drugs, however, careful monitoring is necessary to detect the appearance of any clinically adverse interactions.

REFERENCES

1. American Medical Association Committee on Alcoholism and Addiction, Council of Mental Health (1965): *JAMA,* 193:673.
2. Cohen, S., and Blutt, M. J. (1978): Hypnotic drug therapy. *Drug Abuse Alcohol. Rev.,* 1:6.
3. Cooper, J. R. (1977): *Sedative-Hypnotic Drugs: Risks and Benefits,* p. XII. National Institute on Drug Abuse, Rockville, Maryland.
4. Harvey, S. C. (1975): Hypnotics and sedatives. In: *The Pharmacological Basis of Therapeutics,* edited by L. S. Goodman and A. Gilman, pp. 102–136. Macmillan, New York.
5. Jaffee, J. (1977): Hypnotic and sedative agents. In: *Psychopharmacology in the Practice of Medicine,* edited by M. Jarvik, pp. 327–342. Appleton-Century-Crofts, New York.
6. Nayler, W. G., and Szeto, J. (1972): Effect of sodium pentobarbital on calcium in mammalian heart muscle. *Am. J. Physiol.,* 222:339.
7. Anderson, T. W., and Gravenstein, J. S. (1966): Cardiovascular effects of sedative doses of pentobarbital and hydroxyzine. *Anesthesiology,* 27:272.
8. Hollister, L. (1975): Hydroxyzine hydrochloride: Possible adverse cardiac interactions. *Psychopharmacol. Commun.* 1:61.
9. Thorstrand, C. (1975): Cardiovascular effects of poisoning by hypnotic and tricyclic antidepressant drugs. *Acta Med. Scand.* [*Suppl.*], 583:1.
10. Shubin, H., and Weil, M. H. (1965): The mechanism of shock following suicidal doses of barbiturates, narcotics and tranquilizer drugs, with observations on the effects of treatment. *Am. J. Med.,* 38:853.
11. Schreiner, G. E., and Teehan, B. P. (1972): Dialysis of poisons and drugs: Annual review. *Trans. Am. Soc. Artif. Intern. Organs,* 18:563.

12. Hansen, A. R., Kennedy, K. A., Ambre, J. J., et al. (1975): *Glutethimide poisoning—A metabolite contributes to morbidity and mortality. N. Engl. J. Med.,* 292:250.
13. Chazan, J. A., and Cohen, J. J. (1969): Clinical spectrum of glutethimide intoxication. *JAMA,* 205:837.
14. Pascarelli, E. F. (1973): Methaqualone abuse. The quiet epidemic. *JAMA,* 224:512.
15. Schwartz, H. S. (1976): Acute meprobamate poisoning with gastrotomy and removal of drug containing mass. *N. Engl. J. Med.,* 295:1177.
16. Blumberg, A. G., Rosett, H. L., and Dobraw, A. (1959): Severe hypotensive reactions following meprobamate overdose. *Ann. Intern. Med.,* 57:607.
17. Lhoste, F., Lemaire, F., and Rapin, M. (1977): Treatment of hypotension in meprobamate poisoning. *N. Engl. J. Med.,* 296:1004.
18. Bardodej, Z., Krivucova, M., and Pokorny, F. (1955): A biochemical explanation of alcohol intolerance in trichlorethylene intoxication. *Pracovni Lekarstui (Prague),* 7:263.
19. Sellers, E. M., Carr, G., Bernstein, J. G., et al. (1972): Interaction of chloralhydrate and ethanol in man II. Hemodynamics and performance. *Clin. Pharmacol. Ther.,* 13:50.
20. Klotz, U., Avant, G. R., Hoyumpa, A., et al. (1975): The effect of age and liver disease on the disposition and elimination of diazepam in adult man. *J. Clin. Invest.,* 55:347.
21. Greenblatt, D. J., Allen, M. D., and Shader, R. I. (1977): Toxicity of flurazepam in the elderly. *Clin. Pharmacol. Ther.,* 21:355.
22. Boston Collaborative Drug Surveillance Program (1973): Clinical depression of the central nervous system due to diazepam and chlordiazepoxide in relation to cigarette smoking and age. *N. Engl. J. Med.,* 288:277.
23. Abel, R. M., Reis, R. L., and Staroscik, R. N. (1970): Coronary vasodilatation following diazepam. *Br. J. Pharmacol.,* 38:620.
24. Liebeswar, G. (1972): The depressant action of flurazepam on the maximum rate of rise of action potentials recorded from guinea pig papillary muscles. *Naunyn Schmiedebergs Arch. Pharmacol.,* 275:445.
25. Greenblatt, D. J., and Shader, R. I. (1974): *Benzodiazepines in Clinical Practice,* p. 141. Raven Press, New York.
26. Korttila, K. (1975): The effect of diazepam, flunitrazepam and droperidol with an analgesic on blood pressure and heart rate in man. *Arzneim. Forsch.,* 25:1303.
27. Dalen, J. E., Evans, G. L., Banas, J. S., et al. (1969): The hemodynamic and respiratory effects of diazepam (Valium). *Anesthesiology,* 30:259.
28. Rao, S., Sherbaniuk, R. W., Prasad, K., et al. (1973): Cardiopulmonary effects of diazepam. *Clin. Pharmacol. Ther.,* 14:182.
29. Katz, J., Finestone, S. C., and Pappas, M. T. (1967): Circulatory response to tilting after intravenous diazepam in volunteers. *Anesth. Analg. (Cleve.),* 46:267.
30. McClish, A. (1966): Diazepam as an intravenous agent for general anesthesia. *Am. Anesth. Soc. J.,* 13:562.
31. Coté, P., Gueret, P., and Bourassa, M. G. (1974): Systemic and coronary hemodynamic effects of diazepam in patients with normal and diseased coronary arteries. *Circulation,* 50:1210.
32. D'Amelio, G. D., Volta, S. D., Stritoui, P., et al. (1973): Acute cardiovascular effects of diazepam in patients with mitral valve disease. *Eur. J. Clin. Pharmacol.,* 6:61.
33. Greenblatt, D. J., and Shader, R. I. (1974): *Benzodiazepines in Clinical Practice,* p. 144. Raven Press, New York.
34. Forssell, G., Norlander, R., Nyquist, O., et al. (1975): Diazepam in cardioversion. *Acta Med. Scand.,* 197:255.
35. Rotem, C. E. (1970): Diazepam injectable as premedication for electrical conversion. *Can. Med. Assoc. J.,* 103:381.
36. Zsigmond, E. K. (1972): Causes of ventricular arrhythmias. *JAMA,* 221:712.
37. Nevins, M. A. (1971): Ventricular arrhythmia and diazepam. *JAMA,* 215:643.
38. Barrett, J. S., and Hey, E. B. (1970): Ventricular arrhythmias associated with the use of diazepam for cardioversion. *JAMA,* 214:1323.
39. Ikram, H., Rubin, A. P., and Jewkes, R. F. (1973): Effect of diazepam on myo-

cardial blood flow of patients with and without coronary disease. *Br. Heart J.,* 35:626.

40. Coté, P., Campeau, L., and Bourassa, M. G. (1976): Therapeutic implications of diazepam in patients with elevated left ventricular fllling pressure. *Am. Heart J.,* 91:747.
41. Coté, P., Noble, J., and Bourassa, M. G. (1976): Systemic vasodilatation following diazepam after combined sympathetic and parasympathetic blockade in patients with coronary artery disease. *Catheter. Cardiovas. Diag.,* 2:367.
42. Formanek, A., Korbuly, D., Moore, R., et al. (1976): The effect of valium on myocardial blood flow. *Radiology,* 121:541.
43. Markiewicz, W., Hunt, S., Harrison, D. C., et al. (1976): Circulatory effects of diazepam in heart disease. *J. Clin. Pharmacol.,* 16:637.
44. Benson, W. H. (1971): Comparative evaluation of diazepam (Valium®) and phenobarbital for the relief of anxiety related symptoms in patients hospitalized for acute myocardial infarction. *J. Med. Assoc. Ga.,* 60:276.
45. Hackett, T. P., and Cassem, N. H. (1972): Reduction of anxiety in the coronary care unit: A controlled double blind comparison of chlordiazepoxide and amobarbital. *Curr. Ther. Res.,* 14:649.
46. Greenblatt, D. J., Allen, M. D., and Shader, R. I. (1977): Toxicity of high dose flurazepam by the elderly. *Clin. Pharmacol. Ther.,* 21:355.
47. Linnoila, M., and Viukari, M. (1976): Efficacy and side effects of nitrazepam and thioridazine as sleeping aids for psychogeriatric patients. *Br. J. Psychiatry,* 128: 566.
48. Woody, G. E., O'Brien, C. P., and Greensteiz, R. (1975): Misuse and abuse of diazepam. An increasingly common problem. *Int. J. Addict.,* 10:843.
49. Preskoen, S. H., and Denner, L. J. (1977): Benzodiazepines and withdrawal psychosis. *JAMA,* 237:36.
50. Diazepam (Valium) in hypertension (1974): *Med. Lett. Drug Ther.,* 16:96.
51. Whitehead, W. E., Blackwell, B., and Robinson, A. (1977): Why physicians prescribe benzodiazepines in essential hypertension: A phase IV study. *Biol. Psychiatry,* 12:597.
52. Burrows, G. D., and Davis, B. (1971): Antidepressants and barbiturates. *Br. Med. J.,* 4:113.
53. Silverman, G., and Braithwaite, R. (1972): Interaction of benzodiazepines with tricyclic antidepressants. *Br. Med. J.,* 4:111.
54. Crocker, J., and Morton, B. (1969): Tricyclic (antidepressant) drug toxicity. *Clin. Toxicol.,* 2:397.
55. Abdow, F. A. (1964): Elavil-Librium combination. *Am. J. Psychiatry,* 120:1204.
56. Anon (1969): General practitioner clinical trials. Chlordiazepoxide with amitriptyline in neurotic depression. *Practitioner,* 202:437.
57. Nobel, J., and Matthew, T. (1969): Acute poisoning by tricyclic antidepressants: Clinical features and management of 100 patients. *Clin. Toxicol.,* 2:403.
58. Curry, S. H., Davis, J. M., and Janowsky, D. S. (1970): Factors effecting chlorpromazine levels in psychiatric patients. *Arch. Gen. Psychiatry,* 22:209.
59. Antlitz, A. M., Tolentino, M., and Kosai, M. F. (1968): Effects of butabarbital on orally administered anticoagulants. *Curr. Ther. Res.,* 10:70.
60. Gross, J. E., and Dickhaus, D. W. (1965): Increased bishydroxycoumarin requirements in patients receiving phenobarbital. *N. Engl. J. Med.,* 27:1094.
61. MacDonald, M. G., and Robinson, D. S. (1968): Clinical observations of possible barbiturate interference with anticoagulation. *JAMA,* 204:97.
62. Aggeler, P. M., and O'Reilly, R. A. (1969): Effect of heptabarbital on the response to bishydroxycoumarin in man. *J. Lab. Clin. Med.,* 74:229.
63. Sellers, E. M., and Koch-Weser, J. (1970): Potentiation of warfarin induced hypoprothrombinemia by chloral hydrate. *N. Engl. J. Med.,* 283:827.
64. Boston Collaborative Drug Surveillance Program (1972): Interaction between chloral hydrate and warfarin. *N. Engl. J. Med.,* 286:53.
65. Udall, J. (1974): Warfarin-chloral hydrate interaction. Pharmacological activity and clinical significance. *Ann. Intern. Med.,* 81:341.

66. Griner, P. F., Raisz, L. G., Rickles, F. R., et al. (1971): Chloral hydrate and warfarin interactions. Clinical significance. *Ann. Intern. Med.,* 74:540.
67. Breckenridge, A., and Orme, M. (1973): Interactions of benzodiazepines with oral anticoagulants. In: *The Benzodiazepines,* edited by S. Garattini, E. Mussini, and L. O. Randall, pp. 647–654. Raven Press, New York.
68. Robinson, D. S., and Sylvester, D. (1970): Interaction of commonly prescribed drugs with warfarin. *Ann. Intern. Med.,* 72:853.
69. Jelliffe, R. W., and Blankenhorn, D. H. (1966): Effect of phenobarbital on digoxin metabolism. *Clin. Res.,* 14:160.
70. Hutcheon, D. E. (1975): Cardiovascular drug interactions. *J. Clin. Pharmacol.,* 9:129.
71. Data, J. L., Wilkinson, G. R., and Nies, A. S. (1976): Interaction of quinidine with anticonvulsant drugs. *N. Engl. J. Med.,* 294:699.
72. Tudhope, G. R. (1969): Advances in medicine. *Practitioner,* 203:405.
73. Diamond, W. D., and Buchanan, R. A. (1976): A clinical study of the effect of phenobarbital on diphenylhydantoin plasma levels. *J. Clin. Pharmacol.,* 10:306.
74. Morselli, I., Rizzo, M., and Garatinni, S. (1971): Interactions between phenobarbital and diphenylhydantoin in animals and in epileptic patients. *Ann. N.Y. Acad. Sci.,* 177:88.
75. Kutt, H., Haynes, J., Verebely, K., et al. (1969): The effect of phenobarbital on plasma diphenylhydantoin levels and metabolism in man and rat liver microsomes. *Neurology,* 19:611.
76. Heinonen, J., Takki, S. S., and Jarho, L. (1970): Plasma levels of lidocaine in patients treated with potential inducers of microsomal enzymes. *Acta Anaesthesiol. Scand.,* 14:89.
77. Dunbar, R. W., Boettinger, R. B., Haley, J. V., et al. (1971): The effects of diazepam on the antiarrhythmic response to lidocaine. *Anesth. Analg.,* 50:85.
78. Kaldor, A., Juvancz, P., Demeczky, M., et al. (1971): Enhancement of methyldopa metabolism with barbiturates. *Br. Med. J.,* 3:518.
79. Sjöquist, F. (1965): Psychotropic drugs 2: Interaction between monoamine oxidase (MAO) inhibitors and other substances. *Proc. R. Soc. Med.,* 58:967.

Chapter 7

The Major Tranquilizers

PHENOTHIAZINES

The major tranquilizers are utilized mainly in the treatment of psychoses. Of this group of drugs, the phenothiazines (Table 1) are among the most widely used psychotropic agents in medical practice. Chlorpromazine (Thorazine®) can be considered the prototype of this group.

Pharmacology

Chlorpromazine, when administered orally, is readily absorbed from the intestinal tract at a rate dependent on the dosage form. Although there is considerable intersubject variability, peak plasma levels are usually seen in 2 to 3 hr. The plasma half-life is rather short (less than 6 hr), but excretion of metabolites may occur for up to 6 weeks following discontinuation of medication. Tissue binding is considerable, and various metabolites can be

TABLE 1. *Commonly used major tranquilizers*

Generic name	Trade name
Phenothiazines	
Aliphatics[a]	
Chlorpromazine	Thorazine
Promazine	Sparine
Triflupromazine	Vesprin
Piperazines[a]	
Acetophenazine	Tindal
Butaperazine	Repoise
Carphenazine	Proketazine
Fluphenazine	Prolixin, Permitil
Pherphenazine	Trilafon
Prochlorperazine	Compazine
Thiopropazine	Dartal
Trifluperazine	Stelazine
Piperidines[a]	
Mesoridazine	Serentil
Piperacetazine	Quide
Thioridazine	Mellaril
Rauwolfia alkaloids	
Reserpine	
Butyrophenones	
Haloperidol	Haldol
Thioxanthenes	
Chlorprothixene	Taractan
Thiothixene	Navane

[a] Refers to substitution of the side group on position 10 of the three-ring structure of the phenothiazines.

detected in the urine for up to 6 months after discontinuing the drug in individuals previously on chronic maintenance.

Metabolism occurs in the liver with excretion of metabolites in both urine and feces. Some metabolites may be clinically active (7-hydroxychlorpromazine). Metabolism occurs through hydroxylation and subsequent conjugation with glucuronic acid, sulfoxide formation, or demethylation. Chlorpromazine can cause an induction of the hepatic microsomal system, which can not only affect its own breakdown but can also result in interactions with other drugs metabolized by this system (1).

Hemodynamics

Normal Subjects

The actions of the phenothiazines on the cardiovascular system are complex, relating to its direct effects on the heart and vasculature as well as indirect actions mediated through the autonomic and central nervous systems

(CNS). Chlorpromazine is not only an alpha blocker but can also exert atropine-like effects, resulting in reflex tachycardia and vasodilation. Parasympathetic effects associated with the ability of the drug to depress central vasomotor centers can result in tachycardia and hypotension (2,3). A direct myocardial depressant effect has also been demonstrated experimentally in papillary muscle. Chronic administration has been associated with the development of cardiomegaly, congestive failure, and refractory arrhythmias (4). Paradoxically, chlorpromazine has also been demonstrated to have coronary vasodilator activity equal to and at times greater than that seen with papaverine and nitroglycerin (5). An antiarrhythmic effect on the heart similar to that of quinidine has also been reported (4–6).

Clinically, chlorpromazine can affect the renin-aldosterone axis. Intravenous administration dramatically elevates plasma aldosterone levels and plasma renin activity. This is probably secondary to chlorpromazine activity as an alpha blocker or a beta-adrenergic agonist, although other mechanisms cannot be excluded (7).

Hypotension

Hypotension may occur following parenteral administration of chlorpromazine. Carlsson et al. (8), studying the circulatory response in persons maintained on large doses of chlorpromazine at rest and during exercise, noted a decrease in blood pressure and stroke volume without an increase in heart rate sufficient to maintain resting cardiac output. The hypotension may be secondary to either centrally mediated pressor reflexes or an adrenergic blockade. The ability of phenothiazines to serve as effective alpha blockers is important in the treatment of chlorpromazine-induced hypotension. The use of an agent with both alpha and beta receptor activity, such as epinephrine, might result in an "unmasking" of beta effects with an associated worsening of the hypotension. For this reason, only sympathomimetic drugs with alpha activity should be administered.

Hypotension is more common with chlorpromazine and thioridazine and less so with piperazine derivatives. Oral doses may also be related to a mild hypotensive reaction, which may resolve with time as tolerance develops (9). Orthostatic changes, however, may persist for long periods.

In an attempt to identify those patients on oral phenothiazines at risk for hypotensive reactions, Swett et al. (10) reviewed blood pressure changes in 515 persons in an inpatient setting maintained on varying doses of chlorpromazine. Data were analyzed by multiple regression analysis to determine the independent effect of measured variables. Hypotension, defined as a decrease in blood pressure of 15 mm Hg or more, accompanied by symptoms of dizziness or fainting, was found to be significantly related to smoking, dose of chlorpromazine administered, and initial level of diastolic blood pressure ($p < 0.05$). The incidence of hypotension in nonsmokers was 10%, light smokers ($<$ 21 cigarettes/day) 8%, and intermediate smokers (21 to 40 cigarettes/day) 5%. There was no hypotension observed in heavy smokers ($>$ 40 cigarettes/day). Five percent of patients taking less than 100 mg chlorpromazine/day had hypotension as compared to 10% taking a daily dose of 500 mg or more. Only 6% of persons with initial diastolic pressures of less than 100 mm Hg experienced hypotensive reactions as compared to 26% of those with diastolic pressures of 100 mm Hg or higher. Although an association may be expected of a greater risk of hypotension with increasing chlorpromazine use and the presence of significant diastolic hypertension, the reason for the apparent "beneficial" effects of nicotine remains to be defined. It has been suggested that smokers require greater doses of pentazocine and propoxyphene than nonsmokers (11,12). Similarly, the lower rates of drowsiness in patients receiving benzodiazepines have been reported in smokers versus nonsmokers (13). These actions may result from the ability of nicotine to induce hepatic enzymes responsible for metabolizing these drugs.

Persons With Cardiovascular Disease

The ability of chlorpromazine to dilate the vascular musculature, associated with a decrease in arterial pressure, has suggested its clinical use in altered hemodynamic states. Therapeutic uses might include (a) control of arterial hypertension, (b) alleviation of the generalized vasoconstriction and maldistribution of systemic blood flow after cardiopulmonary bypass or excessive hemorrhage, and (c) reduction of left ventricular afterload in low cardiac output states associated with an elevated systemic vascular resistance. Stinson et al. (14) studied the effectiveness of chlorpromazine compared to nitroprusside, nitroglycerin, and trimethaphan in patients recovering from open heart surgery. The hemodynamic effects of chlorpromazine were found to be similar to those associated with nitroprusside, with the exception that the average increase in heart rate was notably greater with chlorpromazine. This increase in heart rate, however, abrogated any reduction in left ventricular minute work and left ventricular preload or afterload so that there was no net decrease in myocardial oxygen demand.

Electrocardiographic Changes

Electrocardiographic changes, at times quite impressive, are now known to occur in persons on phenothiazines, the degree of abnormality being dose related. The most frequent asymptomatic alterations seen are repolarization abnormalities resembling those produced by quinidine. These changes include depression, widening, notching, inversion, and flattening of T-waves, presence of U-waves, and prolongation of QT intervals (Figs. 1 and 2). Patients receiving thioridazine (Mellaril®) in doses of 150 to 400 mg/day were noted to

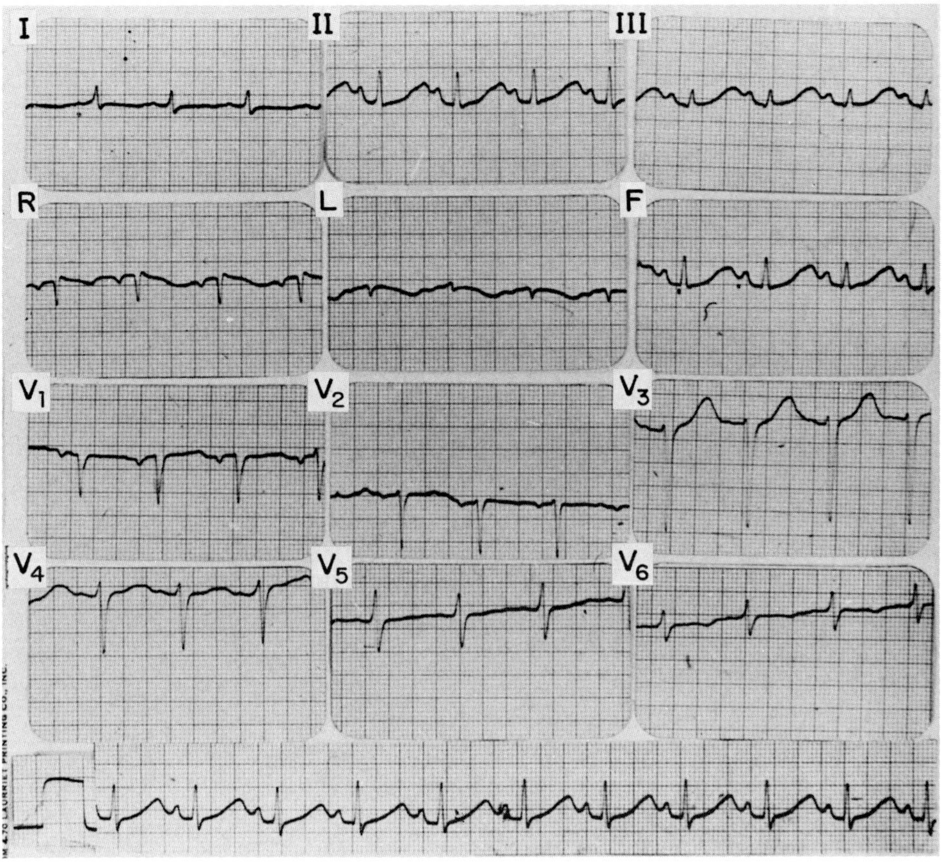

FIG. 1. ECG of an asymptomatic 31-year-old man maintained on 2 g/day chlorpromazine. Note prolonged QTc (0.51 sec) with T-wave deformities in leads II, III, and avf. (Reprinted from Stimmel, ref. 60.)

have low voltage T-waves in 44% and T-wave widening in 23%. Only 32% of these patients had normal electrocardiograms (ECGs) (15). Huston and Bell (16) noted T-wave changes in 50% of 106 hospitalized patients on thioridazine. In persons on 150 to 900 mg/day, this incidence increased to 70%. Similar changes have been noted with chlorpromazine (Thorazine®), trifluoperazine (Stelazine®), mesoridazine (Serentil®) (17–19) and fluphenazine (20).

The presence of first degree atrioventricular block with conduction delay, nonconducted premature atrial beats, and atrial flutter with varying block have also been reported in persons receiving thioridazine therapy (21,22). Recurrent unifocal and multifocal ventricular premature beats, ventricular tachycardia, and ventricular fibrillation have also been described in essentially healthy persons (23–25). Although most of these arrhythmias

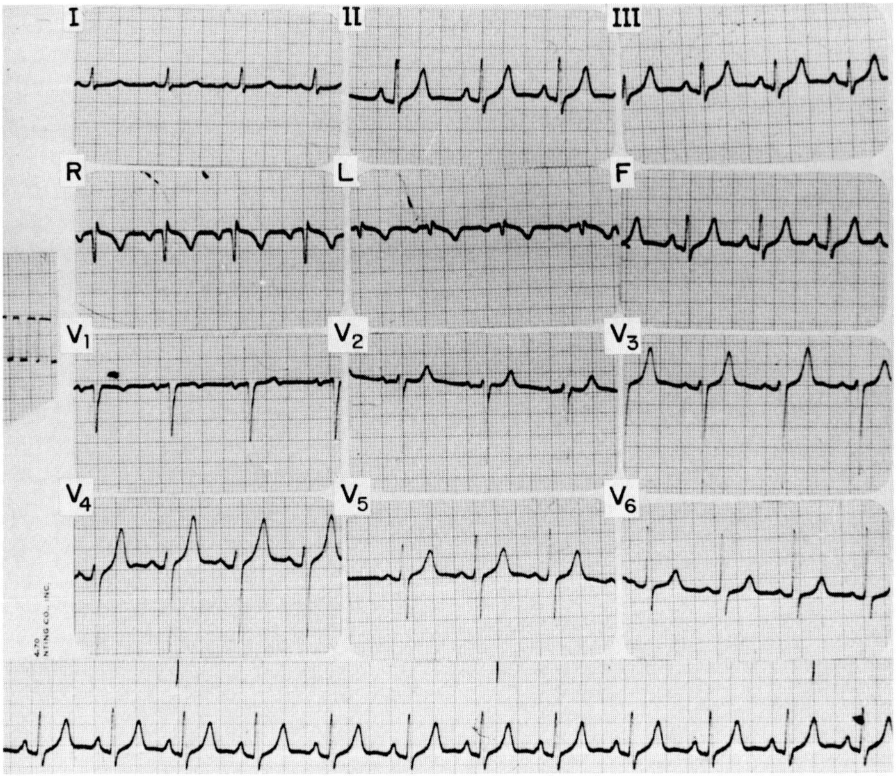

FIG. 2. ECG of patient in Fig. 1 48 hr after discontinuing chlorpromazine. Both QTc and T-wave alterations have normalized. (Reprinted from Stimmel, ref. 60.)

have appeared in patients receiving extremely high doses of thioridazine (1,500 to 3,600 mg), arrhythmias in patients receiving lower doses (less than 800 mg/day) have also been reported. Interestingly, no electrocardiographic changes were reported (23) in children maintained on phenothiazines in doses equivalent to those producing such changes in adults (26).

There is difficulty in assessing the clinical importance of these studies because of an inadequate stratification of patients with respect to the existence of prior cardiovascular disease. In addition, the reported experimental designs infrequently permit administration of the drug in a sequential fashion, with each patient serving as his/her own control. For this reason, the study of Holden and Itil (27) is of particular relevance. These investigators studied chronic schizophrenic patients admitted to a psychiatric institution for intensive treatment. Both male and female and white and black patients under 50 years of age were studied. Only data of patients who were physically well with normal baseline laboratory and electrocardiographic findings were analyzed. All persons were placed on placebo treatment for a minimum of 4 weeks prior to the start of any drug therapy. Electrocardiographic examinations were completed approximately every 3 weeks for each patient during the placebo period, the period on drug therapy, and the post drug or placebo period.

A total of 196 persons were studied on placebo therapy. Of these, 57 (29%) exhibited abnormal records at one time or another during this period. Seventy-five persons were subsequently treated with phenothiazines, with 34 (45%) exhibiting abnormal ECGs. The percentage of abnormal ECGs was found to differ considerably with the specific phenothiazine used. Thioridazine, combined with chlordiazepoxide, was found to give the lowest incidence of abnormal records (31%), whereas fluphenazine, combined in oral and intramuscular form, resulted in the greatest percentage (91%) of abnormal records. The most common abnormalities were T-wave changes, although in four of the 11 patients on combined fluphenazine therapy, sinus bradycardia developed, with atrial ventricular block developing in one. Life-threatening arrhythmias, such as ventricular bigeminy or ventricular fibrillation, were infrequently observed. All the electrocardiographic changes were considered to be unrelated to dose, the dosage range for the development of T-wave changes being quite broad. These findings differed from those of Huston and Bell (16), who noted a dose-related increase in electrocardiographic abnormalities in hospitalized patients maintained on thioridazine.

Similar findings were reported by Backman and Elosuo (17), who administered 159 mg/day chlorpromazine to patients with normal ECGs prior to the start of the study. Significant depression of the T-wave and extension of QT interval were noted after 1 week of therapy. Within 1 week after discontinuing the drug, these changes usually reverted to normal (28,29).

Sudden Death

In the past 13 years, reports of sudden, unexplained death in persons receiving phenothiazines have appeared in the literature, implicating a fatal arrhythmia as the mode of exodus (30–33). The clinical relevance of electrocardiographic alterations in producing sudden death secondary to fatal arrhythmias has not been clearly defined. It must be emphasized that cardiac patients in psychiatric institutions are expected to have an incidence of sudden death owing to their cardiac disease independent of the prescription of phenothiazines or other psychotropic agents. Swett and Shader (34), in a review of 1,932 consecutively monitored psychiatric inpatients, were unable to relate the appearance of serious cardiac effects to any specific drug, although the incidence of these adverse effects was clearly higher in persons with cardiac disease (18.8 versus 1.3%).

Mechanisms for sudden death in persons on phenothiazines, however, can be easily hypothesized. Prolongation of the QT interval for any reason reflects delayed ventricular repolarization and an increase in the duration of the vulnerable period, with the predisposition to development of ventricular arrhythmias. In the presence of QT prolongation, single or multiple ventricular premature beats may lead to fatal ventricular fibrillation. Giles and Modlin (35) described two patients on thioridazine dying with ventricular arrhythmias who had evidence of myocardial atrophy with destruction of cellular cytoplasm at postmortem examination. Thioridazine-induced ventricular tachycardia requiring control with a temporary pacemaker has also been reported (36).

Autopsies in persons dying suddenly while on phenothiazines show lesions in the intramyocardial arterioles and arteriolar capillary bed. Lesions have also been noted in the conduction tissue. Increased pigmentation has been noted with deposits of acid mucopolysaccharide surrounding the altered arterioles (37,38). Most of these patients had electrocardiographic evidence of the repolarization abnormalities described above prior to their demise. These lesions might have significantly affected the conduction system; however, a cause and effect has not yet been demonstrated, and deposition of lipofuscin-staining pigment can be observed in a wide variety of postmortems unrelated to phenothiazine ingestion.

Biochemical Mechanism

The biochemical mechanism responsible for these electrocardiographic alterations has not been elucidated. Phenothiazines can inhibit the adenosine triphosphate enzyme system required for cellular repolarization (16). Landmark (26) demonstrated the ability of phenothiazines to reduce potassium efflux from isolated rat cells accompanied by prolonged repolarization. The ability of phenothiazines to chelate calcium, magnesium, and zinc, ions essential for specific enzyme activity, may be an important factor. Urinary excretion of sodium and magnesium has been shown to increase following oral administration of thioridazine. Clinical studies of serum electrolytes in persons receiving phenothiazines, however, have shown no abnormalities.

Alterations in myocardial catecholamine concentration have also been suggested as an etiologic mechanism (39,40). Phenothiazines, through either a direct effect on the myocardial cell or their action on the autonomic nervous system, may sensitize the heart to a catecholamine effect with subsequent arrhythmia. The quinidine-like effect exerted by phenothiazines may also induce reentry arrhythmias if myocardial suppression occurs unevenly.

Treatment

The alterations in repolarization in persons on phenothiazines can be reversed by (a) overnight fasting, (b) the administration of oral potassium salts, even in the presence of normokalemia, and (c) propranolol (41). To determine the effect on the ECG of a glucose load, Chouinard and Annable (39) administered perphenazine, perphenazine and amitryptyline, and/or placebo to 54 persons. ECGs were obtained in a baseline state, after an overnight fast, and after a 600-calorie meal. Among the drug-treated patients, a statistically significant increase in repolarization abnormalities was noted after eating (32%), whereas no such increase was observed in the placebo group.

These findings suggest that the repolarization abnormalities observed may result from an alteration in intracellular/extracellular potassium ratio. In persons on phenothiazines exhibiting repolarization abnormalities, one of the above procedures may be utilized as a test to distinguish those changes secondary to organic heart disease. In addition, although the clinical relevance of these alterations remains to be determined, it might be helpful to obtain ECGs in both the fasting and postprandial state in patients with heart disease who are to be maintained on phenothiazine therapy.

Overdose Reactions

Treatment of phenothiazine overdose is mainly supportive and directed to therapy of cardiovascular complications, as these drugs are highly bound to plasma proteins. Although elimination by diuresis may be enhanced, conventional dialysis is usually ineffective because of plasma protein binding. Since the anticholinergic effects of phenothiazines result in a delayed gastric emptying time, gastric lavage, even a while after ingestion, may be effective in removing considerable amounts of the drug.

Neurologic complications, such as hypothermia and seizure activity, should be managed appropriately. Extrapyramidal symptoms can be diminished by use of antiparkinsonian medications. Since these agents also have anticholinergic effects, however, they should be used only when extrapyramidal signs are severe.

The presence of ventricular arrhythmias should be managed in a manner similar to quinidine-induced ventricular tachycardia. Lidocaine, which enhances conduction velocity in myocardial fibers, may be effective if reentrant excitation secondary to depressed conduction velocity is the precipitant cause of the arrhythmia. The successful use of lidocaine may result in an underlying sinus node dysfunction, such as sinus bradycardia or sinus arrest with a slow idioventricular response. In such cases, pacemaker insertion becomes mandatory (24).

Hypotension, if present, in the absence of an arrhythmia as a precipitating cause, may be treated with intravenous fluid administration. Too rapid replacement may result in precipitation of acute pulmonary edema and myocardial failure in the face of direct depressant effect of phenothiazines on the myocardium. Pressor agents, without significant beta receptor activity (norepinephrine, methoxamine), may also be used. Agents with primary beta activity (epinephrine) are contraindicated.

With adequate treatment, mortality in the absence of serious underlying disease should be low (42–44). Of 413 reported cases in the literature, there were 11 deaths (2.6%). Mortality rates in children may be somewhat higher.

Drug Interactions

The phenothiazines may induce the hepatic endoplasmic reticulum, affecting metabolism of other drugs detoxified by this system. The alpha-adrenergic blocking activity of the phenothiazines may also result in clinical drug interactions when administered with sympathomimetic agents (Table 2).

TABLE 2. *Selected drug interactions of phenothiazines*

Drug	Effect
Alcohol	Synergistic respiratory depressant effect
Alpha-methyldopa	Exacerbation of hypertension
Amphetamines	Decreased stimulant effect
Barbiturates	Decrease in phenothiazine half-life
Diphenylhydantoin	Enhanced antiarrhythmic effect
Guanidethine	Exacerbation of hypertension
Lithium	Potentiation of phenothiazine-induced hypoglycemia
Propranolol	Enhancement of hypotensive effect
Quinidine	Enhanced antiarrhythmic effect[a]
Sympathomimetics	Increase in plasma catecholamine levels[b]
Tricyclic antidepressants	Inhibition of tricyclic antidepressant metabolism

[a] With phenothiazine overdose may result in depression of myocardial contractility.

[b] Use with agents having both alpha and beta receptor activity, e.g., epinephrine, can enhance beta activity with resulting toxicity.

Mood-Altering Drugs

Combination with alcohol may result in a synergistic CNS depressant effect (45). Metabolism of the tricyclic antidepressants has been shown to be inhibited (46), whereas the use of barbiturates and phenothiazines is associated with an acceleration of phenothiazine metabolism owing to the more potent enzyme-inducing properties of barbiturates (47). Hyperglycemia, known to be associated with both lithium and chlorpromazine administration, might potentially be accentuated with concomitant use of these drugs (48). Concomitant use with amphetamines may interfere with amphetamine uptake into the adrenergic neuron, with a subsequent decreased effect (49).

Cardiac Medications

Use of phenothiazines with sympathomimetic drugs results in a dose-dependent increase in plasma norepinephrine and epinephrine levels. Concomitant use with agents having both alpha and beta receptor activity, such as epinephrine, might result in an unmasking of beta effects with resulting adverse reactions.

Antihypertensives that act through the adrenergic neuron, such as guanethidine and alpha-methyldopa, when administered concomitantly with phenothiazines, may be associated with an exacerbated hypertensive response that may be clinically important (50–52). Conversely, the use of phenothiazines and propranolol may be associated with an enhancement of propranolol-induced hypotension (48).

The use of quinidine or diphenylhydantoin in the presence of phenothiazines may also be associated with a potentiation of antiarrhymic action of either drug. As discussed above, the phenothiazines have a quinidine-like depressant action on the myocardium. Synergistic effects may occur with the combined administration of these agents. Quinidine is contraindicated as an antiarrhythmic in arrhythmias induced by phenothiazine overdose. An enhanced antiarrhythmic response could also conceivably occur with concomitant use of diphenylhydantoin through a phenothiazine inhibition of diphenylhydantoin metabolism (53). The clinical importance of this interaction has not been demonstrated.

RAUWOLFIA ALKALOIDS

The use of the rauwolfia alkaloids as major tranquilizers greatly diminished soon after their discovery with the appearance of the phenothiazines. Of the alkaloids, reserpine is in most frequent use as an antihypertensive rather than a tranquilizing agent. Clinically, after a transient, dose-dependent, sympathomimetic effect, reserpine depletes stores of catecholamine and 5-hydroxytryptamine in the heart and blood vessels, producing a slow fall in systemic blood pressure. The hypotensive action is more marked in hypertensive subjects and is usually accompanied by a bradycardia and a reduced cardiac output (54). Cardiovascular reflexes are only mildly depressed, although postural hypotension may occur. Toxic cardiovascular effects include marked hypotension, congestive heart failure secondary to salt and water retention, flushing, and bradycardia.

Drug Interactions

Reserpine-induced catecholamine depletion results in potential interactions whenever this agent is used with drugs acting on the autonomic nervous system. Accentuation of hypertension may occur with concomitant use with monoamine oxidase inhibitors, whereas a diminished response might occur with ephedrine and a potentiation of sympathetic blockade with propranolol (55). The early release of catecholamine secretion with reserpine could conceivably enhance arrhythmia formation in the patient prone to digitalis toxicity when these two agents are administered simultaneously (56). However, there is little documentation in the literature concerning the clinical importance of this interaction.

BUTYROPHENONES

Haloperidol, the prototype of the butyrophenones, is an effective alternative to the phenothiazines as an antipsychotic agent. It resembles the piperazine group of phenothiazines in its activity and is readily absorbed from the gastrointestinal tract, and concentrated in the liver, with excretion in bile and urine. Haloperidol can be detected in the body weeks following ingestion; therefore, its effects may be cumulative.

The clinical use of the butyrophenones has not been reported to be associated with any specific detrimental cardiovascular effects (57–58). However, tachycardia can occur, and transient hypotensive reactions have been reported. Gerl (59), in a survey of patients maintained on haloperidol, consistently found a small decrease in arterial blood pressure. The relative lack of adverse cardiovascular effects makes these agents most appropriate in patients maintained on an antihypertensive drug acting primarily on the autonomic nervous system.

Drug Interactions

Since haloperidol is metabolized in the liver, an interaction may occur with concomitant use of drugs similarly metabolized, such as oral anticoagulants. The clinical importance of these interactions remains to be defined.

THIOXANTHENES

The two thioxanthenes commonly used in psychiatric practice are thiothixene (Navane®), a piperazine phenothiazine analog, and chlorprothixene, the analog of chlorpromazine. The hemodynamic changes induced with therapeutic use of thiothixene in schizophrenic patients have been found to be minimal and of little clinical significance (57). The number of published studies, however is rather limited. The structural similarities of chlorprothixene with chlorpromazine should warrant caution in the use of this agent in persons with severe cardiovascular disease.

REFERENCES

1. Byck, R. (1975): Drugs and the treatment of psychiatric disorders. In: *The Pharmacological Basis of Therapeutics, 5th Edition,* edited by L. S. Goodman and A. Gilman, p. 163. Macmillan, New York.

2. Pletscher, A. (1967): A pharmacological and biochemical basis of some somatic side effects of psychotropic drugs. In: *Neuropsychopharmacology,* edited by H. Brill, pp. 551–577. Exerpta Medica, Amsterdam.
3. Ebert, M., and Shader, R. (1963): Cardiovascular effects of psychotropic drug side effects. In: *Chemical and Theoretical Perspectives,* edited by R. Shader and A. D. Masco, p. 152. Williams & Wilkins, Baltimore.
4. Alexander, C. S. (1968): Cardiotoxic effects of phenothiazines and related drugs. *Circulation,* 38:1014.
5. Shamsi, M. A., Kulshrestha, V. K., Dhawan, K. N., et al. (1971): Correlation of chemical structure of phenothiazines with their coronary dilator and antiarrhythmic activities. *Jpn. J. Pharmacol.,* 21:747.
6. Alexander, C. S., and Nino, A. (1969): Cardiovascular complications in young patients taking psychotropic drugs. *Am. Heart J.,* 78:757.
7. Robertson, D., and Michelakis, A. M. (1975): The effect of chlorpromazine on plasma renin activity and aldosterone in man. *J. Clin. Endocrinol. Metab.,* 41:1166.
8. Carlsson, C., Dencker, S. J., Grimby, G., et al. (1968): Circulatory studies during physical exercise in mentally disordered patients. I effects of large doses of chlorpromazine. *Acta Med. Scand.,* 184:499.
9. Sakalis, G., Curry, S. H., Mould, G. P., et al. (1972): Physiologic and clinical effects of chlorpromazine and their relationship to plasma level. *Clin. Pharmacol. Ther.,* 13:1931.
10. Swett, C., Cole, J. O., Hartz, S. C., et al. (1977): Hypotension due to chlorpromazine: Relation to cigarette smoking, blood pressure and dosage. *Arch. Gen. Psychiatry,* 34:661.
11. Boston Collaborative Drug Surveillance Program. Decreased clinical efficacy of propoxyphene in cigarette smokers. (1973) *Clin. Pharmacol. Ther.,* 14:259.
12. Kerri-Szanto, M., and Pomeron, J. R. (1971): Atmospheric pollution and pentazocine metabolism. *Lancet,* 1:947.
13. Boston Collaborative Drug Surveillance Program. (1973) Clinical depression of the central nervous system due to diazepam and chlordiazepoxide in relation to cigarette smoking and age. *N. Engl. J. Med.,* 288:277.
14. Stinson, E. B., Holloway, E. L., Derby, G., et al. (1975): Comparative hemodynamic responses to chlorpromazine, nitroprusside, nitroglyerin and trimethaphan immediately after open heart operations. *Circulation* [*Suppl.*], 51–52, I–26–33.
15. Grauaner, K. F., and Murphree, D. D. (1964): Electrocardiographic changes associated with thioridazine. *J. Neuropsychiatry,* 5:344.
16. Huston, J. R., and Bell, G. E. (1966): The effect of thioridazine hydrochloride and chlorpromazine on the electrocardiogram. *JAMA,* 198:134.
17. Backman, H., and Elosuo, R. (1968): The effect of nemoleptics on the electrocardiogram. *Acta Med. Scand.,* 183:543.
18. Ban, T. A., and St. Jean, A. (1975): Electrocardiographic changes induced by phenothiazine drugs. *Am. Heart J.,* 70:2575.
19. Dillenkoffer, R. C., Gallant, D. M., and Phillips, J. H. (1972): Electrocardiographic evaluation of mesoridazine (Serentil). *Curr. Ther. Res.,* 14:71.
20. Quitkm, F., Rifkin, A., and Klein, D. (1975): Very high dosage vs. standard dosage. Fluphenazine in schizophrenics. *Arch. Gen. Psychiatry,* 32:1276.
21. Fletcher, G. F., and Wenger, N. K. (1969): Cardiotoxic effects of mellaril: Conduction disturbances and supraventricular arrhythmias. *Am. Heart J.,* 78:135.
22. Levine, D. G., and Marshall, A. J. (1975) Cardiac arrhythmias induced by phenothiazine. *Lancet,* 3:990.
23. Desautels, S., Filteau, C., and St. Jean, A. (1964): Ventricular tachycardia associated with administration of thioridazine hydrochloride. *Can. Med. Assoc. J.,* 90: 1030.
24. Fowler, N. O., McCall, D., Chou, T., et al. (1976): Electrocardiographic changes and cardiac arrhythmias in patients receiving psychotropic drugs. *Am. J. Cardiol.,* 37:223.
25. Wolpert, A., and Farr, D. (1975): Psychotropics and their effect on the EKG in children. *Dis. Nerv. Syst.,* 36:435.
26. Landmark, K. H. (1970): Cardiac effects of phenothiazines. *Nord. Med.,* 83:617.

27. Holden, M., and Itil, T. (1977): Electrocardiographic changes with psychotropic drugs. In: *Stress and the Heart,* edited by D. Wheatley, pp. 87–96. Raven Press, New York.
28. Chouinard, G., Annable, L., Melamçon, J. et al. (1975): Chlorpromazine induced electrocardiogram abnormalities. *Int. J. Clin. Pharmacol.,* 11:327.
29. Wendkos, M. H. (1967): Cardiac changes related to phenothiazine therapy with special reference to thiordiazine. *J. Am. Geriatr. Soc.,* 15:20.
30. Leestma, J. E., and Koenig, K. L. (1968): Sudden death and phenothiazines. A current controversy. *Arch. Gen. Psychiatry,* 18:137.
31. Kelly, H. G., Fay, J. E., and Laverty, S. G. (1963): Thioridazine hydrochloride (Mellaril): Its effects on the ECG and a report of two fatalities with ECG abnormalities. *Can. Med. Assoc. J.,* 89:546.
32. Hollister, L. E., and Kosek, J. C. (1968): Sudden death and phenothiazines. *Arch. Gen. Psychiatry,* 8:137.
33. Peel, R., and Von Loetzen, I. S. (1973): Phenothiazine deaths, a critical review. *Am. J. Psychiatry,* 130:306.
34. Swett, C. P., and Shader, R. I. (1977): Cardiac side effects and sudden death in hospitalized psychiatric patients. *Dis. Nerv. Syst.,* 38:69.
35. Giles, T. D., and Modlin, R. K. (1968): Death associated with ventricular arrhythmia and thioridazine hydrochloride. *JAMA,* 205:108.
36. Schoonmaker, F. W., Osteen, R. T., and Greenfield, J. C. (1966): Thioridazine (Mellaril) induced ventricular tachycardia controlled with an artificial pacemaker. *Ann. Intern. Med.,* 65:1076.
37. Richardson, H. L., Graupner, K. I., and Richard, M. E. (1966): Intramyocardial lesions in patients dying suddenly and unexpectedly. *JAMA,* 195:254.
38. Alexander, S., Shader, R., and Grinspoon, L. (1967): Electrocardiographic effects of thioridazine hydrochloride (Mellaril). *Lahey Clinic Found Bull.,* 16:207.
39. Chouinard, G., and Annable, L. (1977): Phenothiazine induced ECG abnormalities. *Arch. Gen. Psychiatry,* 34:951.
40. Giles, T. D., and Modlin, R. K. (1968): Death associated with ventricular arrhythmias and thioridazine hydrochloride. *JAMA,* 205:108.
41. Alvarez-Mena, S. C., and Frank, M. J. (1973): Phenothiazine induced T wave abnormalities. Effects of overnight fasting. *JAMA,* 224:1730.
42. Donlon, P. T., and Tupin, J. P. (1977): Successful suicides with Thioridazine and Mesoridazine. *Arch. Gen. Psychiatry,* 34:955.
43. Davis, J. N., Bartlett, E., and Termini, B. A. (1968): Overdosage of psychotropic drugs: A review. *Dis. Nerv. Syst.,* 29:157.
44. Joubert, P. H., and Oliver, J. A. (1974): Fatal suicidal ingestion of thioridazine. *Clin. Toxicol.* [*Suppl.*], 7:133.
45. Milner, G., and Landaver, A. A. (1971): Alcohol, thioridazine and chlorpromazine effects on skills related to driving behavior. *Br. J. Psychiatry,* 118:351.
46. Gram, L. F., and Overo, K. F. (1972): Drug interaction: Inhibitory effects of neuroleptics on metabolism of tricyclic antidepressants in man. *Br. Med. J.,* 1:463.
47. Curry, S. H. (1970): Factors effecting chlorpromazine plasma levels in psychiatric patients. *Arch. Gen. Psychiatry,* 22:209.
48. Hansten, P. D. (1976): *Drug Interactions: Third Edition.* Lea & Febiger, Philadelphia.
49. Espelin, D. E., and Done, A. K. (1968): Amphetamine poisoning: Effectiveness of chlorpromazine. *N. Engl. J. Med.,* 278:1361.
50. Westervelt, F. B., and Atuk, N. O. (1974): Methyldopa induced hypertension. *JAMA,* 227:557.
51. FDA Reports of Suspected Adverse Reactions to Drugs (1970): No. 700201–058–00101.
52. Fann, W. E. (1971): Chlorpromazine reversal of antihypertensive action of quanethedine. *Lancet,* 2:436.
53. Kutt, H., and Verebely, K. (1970): Metabolism of diphenylhydantoin by rat liver microsomes I. Characteristics of the reaction. *Biochem. Pharmacol.,* 19:675.
54. Cohen, S. I., Young, M. W., Lau, S. H., et al. (1968): Effect of reserpine therapy

on cardiac output and atrioventricular conduction during rest and controlled heart rates in patients with essential hypertension. *Circulation,* 37:738.
55. Hansten, P. D. (1976): In: *Drug Interactions: Third Edition,* pp. 17,80,81. Lea & Febiger, Philadelphia.
56. Dick, H., McCawley, E. J., and Fisher, W. A. (1962): Reserpine-digitalis toxicity. *Arch. Intern. Med.,* 109:503.
57. Carlsson, C., Dencker, S. J., Grimby, G., et al. (1976): Hemodynamic effects of thiothixene and chlorpromazine in schizophrenic patients at rest and during exercise. *Int. J. Clin. Pharmacol.,* 13:262.
58. Aman, M. G., and Werry, J. S. (1975): The effect of methylphenidate and haloperidol on the heart rate and blood pressure of hyperactive children with special reference to time of action. *Psychopharmacologica,* 43:163.
59. Gerl, B. (1974): Clinical observations of the side effects of haloperidol. *Acta Psychiatr. Scand.,* 40:60.
60. Stimmel, B. (1975): The effects of mood altering drugs on the heart. In: *Current Cardiovascular Topics. Vol. 1: Drugs in Cardiology,* edited by E. Donoso, pp. 212–213. Stratton Intercontinental, New York.

Chapter 8

Drugs Used for Affective Disorders

TRICYCLIC ANTIDEPRESSANTS

The tricyclics (Table 1) are widely used for the treatment of depressive states. Their effectiveness is reflected by the observation that in 1973, American physicians wrote more than 24 million prescriptions for these agents alone or in combination with other drugs (1). Other countries have experienced a similar increase in use, with the incidence of toxicity due to self-poisoning consistently increasing. As an example, in Scotland in 1965, 1% of all suicide attempts involved tricyclic overdose. This figure rose to 7% in 1967 and more than 10% in 1973 (2).

Pharmacology

Imipramine, synthesized in 1948 by Hafliger, is the prototype of the tricyclics. It is a dibenzazepine differing structurally from the phenothiazines

TABLE 1. *Drugs used for affective disorders*

Generic name	Trade name
Tricyclic antidepressants	
Amitriptyline	Elavil, Endep
Desipramine	Norpramin, Pertofrane
Doxepin	Adepin, Sinequan
Imipramine	Imavate, Janimine, Presamine, SK Pramine, Tofranil
Nortriptyline	Aventyl, Pamelor
Protriptyline	Vivactil
Amitriptyline and perphenazine	Triavil, Etrafon
Lithium salts	Eskalith, Lithane, Lithonate, Lithotabs
MAO inhibitors	
Phenelzine	Nardil
Isocarboxazid	Marplan
Tranylcypromine	Parnate

by replacement of the sulfur with a methylene linkage. Generically, the term tricyclics is applied to all agents in this group because of the general structure of these drugs, which consist of a linkage of two benzene rings to form a third central ring.

Mechanism of Action

The mechanism of action of the tricyclics is complex. Their basic effect is to prevent the reuptake of serotonin and norepinephrine (NE) at adrenergic neurons, thereby raising the concentration of NE at the receptors. This activity is selective for adrenergic nerve terminals with little or no effect being noted at dopamine receptors (3). Since this action is of great importance in understanding not only the effects of tricyclics on the cardiovascular system but also the mechanism by which interaction with other drugs occurs, a brief review of the function of the adrenergic neuron is appropriate (4).

NE is synthesized within the granule of the nerve terminal through the conversion of tyrosine to dihydroxyphenalanine (dopa) and then to dopamine (Fig. 1). Synthesis of dopa and dopamine occurs within the cell cytoplasm. Dopamine subsequently enters storage vesicles and is converted to NE. NE is discharged to the exterior by initiation of the nerve action potential, which may occur either spontaneously or after administration of sympathomimetic drugs. Following NE release and subsequent combination at the alpha or beta adrenoceptor sites of the effector cells, excess NE either reenters the nerve terminal where it may be metabolized by monoamine oxidase (MAO) or is metabolized extracellularly by catechol-O-methyltransferase (COMT). NE that is not metabolized is stored in vesicles until subsequent release. Compounds with similar structures are also taken up into the vesicle through this system. Noncatechol sympathomimetic amines exert a pharmacologic effect partially through a direct action on adrenergic receptors and partially through an indirect effect, resulting in a release of NE from the storage granules. Drugs exerting a predominantly indirect effect enter the adrenergic neuron by the same uptake mechanism (5).

The tricyclics prevent the reuptake of NE, thereby potentiating the normal response of NE as a neurotransmitter simulating the effects of excessive exogenous NE. This adrenergic potentiation can be eliminated or even reversed when high doses of tricyclics are administered (6,7). In addition, when tricyclics are administered concomitantly with indirect-acting sympathomimetic agents, uptake of these drugs is prevented, resulting in an antagonism of the intended drug action (8,9). The effects of direct-acting agents, however, are enhanced by tricyclics as the increased concentration of NE at the receptor site would be associated with a diminished NE uptake.

The tricyclics have also been demonstrated to have an anticholinergic effect when administered in moderate or large doses, manifested by a diminished response to acetylcholine-induced bradycardia in dogs and cats

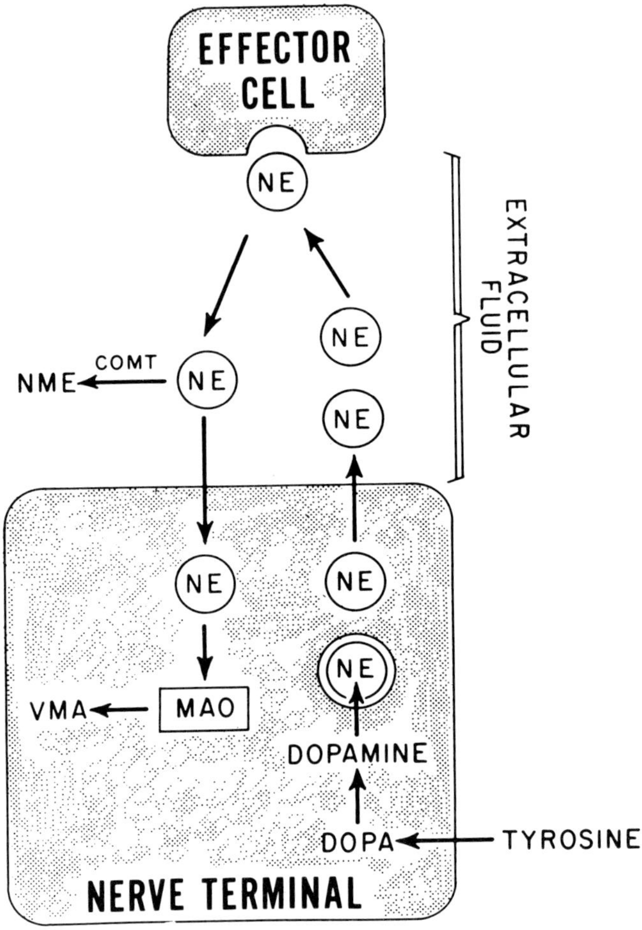

FIG. 1. Synthesis, uptake, and metabolism of norepinephrine (NE). NE is synthesized within the nerve terminal from tyrosine through formation of dopa and dopamine. It is then stored in granules until released by incoming nerve impulses. The NE released in the extracellular fluid may attach to adrenergic receptors on effector cells or diffuse into the circulation. NE stores in the nerve terminal are replenished by biosynthesis and the amine transport system of the axonal membrane. Degradation of NE occurs through catechol-O-methyl transferase (COMT) and monoamine oxidase (MAO).

(10,11). Smaller doses may potentiate acetylcholine-induced hypotension through either a central action or an inhibition of acetylcholine hydrolysis (12,13). At higher dosages, depression of myocardial contractility and heart rate are frequent.

Absorption and Biotransformation

The tricyclics are quickly absorbed from the gastrointestinal tract after oral administration. Imipramine is rapidly distributed and metabolized by N-demethylation to form desmethylimipramine (DMI). Both imipramine and

DMI are fat soluble and readily cross the blood-brain barrier. DMI undergoes subsequent hydroxylation with O-glucuronidation. N-oxidation also occurs to a variable degree.

Protein binding is considerable, with more than 90% of amitryptyline and its active metabolite nortriptyline present in plasma in the bound state. Since metabolism occurs primarily in the liver, plasma levels can be increased by concomitant administration of drugs that inhibit the hepatic enzyme systems. Clinically, there is also a genetically determined individual variation in steady state plasma concentrations of tricyclics after single dose administration. A standard dose of 150 mg amitriptyline can result in an interpatient variation of up to 30-fold in steady state plasma concentration. A significant, positive correlation between plasma concentration of either amitriptyline or its active metabolite and the therapeutic response has been reported but not consistently confirmed (12).

Although a long latency of onset of action exists, with therapeutic effects not evident until several weeks of therapy, excretion is relatively rapid. Forty percent of a radioactive dose of imipramine appears in the urine within 24 hr, with 70% excreted within 72 hr. Fecal excretion accounts for a small portion of eliminated imipramine (13).

Hemodynamic Effects

Laboratory Studies

Jefferson (14), in an excellent review of hemodynamic effects of tricyclics on laboratory animals, noted small doses to be associated with an increase in blood pressure, heart rate, cardiac contractility, and coronary blood flow. Higher doses had reverse effects. Intravenous administration in dogs, rats, and guinea pigs results in a decrease in the maximal rise of left ventricular pressure and a reduced cardiac output (15). Blood pressure is usually maintained through a compensatory increase in peripheral vascular resistance. Administration of high dose tricyclic metabolites may also have a markedly adverse effect, with infusion of 5 mg/kg hydroxyimipramine associated with cardiac arrest.

The response to interactions between sympathomimetics and tricyclics in laboratory animals varies not only with tricyclic dosage but also with the specific sympathomimetic amine. A dual dose-related effect exists with NE and epinephrine. Little if any positive response occurs with isoproterenol, and an antagonist or inhibitory effect is seen with those amines having a predominantly indirect action on the adrenergic neuron.

Clinical Studies

Clinically, the use of tricyclics has been associated with tachycardia and alterations in blood pressure that vary with the specific tricyclic, age of the subject, time of measurement, and the presence of preexisting cardiac disease

(Table 2). Administration of therapeutic doses of tricyclics to depressed subjects without evidence of cardiac disease showed the heart rate to increase, with minimal changes in blood pressure. No relationship was demonstrated between plasma levels of nortriptyline and resulting tachycardia (17). Freyschuss et al. (18) were also unable to demonstrate significant orthostatic changes with nortriptyline in healthy young adults 3 weeks after initiating therapy.

The direct effect of amitryptyline on the arterial system has been studied by Thorstrand and Lindblad (19). Intraarterial administration of amitriptyline in the forearm of healthy volunteers at rates varying from 0.05 to 0.20 mg/min resulted in a dose-dependent increase in blood flow in the ipsilateral forearm to a maximum of 73% when the infusion exceeded 0.10 mg/min. No changes were noted in heart rate, blood pressure, or blood flow in the contralateral arm. These findings suggest a peripheral dilatory effect on resistance vessels at high dose levels, possibly through blockage of alpha-mediated constrictor tone or through a direct myogenic action. The peripheral action of high dose tricyclic in inducing vasodilation may be of clinical importance in the hyperkinetic vasodilatory state seen with tricyclic poisoning.

The administration of tricyclics to geriatric patients, especially those with preexisting cardiovascular disease, is associated with clinically important orthostatic hypotension. Muller et al. (20), comparing hypotensive changes in 82 patients with ($N = 41$) and without ($N = 41$) cardiac disease, found postural hypotension to be severe in 24%, moderate in 14%, and mild in 37% of persons with cardiovascular disease. On those without cardiac disease, none had severe, 7% had moderate, and 29% had mild orthostatic changes. Kantor et al. (21), in a study of seven persons with a history of cardiovascular disease given therapeutic doses of imipramine, noted significant, sustained orthostatic changes to develop in all. Although subjective complaints associated with hypotension, such as dizziness and lightheadedness, improved with time, the hypotension did not resolve during a 5-week period.

TABLE 2. *Clinical responses to tricyclic antidepressants in selected population groups*

Parameter	Healthy persons	Cardiac disease	Geriatric populations
Blood pressure	↓/NC	↓	↓
Heart rate	↑	↑	↑
Electrocardiogram			
Repolarization alterations	+	+	+
HV interval	↑	↑	NM
AH interval	NC	NC	NM
Arrhythmias	±	+	NM

NC, no change; NM, not specifically measured; ↑, increase; ↓, decrease; +, present.

The degree of hypotension is dependent on the specific tricyclic administered. Doxepin has been associated with a lower incidence of hypotension (2.6%) and tachycardia (2.9%) than amitriptyline (8.6% and 30%, respectively) (22). Both agents are less likely to produce orthostatic changes than imipramine. Maprotiline (Ludiomil®), a tetracyclic, is associated with the least hemodynamic effects. Controlled studies with randomization of tricyclic therapy, however, have yet to be performed. Existing evidence regarding the efficacy of one agent over the other in the elderly and/or cardiac patient remains inconclusive.

The mechanisms involved in the production of orthostatic hypotension have not been clearly defined. Current hypotheses include: (a) a decrease in myocardial contractility (23,24), (b) an interference of central adrenergic reuptake of NE with a paradoxical hypotensive response (25), (c) a potentiation of the cholinergic effects seen at low dose tricyclic therapy, and (d) a local vasodilatory effect on the constrictor arterioles. It should also be noted that hypertension secondary to tricyclic administration has occasionally been reported in the literature; in the absence of concomitant administration of a sympathomimetic drug, however, such reactions are rather unusual.

Other hemodynamic complications in patients with cardiac disease include congestive heart failure and myocardial infarction (20,25–28). In most instances, these events have been associated with tricyclic poisoning rather than appropriate clinical use.

Effects on Rhythm and Conduction

Animal Studies

The cardiotoxic effects of these agents were first described in 1963 by Sigg et al. (7). Bradycardia and an increase in ventricular contractility occurring at low infusion rates could be reversed when the infusion rates exceeded 1 mg/kg. Nortriptyline infusion in guinea pigs has been associated with alteration in repolarization and intraventricular conduction and the appearance of right axis deviation, arrhythmias, and variable degrees of A-V block (29).

Imipramine and the metabolites DMI, 2-hydroxyimipramine (OH-IMI), and 2-hydroxy-DMI (OH-DMI) have been shown to be cardiotoxic in dogs at doses considered to be therapeutic (30). Serious arrhythmias in animals, however, are usually produced by intravenous infusions, resulting in concentrations considerably in excess of those seen clinically. The magnitude of these changes is dose related (28–30). The basal hemodynamic state of the animal has also been demonstrated to be of importance. Dogs made hypertensive have exhibited electrocardiographic changes at lower doses of imipramine than control animals (31). The combined effects of stress and tricyclics in inducing ventricular fibrillation in cardiomyopathic rats has been discussed in Chapter 3.

Mechanism of Action

The mechanisms of the electrocardiographic changes remain to be clearly defined. The anticholinergic activity of the tricyclics may result in an atropine-like effect on cardiac conduction. These agents have been demonstrated to have an affinity for rabbit and rodent cardiac muscle (32,33). In the isolated rabbit heart, neuronal uptake of exogenous NE is inhibited, and in the presence of NE infusion, ventricular arrhythmias are frequent (34). Lidocaine, diphenylhydantoin, or quinidine have little effect on the arrhythmic activity. Propranolol is an effective inhibitor, emphasizing the prominence of an adrenergic mechanism. The potency of the individual tricyclics in inhibiting NE uptake varies with doxepin > amitryptyline > nortriptyline > protriptyline (34).

Recently, imipramine has been shown to have a direct effect on cardiac Purkinje fibers unrelated to its general effects on the autonomic system (35, 36). Intracellular imipramine injection results in a decrease in dpdt action potential duration and conduction velocity. These actions demonstrate both a similarity to the actions of quinidine and distinct differences with respect to duration of the action potential and may be responsible for the electrocardiographic changes observed clinically.

Production of arrhythmias may be related to interference with ionic transport through cell membranes. In isolated animal heart tissue, imipramine has been shown to cause changes in transmembrane potential as well as a dose-dependent decrease in potassium ion flux (37–39). Imipramine inhibition of enzymes involved in cellular transport has been reported (31). The clinical relevance of these findings is unknown, as imipramine-induced electrocardiographic changes have not been found to be clinically correlated with either plasma potassium or levels of potassium excretion (40).

Electrocardiographic alterations may also develop as a result of interactions of the tricyclics with other agents. Experimental A-V block is associated with an increased toxicity of digoxin in the stressed rat pretreated with large doses of tricyclics (41). Toxic levels of tricyclics may also accumulate in the presence of administration of another drug that acts as a competitive metabolic inhibitor.

The data concerning the mechanism of action, however, have all been derived from animal models. Since considerable interspecies variation exists with respect to tricyclic metabolism, extrapolation to humans must be performed cautiously.

Clinical Studies

Healthy Subjects

Cardiovascular effects secondary to the clinical use of these agents have been described in the literature in patients taking therapeutic as well as toxic doses. Asymptomatic electrocardiographic changes consisting of prolongation of the QT interval, widening of QRS complexes, and ST- and T-wave changes, are similar to those seen with the phenothiazines (41–44) and have been noted in up to 20% of persons (Table 2) (Figs. 2 and 3). T-wave changes may occur at therapeutic serum levels, and prolonged PR and QRS intervals may occur. Even in patients without known cardiac disease, these changes may be followed by conduction disturbances or arrhythmias of clinical importance.

Effects on cardiac conduction have been studied. Tricyclics lengthen the PR interval through prolongation of the H-V interval. The A-H nodal conduction system remains relatively unchanged, even in the presence of tricyclic-induced A-V heart block. Widening of the QRS is secondary to a marked slowing of conduction in the ventricle rather than nodal system dysfunction (36,45).

Boakes et al. (46) have precipitated arrhythmias in healthy volunteers administered imipramine for 5 days. However, Moir (47) and co-workers

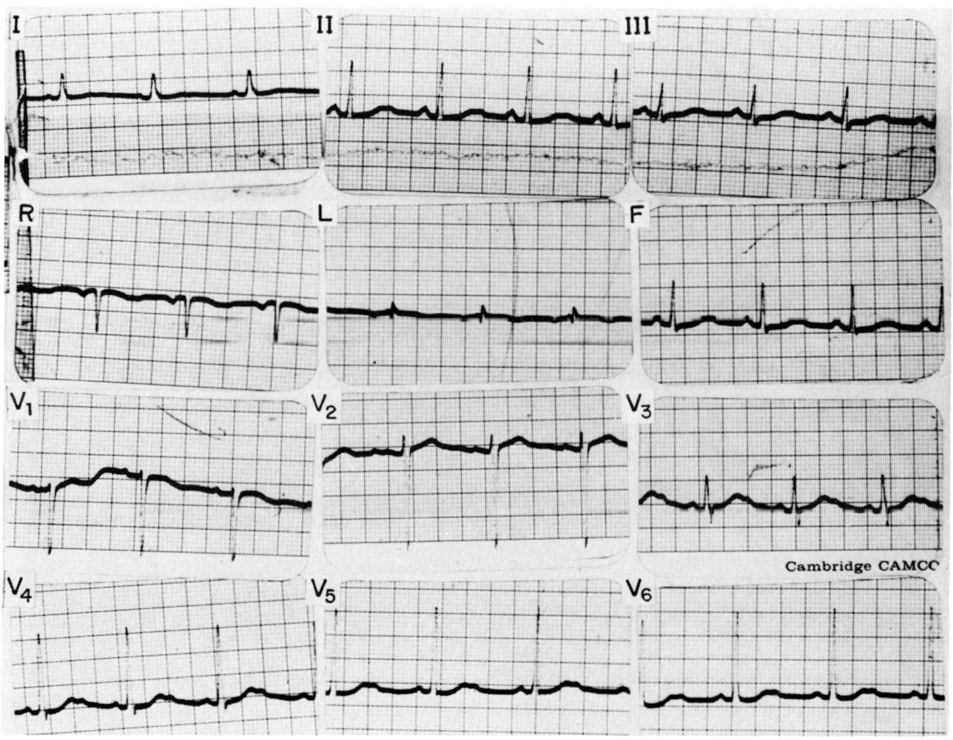

FIG. 2. ECG of an asymptomatic 20-year-old woman taking 100 mg/day amitryptyline. Note ST segment depression in leads II, III, avF. Prominent U-wave exists in V3-V5 and QTc is prolonged. (Reprinted from Stimmel, ref. 128.)

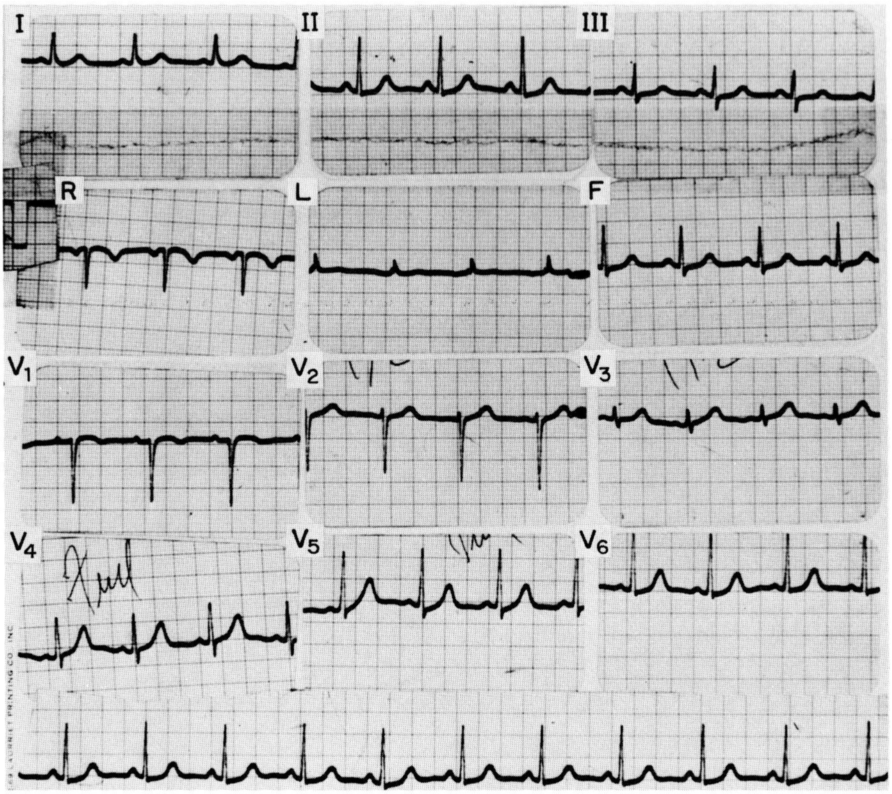

FIG. 3. ECG of the woman in Fig. 2 24 hr after discontinuing amitryptyline. T-wave morphology is normal; U-waves are no longer present. (Reprinted from Stimmel, ref. 128.)

were unable to demonstrate an increased incidence of arrhythmias in patients on tricyclics undergoing electroconvulsive therapy as compared to a group of subjects not taking these medications. Furthermore, as discussed below, it has been suggested that imipramine may actually have value as an anti-arrhythmic agent.

Most of these studies have not been associated with simultaneous measurements of tricyclic plasma levels. Since steady state plasma levels vary greatly on an individual basis, and serum levels are not always reflective of the oral dose, measurement of plasma levels becomes of considerable importance. Zeigler et al. (11), in a study of young, healthy subjects given nortriptyline, found plasma concentrations within a therapeutic range to be unassociated with any conduction disturbances. Similar findings were reported by Freyschuss et al. (18).

Other investigators have noted electrocardiographic alterations (26). Kristiansen (27) demonstrated electrocardiographic changes in subjects given antidepressants and then subjected to physical exercise. Kantor et al. (48) described a longitudinal study of a 74-year-old man with asymptomatic right bundle branch block in whom 2:1 A-V block developed while on imipramine. The A-V block appeared at a plasma level of imipramine within the therapeutic range. Both the clinical response of the drug and the cardiac effect were noted at the same plasma level, disappearing when therapy was discontinued. In addition, the rate of disappearance and clinical relapse of the depression were compatible with the known half-life of imipramine. Other individual case reports have also been published documenting the ability of tricyclics to cause conduction delays in individuals presumably free of clinical cardiac disease (49–51).

In an attempt to better elucidate the cardiovascular effects of these agents in the absence of obvious cardiac disease, Burckhardt et al. (52) carried out a prospective study in 143 patients receiving treatment with either tricyclic or tetracyclic antidepressants. Although no alterations in orthostatic regulation of blood pressure between control and treatment periods were observed, changes in the electrocardiogram (ECG) and systolic time intervals (STI) did occur. Significant increases in heart rate, PR interval, and T-wave amplitude ($p < 0.05$) were noted. Prolongations of QTc interval and QRS duration also occurred but did not reach statistical significance. With prolonged treatment, all these alterations, with the exception of heart rate, reverted toward control values. Measurements of STI revealed a significant prolongation of preejection period (PEP) and PEP/left ventricular ejection time ratio ($p < 0.005$) during the period of administration, indicating a depression of myocardial contractility. These changes reverted to normal upon discontinuation of therapy.

Plasma levels of tricyclic antidepressants above the therapeutic range are frequently associated with electrocardiographic changes. Vohra et al. (17, 53) administered nortriptyline or doxepin to subjects free of heart disease. Increases in PR interval and QTc intervals were noted in patients on nortriptyline but not in those taking doxepin. Burrows et al. (54) also found nortriptyline but not doxepin to produce significant prolongation of the QRS. In both these studies, plasma levels of nortriptyline were in excess of therapeutic levels, whereas plasma levels of doxepin were either not determined or found to be below the therapeutic window.

Persons With Cardiac Disease

The importance of the cardiac effects of the tricyclics received new emphasis when Coull (55) noted an association with sudden death and ingestion of these drugs. Six of 53 patients with cardiac disease died suddenly after administration of amitryptyline (Elavil®) as compared with none in 53 control patients matched for age, sex, and diagnosis. Sudden death was not reported in either persons receiving imipramine (Tofranil®) or noncardiac patients on amitryptyline. This finding was not confirmed by a subsequent study by the Boston Collaborative Drug Surveillance Program (56). Moir et al. (41), however, subsequently demonstrated 13 unexpected deaths in 119 patients with cardiac disease receiving amitryptyline as compared to three deaths in a carefully matched control group. The prognosis of both groups after discharge revealed subsequent mortality rates in both the original test and control groups to be quite similar, suggesting that amitryptyline may have indeed precipitated inevitable sudden death by months or years (47).

The reasons for the discrepant findings are not readily apparent but may be related to the characteristics of the groups studied. Jicks in the Boston survey (56) included all persons with cardiovascular disease without distinguishing between those receiving amitryptyline and those receiving other tricyclic antidepressants. In Moir's study, only those patients with cardiac disease taking amitryptyline were included.

In an attempt to more closely monitor the effects of imipramine in elderly patients with cardiac disease, Kantor et al. (21) studied the effects of this drug on seven depressed patients, six of whom had electrocardiographic abnormalities and four of whom had hypertensive or ischemic heart disease prior to initiation of therapy. The patients were monitored for 1 week under the control settings and then started on doses of imipramine of 3.5 mg/kg/day adjusted upward, as indicated, to obtain therapeutic plasma concentrations. A clinical effect with respect to recovery from depression was noted in all patients. Mean heart rate increased slightly, but this was of questionable clinical importance. Clinically significant intraventricular conduction delays appeared in all patients.

Hemodynamic effects of imipramine were assessed in 12 patients with coronary heart disease by Biamino et al. (57) through measurement of left ventricular, arterial, and pulmonary pressures. Left ventricular end-diastolic pressure (LVEDP) was found to significantly increase 30 min after injection of 25 mg imipramine, associated with an increase in peripheral resistance and mean arterial blood pressure. An augmentation of stroke work index and stroke volume index was also observed. These findings suggest a negative inotropic effect which, when combined with an increase in catecholamine levels, may present a risk to patients with cardiac disease predisposed to congestive heart failure.

Finally, it should be noted that although the presence of ventricular or atrial arrhythmias may warrant cautious use of the tricyclics, it has been suggested that imipramine, when administered in therapeutic doses, may in fact have a beneficial suppressive effect in patients with atrial and ventricular premature contractions. Since the tricyclics prolong both intraventricular conduction and repolarization, their action is similar to quinidine and pronestyl. In one study, which included 11 persons with more than 10 ventricular premature contractions per hour, imipramine administered at a dose of 3.5 mg/

kg/day was associated with a 75% or greater reduction in ventricular premature contractions in 10 patients (45). These findings have not yet been confirmed by other investigators; further studies are needed before routine use of imipramine in patients with underlying arrhythmias can be recommended. Persons receiving tricyclics in whom ventricular premature contractions requiring treatment are present should not be treated with quinidine or pronestyl, as the drug interaction might be hazardous.

Summary

In view of the known effects of the tricyclics on cardiac conduction, the use in persons with known cardiac disease should be carefully considered. Evidence has recently been presented suggesting that persons with coronary heart disease succumbing to ventricular fibrillation or sudden death have QTc intervals significantly longer than either controls or those persons with a myocardial infarction uncomplicated by ventricular fibrillation (57a,57b). Among one group of 55 persons surviving a myocardial infarction, the QTc interval was prolonged in 2% of control subjects, 18% of survivors, and 57% of persons who succumbed to sudden death ($p < 0.01$). Since QTc prolongation frequently accompanied tricyclic antidepressant use, these agents should be avoided in those persons who already have prolonged QTc following myocardial infarction. If antidepressant therapy is indicated, the use of tricyclics other than amitryptyline is probably prudent. In the presence of bundle branch block, serious thought should be given to the real need for these agents. If treatment is essential, preliminary evidence suggests that doxepin is preferable. Close observation with frequent electrocardiographic monitoring, however, is mandatory, regardless of the agent prescribed. Measurement of plasma levels to maintain a level less than 200 mg/ml may also be helpful in preventing further electrocardiographic alterations.

Overdose Reactions

Tricyclic poisoning or overdose, although not as prevalent as that seen with other mood-altering drugs, is nonetheless not infrequent. Overdoses are of particular concern in children, who appear to be more susceptible to toxicity. This is related to children exhibiting (a) a lesser percentage of protein-bound drug, (b) higher rates of hepatic biotransformation, and (c) a greater lean body mass than adults. This last factor is associated with relatively less drug being taken up by fatty tissues and more being available to reach the brain (58–60). The importance of an awareness of the increased susceptibility of children to these agents is emphasized by the finding that in the United Kingdom imipramine is the second most common cause of self-induced poisoning among children.

Manifestations

In instances of tricyclic overdose, hypotension and tachycardia are frequently observed (Table 3) (61). These findings may be accompanied by impaired cardiac conduction manifested by repolarization abnormalities, prolongation of the PR interval, widening of the QRS complex, bundle branch blocks, complete heart block, supraventricular and ventricular arrhythmias, and bradycardia and asystole (48,62,63) (Figs. 4 and 5). Elevations of serum enzymes associated with myocardial damage and congestive heart failure have also been reported.

Thorstrand (64) reviewed 153 consecutive patients admitted with tricyclic antidepressant poisoning over a 4-year period. The most common drug ingested was amitryptyline, taken as the sole agent in 41 cases and combined

TABLE 3. *Manifestations of tricyclic antidepressant overdose*

Hypotension
Electrocardiographic alterations
Repolarization alterations
Widening of QRS
Heart block
Arrhythmias
Sinus tachycardia
Ventricular tachycardia
Bradycardia and heart block
Congestive heart failure

with other drugs in 71 cases. The most characteristic electrocardiographic finding, beside an increased heart rate (noted in 73%), was a widening of the QRS complex, greater than 0.11 sec in 42%. Prolongations of the PQ interval were noted in 28% and QT interval in 49%. Despite the presence of decreased intraventricular conduction, there was evidence in some patients of a hyperkinetic circulation. This finding may be related to the presence of increased adrenergic stimulation or peripheral vasodilation, both common effects of tricyclic antidepressants. Hypotension was seen frequently (26%), being inversely correlated with dose. In those persons ingesting large doses, signs of myocardial depression were evident. Mortality rate was 3%.

Treatment

Treatment of cardiac toxicity or actual overdose is mainly supportive since tissue and protein binding do not allow for effective peritoneal or extracorporeal dialysis (Table 4). Diuretic agents are relatively ineffective because of a low renal excretory rate of the drug (65–68). If intervention oc-

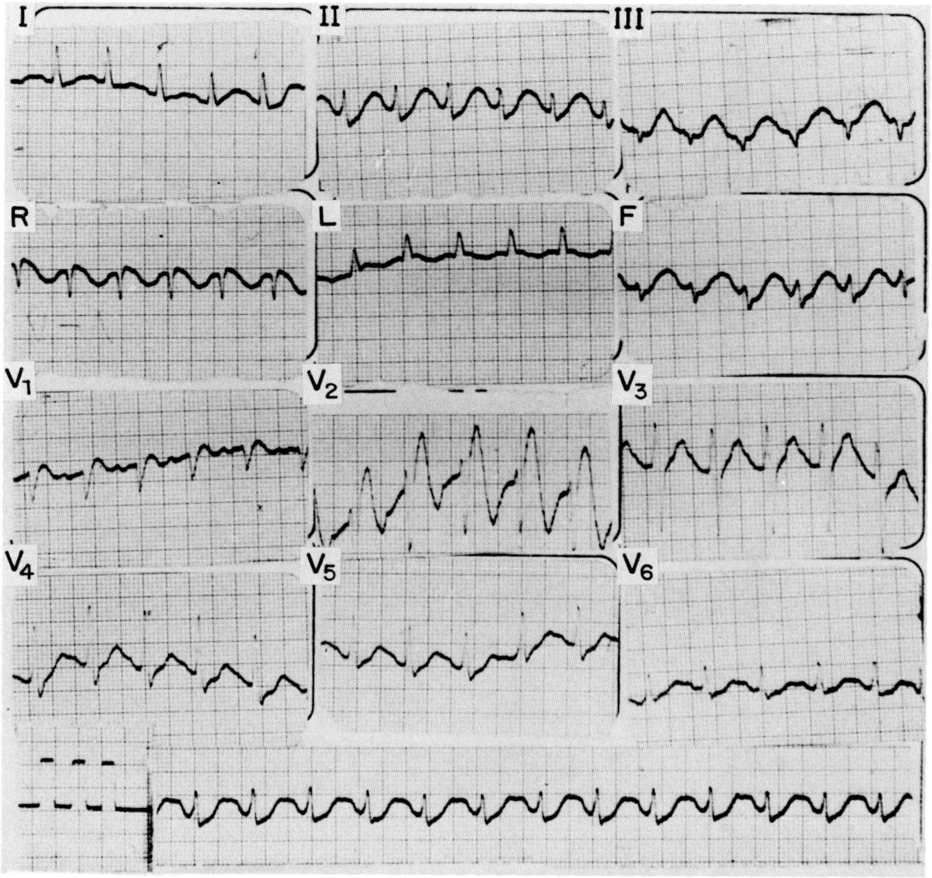

FIG. 4. ECG of a 50-year-old woman who ingested 500 mg amitryptyline in a suicide attempt. Sinus tachycardia at 136 per/min with a right bundle branch block is present. T-waves are broad, merging with the p-waves in all leads. (Reprinted from Stimmel, ref. 128.)

curs early, minimization of absorption by induced emesis with syrup of ipecac and/or administration of activated charcoal may be useful. Evidence has been presented indicating the ability of activated charcoal, when given 30 min after a 75-mg dose of nortriptyline, to lower peak plasma levels by 60%, with multiple doses producing a 70% mean reduction in peak levels. *In vitro* studies have demonstrated that a 10-g packet of a commercial preparation containing 5 g activated charcoal can absorb 3 g nortriptyline, a dose rarely exceeded in overdose reactions (69). Saline cathartics may also facilitate fecal elimination.

It should be emphasized that the half-lives of the tricyclics are quite long, with plasma levels remaining elevated for several days. Sudden deterioration in clinical state may occur, and patients should be closely monitored in the

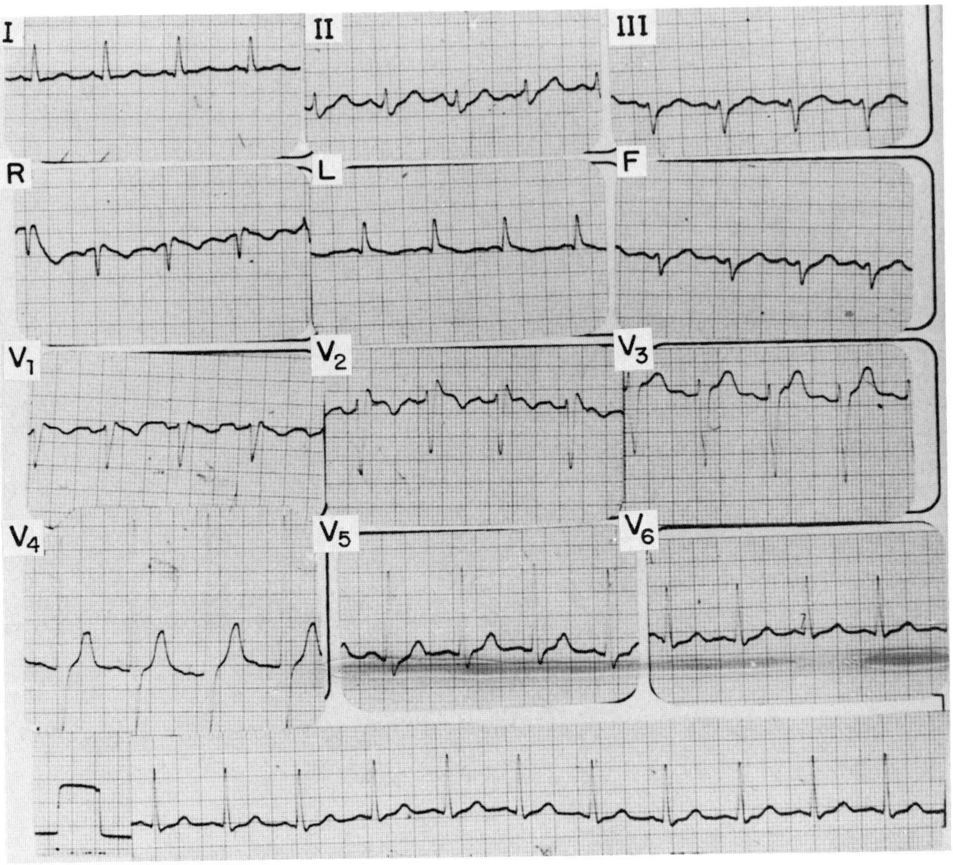

FIG. 5. ECG of woman in Fig. 4 taken 34 hr after amitryptyline ingestion. T-wave morphology has reverted to normal. (Reprinted from Stimmel, ref. 128.)

TABLE 4. *Principles of treating tricyclic antidepressant overdose*

Hasten elimination of agent[a]
Emesis
Activated charcoal
Saline cathartics
Prolonged cardiac monitoring
Treatment of serious arrhythmias[b]
Pharmacologic therapy[c]
Sodium bicarbonate
Physostigmine

[a] In an alert patient.

[b] Type 1 antiarrhythmic agents contraindicated. See text.

[c] Only in cases that cannot be treated adequately by general supportive measures.

intensive care unit for several days in instances of severe overdose (ingested dose greater than 1 g), even in the absence of initial cardiac findings.

Value of Plasma Levels of Tricyclics

Spiker and Biggs (70), in a study of serious tricyclic overdose (plasma levels greater than 1,000 ng/ml), found the half-life to range from 25.3 to 81.4 hr. The only reliable clinical correlate of severe overdose was the duration of the QRS interval. All persons having plasma levels of tricyclics of 1,000 ng/ml or more had a QRS interval of 100 msec or greater, with the plasma levels exhibiting a good correlation with QRS duration. In a subsequent series of 40 patients hospitalized with tricyclic overdose, these authors demonstrated that although a correlation also existed between the amount of drug ingested and the measured plasma level ($p < 0.001$), individual inconsistencies made this information of little clinical use. Plasma levels, however, were of great help. Tricyclic plasma levels of 1,000 ng/ml or more were associated with a significantly greater frequency of need for respiratory support, development of unconsciousness, seizures, presence of ventricular rate greater than 120/min, cardiac arrhythmias, QRS duration 0.1 sec or more, and episodes of cardiac arrest. Several measurements of plasma tricyclic levels revealed a direct relationship between decreasing levels and narrowing of the QRS. Only one-third of patients admitted were found to have severe overdose. Although suggestions have been made with respect to the different toxicities of individual tricyclics, the authors found no difference in plasma levels noted between those taking amitryptyline and those taking other agents.

This correlation was not observed by Thorstrand (64), who found that although the QRS duration was closely related to the severity of the poisoning, concentrations of tricyclic antidepressant in the blood or urine did not show a relationship to either the dose reported to be ingested or the electrocardiographic changes observed. However, plasma concentrations of tricyclics were determined in only 17 of 153 patients. Other investigators have also reported conflicting findings (71–75) with respect to the usefulness of the relationship between plasma tricyclic antidepressant levels and clinical effects. The reason for this conflict may be in the technique of measuring plasma tricyclic antidepressant levels. Tissue concentrations of the tricyclics are considerably higher than in the plasma, with the unbound drug accounting for 7 to 13% of total plasma tricyclics. As a result, in performing correlative studies, determination of free tricyclics in the plasma would be of greater value and be associated with a higher correlation with physiologic response than total tricyclic levels. At present, the available data concerning the significance of this relationship are inconclusive.

Antiarrhythmic Agents

Treatment of arrhythmias should occur when clinically important symptoms develop. It should be emphasized that the prolonged half-life of amitryptyline mandates continuous cardiac monitoring for 5 to 6 days, regardless of presence of symptoms. The relationship of the tricyclics to the type 1 antiarrhythmic drugs warrants cautious administration of agents, such as quinidine and procainamide, to control arrhythmias. If these drugs are used, they should be prescribed in decreased dosage. Beta blockers, e.g., propranolol (Inderal®), are advantageous in offsetting the adrenergic effects. However, these drugs may potentiate tricyclic-induced negative inotropic and chronotropic action. In the presence of hypotension and congestive heart failure, propranolol should be used cautiously, if at all. The use of other beta blockers devoid of negative effects on myocardial contractility, such as practolol or sotalol, may be of value. Diphenylhydantoin (Dilantin®) may also be helpful in preventing both cardiac and cerebral dysrhythmias (47).

Digitalis

Digitalis may be used with caution in the absence of A-V block when congestive heart failure exists. Cardioversion and atrial pacing may also be of value in the presence of refractory arrhythmias or heart block.

Sodium Bicarbonate

Sodium bicarbonate has been reported to be an effective therapeutic agent in children. Brown et al. (76) found that the administration of sodium bicarbonate to 12 children with tricyclic-induced arrhythmias resulted in a rapid reversion to regular rhythm. Although the mechanism of action has not been clearly defined, it may relate to the correction of an existing acidosis or to an increase in plasma tricyclic protein binding.

Physostigmine

The use of physostigmine salicylate, a cholinesterase inhibitor, has been shown to be beneficial in reversal of the central nervous system (CNS) effects of the tricyclics and has a salutary peripheral effect on tachycardia (77–80). The mechanism is related to augmented cholinergic effects as well as to the postulated ability of physostigmine to reverse the tricyclic-induced competitive inhibition of acetylcholine at receptor sites. This drug may be useful in slowing the sinus tachycardia and may be of special value in older patients with myocardial ischemia or bundle branch disease suffering from tricyclic toxicity.

Tobias and Das (80) have reported the effectiveness of physostigmine in reversing abnormal conduction, atrioventricular dissociation, tachycardia, and ventricular arrhythmias in a 22-year-old patient treated for drug overdose. The recommended dose is 2 mg i.v. by slow infusion followed by another 2 mg in 20 min if the first dose is ineffective. If a beneficial response is obtained, 1 to 4 mg should be given every 60 min as necessary (77). The use of physostigmine, however, is not without hazard; severe bradycardia and hypersalivation may occur, which can be quite dangerous in a comatose patient. Convulsions have also been reported (77). Since most patients have only mild anticholinergic symptoms, treatment of cardiac complications with physostigmine should be performed cautiously, accompanied by careful monitoring, only in those patients who cannot be adequately treated supportively.

Drug Interactions

Experimentally, the tricyclics have been shown to inhibit the hepatic microsomal system (81). This in turn can result in a decreased metabolism of drugs normally detoxified through this pathway, with attendant increase in toxic effects. *In vitro* studies have revealed treatment with tricyclics to result in a marked inhibition of metabolism of propranolol, amphetamines, guanethidine, and pentobarbital (14). Clinically, nortriptyline has been shown to increase the plasma half-life of bishydroxycoumarin by a factor of three in normal volunteers (81). It should also be emphasized that concomitant administration of tricyclics and drugs that induce the hepatic microsomal system, such as barbiturates, or inhibit the system, such as methylphenidate, can cause either striking decreases or increases in tricyclic steady state plasma levels.

Interference of metabolism of phenothiazines and tricyclic antidepressants, when both agents are used concomitantly, has also been reported (82). The known effects of phenothiazines on the heart, combined with the cardiovascular actions of the tricyclic antidepressants, could result in a greater likelihood of cardiac toxicity, since both drugs adversely effect cardiac repolarization (83). Frequently, patients presenting with a picture of complex depression are treated with a combination of those two groups of drugs. In such cases, especially in geriatric patients or in those with cardiac disease, serious consideration should be given to an alternate therapeutic approach. If this combination is desired, essential, careful, sequential electrocardiographic monitoring is mandatory.

Synergistic interactions can occur between tricyclic antidepressants and drugs displaying anticholinergic effects, such as glutethimide (Doriden®) and meperidine (Demerol®). The combination with meperidine may result in a potentiation of the narcotic-induced respiratory depression (84).

Sympathetic and Sympathomimetic Agents

Numerous interactions occur between the tricyclic antidepressants and cardiac medications (Table 5). The actions of the tricyclics on the adrenergic neuron not unexpectedly result in an interference with sympathomatic amines

TABLE 5. *Interactions between antidepressants and commonly used cardiac drugs*

	Tricyclic antidepressants				MAO inhibitors			
Drug	HR[a]	BP	ECG	Other	HR	BP	ECG	Other
Antiarrhythmics								
Quinidine	—	—	+		—	—	—	—
Procainamide	—	—	+		—	—	—	—
Lidocaine	—	—	—		—	—	—	—
Diphenylhydantoin	—	—	—		—	—	—	—
Propranolol	↓	↓	—	+[a]	↓	—	—	—
Antihypertensives								
Reserpine	↓/—	—	—	+[b]		↑ ↓		NM
Alpha-methyldopa	↑/—	↑/—	NM	+[e]		↑ ↓		+[c]
Clonidine	NM	↑	NM	+[b,e]		NM		NM
Guanethidine	NM	↑	NM	—		↑		—
Hydralazine	NM	↓	NM	—		↓/—		—
MAO inhibitors	↑	↓	NM	+[f]				
Sympathomimetics	↑	↑	NM	—	↑	↑	±	+[d]
Parasympathomimetics	↓	↓	±	—	NM	NM	NM	NM
Digitalis	↑/—	—	+	NM		—	NM	NM

[a] HR, heart rate; BP, blood pressure; ECG, electrocardiogram.
+, Positive; —, no effect; ±, occasional; NM, not measured.
[a] May accentuate negative ionotropic effects if present.
[b] Accentuate depression.
[c] Hallucinations.
[d] CNS stimulation.
[e] CNS depression.
[f] Reaction quite severe with fatal outcomes reported.

that predominantly act by releasing NE from storage granules (Table 6). These drugs include ephedrine, metaraminol, and mephentermine. Concomitant administration results in an inhibition of the pressor response caused by these drugs. Sympathomimetic drugs having a predominantly direct action on the adrenergic neuron have an enhanced pressor effect in the presence of tricyclics owing to an increased concentration of NE at the receptor site. Clinically, this interaction may result in an augmented sympathetic effect of several-fold in the presence of the tricyclics. Adverse symptoms have also been

TABLE 6. *Interactions between tricyclic antidepressants and sympathomimetic drugs*

Pressor response	
Enhanced	Inhibited
Amphetamines	Ephedrine
Epinephrine	Metaraminol
Norepinephrine	Mephentermine
Phenylephrine	

reported in patients maintained on tricyclics receiving local anesthetics containing epinephrine (85).

Antihypertensives

Clonidine

Antihypertensive agents (Fig. 6) must be used with great caution in persons maintained on tricyclics. Clonidine (Catapres®, ST155) has recently become available as an antihypertensive agent. This drug acts predominantly on the sympathetic cardiovascular medullary centers, decreasing the sympathetic neural activity of the heart, peripheral vasculature, and kidney, with resultant suppression of renin release (86). Clonidine, similar to methyldopa when utilized with a vasodilator and beta blocker combination, results in an additive therapeutic effect in persons with severe hypertension. The tricyclic antidepressants may inhibit the antihypertensive action of clonidine through interaction in the CNS. Briant et al. (87) have demonstrated a rise in blood pressure in four of five patients maintained on clonidine when desipramine was added to the treatment regimen.

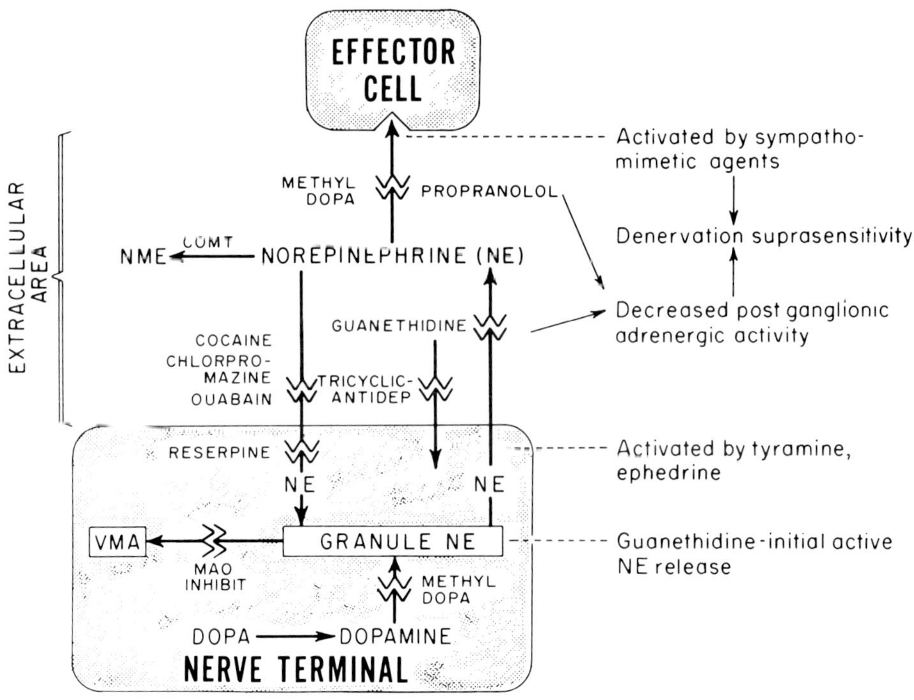

FIG. 6. Action of antihypertensives and tricyclic antidepressants on the sympathetic nervous system. COMT, catechol-O-methyl transferase; MAO inhibit = monoamine oxidase inhibitors; Tricyclic antidep, tricyclic antidepressants; ⩔, interference with normally occurring reactions.

Guanidinium Derivatives

Guanidinium derivatives, such as guanethidine and bethanidine, inhibit NE release and progressively deplete NE by competing with it for reentry into the nerve terminal and by causing a partial release of NE from the granule. This can result in an inhibition of postganglionic adrenergic nerve activity of both alpha and beta receptors. The response of effector receptor cells to catecholamines, however, is heightened.

The coadministration of tricyclic antidepressants can abolish the antihypertensive effect of guanethidine (88,89). The mechanism of this inhibition is secondary to the ability of imipramine and related drugs to block the active transport of guanethidine across axonal membranes and the subsequent uptake of guanethidine by the NE pump, which is essential for its antihypertensive effect.

Hypertension will recur, however, with an increased maintenance dose being required. In one instance, death resulted from this interaction (90). Discontinuing tricyclic therapy is associated with a gradual resumption of guanethidine effectiveness in approximately 5 days, although up to 2 weeks may be required. It should be emphasized that discontinuation of doxepin may be associated with an initial rebound hypertensive response. Hypotensive reactions of considerable severity may also occur if tricyclic therapy is suddenly discontinued without adjusting the guanethidine dose.

Reserpine

Reserpine and related rauwolfia alkaloids deplete catecholamines and 5-hydroxytryptamine through blocking uptake of both NE and dopamine in the granules. This results in an interference at the postganglionic adrenergic nerve ending with a decrease in peripheral vascular resistance. In the CNS, the catecholamines are also depleted, with subsequent metabolization by MAO. In addition, a direct action on the hypothalamus and vasomotor centers in the brainstem results in an inhibition of sympathetic discharge, although the antihypertensive effect of these agents is primarily related to their peripheral effects (91). Since reserpine does not competitively enter the cell, its antihypertensive effect is not specifically antagonized by tricyclics. In the laboratory animal, interactions of tricyclics with reserpine have been reported, but the clinical relevance of these findings is questionable. Since depression is not an unknown reaction to reserpine, however, combination with tricyclics would probably be unwise.

MAO Inhibitors

The MAO inhibitors have complex pharmacologic actions that may be related to enzyme inhibition of other enzymes in addition to MAO. Their basic effect is to increase concentration of dopamine and NE in the nerve endings by preventing their inactivation. Pargyline is the agent in this group most frequently used in the treatment of hypertension. Adverse effects with concomitant use of tricyclics have been well documented and may be quite severe, progressing to circulatory collapse and even death (90,92).

Methyldopa

Alpha-methyldopa acts through inhibiting the decarboxylation of both dopamine and 5-hydroxytryptophan. This is accompanied by a decreased concentration of 5-hydroxydopamine and NE in the CNS and other tissues, with the exception of the adrenal medulla. Methyldopa also depletes NE through the formation of false neurotransmitter (methylnorepinephrine), which displaces NE in the granule and prevents its uptake in the tissues (93). A mild CNS depressant effect also occurs, which reduces sympathetic outflow. The increase in NE secondary to displacement makes it quite hazardous to use this drug in combination with MAO inhibitors. Severe reactions with concurrent use of both these agents have been reported (94). Similarly, the concomitant use of sympathomimetic amines may result in an enhanced sympathomimetic effect with hypertension, tachycardia, and arrhythmias (93). Methyldopa is one of the few autonomic antihypertensives that does not clinically interfere with the tricyclic antidepressants; it is therefore appropriate therapy in patients taking tricyclics when hypertension cannot be controlled by a diuretic agent alone (95,96). However, hypertension and tachycardia have been observed with combined use of alpha-methyldopa and tricyclics (97). Large fluctuations in blood pressure associated with hypotension and tachycardia may occur when administered with ganglion-blocking agents. Simultaneous administration with alpha-methyldopa can result in stimulation of the CNS and hypertensive reactions.

Antiarrhythmics

The similar action of some of the tricyclics to type 1 antiarrhythmic drugs might allow for a potentiation of drug action with enhancement of toxicity when these agents are used concomitantly. Similarly, the concomitant use of any drug having myocardial depressant effect might result in a synergistic action with respect to myocardial depression.

Digitalis

Experimentally, an increased lethality to digoxin has been demonstrated in stressed rats pretreated with large doses of tricyclics (41). Ouabain has been shown to be effective in reducing tricyclic-induced myocardial depression in anesthesized dogs (24). The clinical relevance of these findings remains to be determined, and, when clinically indicated, digoxin should be administered in patients maintained on tricyclic agents, unless heart block is present.

LITHIUM CARBONATE

Lithium has been known to be efficacious in the treatment of manic depression since 1949. The synthesis of newer agents resulted in a diminution of lithium use during the following years. Enthusiasm for this agent has recently increased considerably. At present, lithium is the treatment of choice for control of chronic manic states and has also been used with varying degrees of effectiveness in other psychiatric disorders.

In the 1940s, the use of this agent, most prominently as a salt substitute, was followed by reports of lithium toxicity (97,98). These cases mainly involved persons with preexisting hypertension and cardiomegaly whose dietary salt intake was quite restricted. The adverse publicity resulted in a withdrawal of lithium from the market until 1970, when it was officially released by the Food and Drug Administration for use in the treatment of manic episodes in the manic-depressive psychoses. At that time, the accompanying release warned against the use of lithium in persons with cardiovascular or renal disease (99).

Pharmacology

Lithium is absorbed from the intestinal tract within 8 hr after oral administration. Peak plasma levels occur within 1 to 3 hr, with a plasma half-life of approximately 24 hr. Renal excretion is the predominant route of elimination. Lithium is distributed in the body water with varying degrees of concentration in different tissues. Diminished body sodium is associated with a slower excretion of lithium and potential for lithium toxicity. In the presence of salt restriction, lithium should be used with extreme caution, if at all.

Effects on Rhythm and Conduction

Animal Studies

Experimentally, as early as 1875, the ability of lithium chloride injected intravenously to cause diastolic arrest of the hearts of frogs, rabbits, and doves was observed (100). Other investigators subsequently demonstrated that this effect was related to the production of hyperkalemia, which in turn resulted in a decrease of the intracellular/extracellular potassium ratio with cardiac arrest and ventricular fibrillation (101,102). More recent experimental studies have revealed lithium to exert an antiarrhythmic effect when administered in the presence of ouabain-induced arrhythmias in dogs or chloroform-induced apnea in mice (103,104). Lithium has been shown to diminish spontaneous depolarization, induce decremental conduction, and slow conduction through the AV node and ventricle (105). In all these studies, however, the dose of lithium administered was excessive so as to make the relevance of these findings to humans questionable.

Mechanism of Action

The mechanism of action of lithium remains to be clarified. Singer and Rotenberg (106) hypothesized that lithium serves as a substitute for other cations participating in ionic transfer and distribution. In addition, an effect on the cellular microenvironment may also be prominent. Lithium replacement of intracellular potassium can result in hyperkalemia and a decrease in the resting membrane potential associated with impaired impulse conduction. This may explain its effect on the cardiac conduction system in animal and tissue experiments and may be relevant to its observed antiarrhythmic activity and its ability to produce T-wave changes in ECGs in patients on lithium therapy.

Lithium inhibits release of NE and 5-hydroxytryptamine, partially through its inhibitory effect on adenylate cyclase. It also increases the reuptake of NE and turnover rate of 5-hydroxytryptamine. This may result in an interference with the catecholamine effect on cardiac cells, preventing asynchronous electrical activity and providing another explanation for its antiarrhythmic action.

Clinical Effects

The most frequent complications of lithium carbonate intoxication are impaired consciousness, slurred speech, fatigue, and muscle weakness, sometimes associated with effects on the cardiovascular system. Schou et al. (98) and Horowitz and Fisher (107) reported prolonged QT intervals and T-wave inversion or flattening in patients with lithium carbonate poisoning. These changes were reversed with discontinuation of lithium. Sinus bradycardia, ventricular contractions, and idioventricular rhythm have also been reported, subsiding when the drug is discontinued (108).

Tseng (109) described autopsy findings in an elderly woman maintained on 300 mg/day lithium carbonate in whom right bundle branch block, atrioventricular dissociation with idioventricular rhythm, and multiple premature ventricular contractions developed. On discontinuation of lithium, the electrocardiographic findings reverted to normal, with the exception of the right bundle branch block. Several weeks later, the patient suddenly expired. On postmortem examination, the myocardium revealed a lithium concentration of 1.5 mg/g tissue. A diffuse interstitial myocarditis was present.

A second case of fatal idiopathic myocarditis has also been reported

(110). Unfortunately, the first patient had been on multiple psychoactive agents for several months prior to her death, making a direct causal relationship between lithium and the observed electrocardiographic changes difficult to document. In the second patient, the possibility existed of unexplained heart failure prior to initiating lithium therapy. The high concentration of lithium carbonate detected in the myocardium, associated with undetectable levels in the brain, suggests an affinity of this drug for heart tissue. Subsequent reports of myocarditis in patients maintained on lithium have also appeared in the literature (111).

Abnormalities of the sinus node, consisting of bradycardia, sinoatrial block, and sinus arrest, have also been described (112–114). Tilkian et al. (115) have reviewed all cases of nonfatal lithium toxicity reported in the literature. There were no described residual cardiac effects in patients who recovered from the drug effect, either in the form of arrhythmias or in a worsening of preexisting congestive heart failure. During the past 6 years when lithium was used more frequently, of the 25 cases reviewed in 11 studies, the only cardiovascular effects noted have been T-wave abnormalities and borderline hypertension, the latter occurring in the setting of dehydration and coma.

Two prospective studies analyzing electrocardiographic changes in persons maintained on lithium have recently been reported. Wren and Dana (116) monitored electrocardiographic changes in 38 chronic alcoholics administered lithium as compared to a control group of 40 chronic alcoholics given a placebo. None of the subjects had any evidence of cardiovascular, renal, or hepatic disease. Changes in the ECG were confined to the T-waves. Lowering of T-wave amplitude was noted in the limb leads in 8% and in the precordial leads in 35% of treated patients as compared to 1.9 and 18% of controls ($p < 0.001$). Changes in T-wave contour, consisting of rounding or flattening, were also noted. These changes were found to be unrelated to serum lithium level but correlated with duration of therapy, the highest incidence noted after 28 days of treatment. No symptoms developed in treated patients, and the alterations were reversible upon discontinuing therapy.

Tilkian et al. (115) performed extended ambulatory monitoring and submaximal exercise testing in 12 persons before and during lithium therapy. Advanced coronary artery disease was present in three persons and evidence suggestive of coronary disease in two. Two patients had premature ventricular contractions in the absence of detectable coronary artery disease, and the remaining four were free of any signs of cardiac disease. Long-term lithium administration was found to both induce and aggravate preexisting ventricular arrhythmias on ambulatory electrocardiographic monitoring in the absence of any electrolyte abnormalities. Exercise performance was not adversely affected. Premature atrial contractions were abolished during exercise, and ventricular arrhythmias, if present, did tend to decrease. Repolarization changes in the form of T-wave inversion were noted in the ECG but were not associated with resting or exercise-induced ST segment changes.

Drug Interactions

The salt-depleting effects of lithium make it important that lithium be administered to persons in normal salt balance. High salt intake or ingestion of sodium bicarbonate is associated with an increased renal excretion of lithium. If lithium is prescribed to persons in congestive heart failure or being maintained on diuretic therapy, salt intake must be carefully monitored.

The chronic use of thiazide diuretics is associated with a decrease in lithium clearance by up to 24% and the potential for lithium toxicity (117). Other sodium-depleting diuretics, such as ethacrynic acid and furosemide, may also inhibit lithium excretion. Acute administration of these diuretics, however, has not been found to affect lithium clearance (117,118). Conversely, aminophylline administration has been associated with an enhanced excretion of lithium, although the clinical significance of this finding remains to be determined (118).

Combined use of lithium with other mood-altering drugs may result in relevant drug interactions. Urinary retention seen with the tricyclic antidepressants may become more severe with concomitant lithium administration because of the diuretic action of lithium. Early symptoms of lithium toxicity, such as nausea, may be attenuated by simultaneous administration of phenothiazines (119).

In the absence of mitigating factors, lithium may be utilized by the elderly in the presence of severe manic states, but it should be accompanied by careful monitoring. Since arrhythmias related to lithium may give rise to nonspecific complaints, as well as dizziness and syncope that may erroneously be attributed to the existing psychosis, such symptoms must be carefully evaluated.

Summary

As a result of the above reports, there has been some hesitation to use lithium in patients with cardiovascular or renal disease. Although much of this reluctance had been based on the early experience with the use of lithium as a salt substitute, documented evidence of isolated effects on the cardiovascular system have been demonstrated, especially in patients with ventricular arrhythmias or sinus node dysfunction. In addition, the use of this drug in the presence of a decreased glomerular filtration rate, active heart failure, or the concomitant administration of diuretics, with or without active salt restriction, may result in an interference in renal clearance of lithium with toxic accumulation.

MAO INHIBITORS

The MAO inhibitors were among the first antidepressant drugs to appear for the clinical treatment of depression. Their potential for toxicity and adverse drug interactions limited their effectiveness. The development of the tricyclic antidepressants resulted in a marked decrease in prescription of MAO inhibitors for anxiety.

Pharmacology

The MAO inhibitors consist of two main groups: the hydrazines (phenelzine, isocarboxozide) and the nonhydrazines (tranylcypromine). Similar to the tricyclic antidepressants, they act to potentiate central noradrenergic function. Unlike the tricyclics, however, they prevent the oxidative deamination of biogenic amines, which in turn results in large amounts of NE accumulating at the nerve ending. It should be emphasized that MAO inhibitors act not only on the organ systems affected by catecholamines and hydroxytryptamine but also on multiple other enzyme systems.

The MAO inhibitors are rapidly absorbed from the intestinal tract. The hydrazide MAO inhibitors are inactivated primarily by acetylation, whereas the nonhydrazide MAO inhibitors combine directly with MAO.

Clinical Effects

The MAO inhibitors have very marked effects on the cardiovascular system. The exact mechanism by which these drugs act on the heart is unclear. It is likely that the general capacity to inhibit enzyme systems is at least partly responsible. Orthostatic hypotension, which may develop slowly, is a common reaction. This effect, when mild and occurring in persons with coronary disease, may be accompanied by a relief of angina in 50% of subjects, although these findings have not been entirely consistent (120–122).

Drug Interactions

As discussed above, the ability of the MAO inhibitors to interfere with enzyme systems has resulted in interactions with multiple other agents to produce severe and at times fatal side-effects. Instances of acute hypertension, precipitated by the use of these agents and simultaneous ingestion of substances containing tyramine (Table 7), have appeared sporadically in the literature. Although ingestion of tyramine is ordinarily without effect because of its rapid metabolism by MAO located in the intestinal wall and liver, once the MAO inhibitors are administered, this reaction no longer occurs. Tyramine may replace NE from its storage granules with subsequent hypertension. Although recovery from such a reaction is usually the rule, severe

TABLE 7. *Tyramine-containing foods*

Avocado pear	Eggplant
Broad (fava) beans	Game meats
Bananas	Herring, kippered and pickled
Beer	Meat extracts
Canned figs	Orange pulp
Cheeses, aged (cheddar, gruyere, camembert, stilton, brie, emmenthal)	Red wines
	Tomato
Chicken livers	Yeast extracts
Chocolate	Yogurt

complications, such as pulmonary edema and intracranial hemorrhage, have been reported (123,124).

Sympathetics and Sympathomimetics

Adverse reactions with sympathomimetic agents and MAO inhibitors will also occur secondary to the excess release of catecholamines. These reactions are marked by a sudden onset of headache, associated with hypertension of varying severity and accompanied at times by pulmonary edema. In cases terminating fatally, cerebral edema and subarachnoid hemorrhage have been demonstrated at postmortem examination (125). The clinical importance of this interaction has been underscored by Villiers (125), who noted 13 of 883 patients admitted to a neurosurgical unit with subarachnoid hemorrhage to be taking these two drugs. It should be emphasized that many sympathomimetic amines are present in over-the-counter medications, such as nasal decongestants and diet pills. The use of these drugs in persons on MAO inhibitors must be proscribed.

Other Drug Interactions

Adverse reactions have also been reported with MAO inhibitors and sedatives, narcotic analgesics, hypoglycemic agents, and antihypertensive agents affecting the autonomic nervous system (Table 5), resulting in a decrease in clinical effect of these drugs with a greater potential for toxicity (126,127).

When MAO inhibitors are combined with diuretics, impressive hypotension may develop, as has recently been emphasized by Shamsie and Barriga (123) in a study concerning the use of these agents in adolescents.

Finally, as stated earlier, use of tricyclics with or soon after MAO inhibitors may produce severe systemic reactions. Several days should elapse before a MAO inhibitor is initiated, and up to 16 days should pass before tricyclic administration to a person previously on MAO inhibitors.

REFERENCES

1. National Disease and Therapeutic Index: Listings from October 1973–September 1974. IMA America, Ambler, Pennsylvania.

2. Newton, R. W. (1975): Physostigmine salicylate in the treatment of tricyclic antidepressant overdosage. *JAMA,* 231:941.
3. Schildkraut, J. J. (1973): Neuropharmacology of the affective disorders. *Ann. Rev. Pharmacol.,* 13:427.
4. Koelle, G. B. (1975): Neurohumoral transmission and the autonomic nervous system. In: *The Pharmacologic Basis of Therapeutics, Fifth Edition,* edited by L. S. Goodman and A. Gilman, pp. 405–445. Macmillan, New York.
5. Iversen, L. L. (1967): *The Uptake and Storage of Noradrenalin in Sympathetic Nerves.* Cambridge University Press, London.
6. Cairncross, D. D. (1965): On the peripheral pharmacology of amitriptyline. *Arch. Int. Pharmacol.,* 154:438.
7. Sigg, E. B., Osborne, M., and Korol, B. (1963): Cardiovascular effects of imipramine. *J. Pharmacol. Exp. Ther.,* 141:237.
8. Borga, O., Azarnoff, D. L., Forshell, G. P., et al. (1969): Plasma protein binding of tricyclic antidepressants in man. *Biochem. Pharmacol.,* 18:2135.
9. Braithwaite, R. A., Goulding, R., Theano, G., et al. (1972): Plasma concentration of amitriptyline and clinical response. *Lancet,* 1:1297.
10. Ziegler, V. E., Co, B. T., Taylor, J. R., et al. (1976): Amitriptyline plasma levels and therapeutic response. *Clin. Pharmacol. Ther.,* 19:795.
11. Ziegler, V. E., Clayton, P. J., Taylor, J. R., et al. (1976): Nortriptyline plasma levels and therapeutic response. *Clin. Pharmacol. Ther.,* 20:458.
12. Copper, A., Montgomery, S., Ghose, K., et al. (1978): Amitriptyline plasma concentration and clinical effect. *Lancet,* 1:63.
13. Byck, R. (1975): Drugs and the treatment of psychiatric disorders. In: *The Pharmacological Basis of Therapeutics,* edited by L. S. Goodman and A. Gilman, p. 178. Macmillan, New York.
14. Jefferson, J. W. (1975): A review of the cardiovascular effects and toxicity of tricyclic antidepressants. *Psychosom. Med.,* 37:160.
15. Van de Ree, J. K., Zimmerman, A. N. E., and Van Heijst, A. N. P. (1972): Intoxication with tricyclic antidepressants. Hemodynamic consequences. *Eur. J. Toxicol.,* 5:302.
16. Langslet, A., Johansen, W. A., Ryg, M., et al. (1971): Effects of dibenzepine and imipramine on the isolated rat heart. *Eur. J. Pharmacol.,* 14:333.
17. Vohra, J., Burrows, G. D., and Sloman, G. (1975): Assessment of cardiovascular side effects of therapeutic doses of tricyclic antidepressant drugs. *Aust. N.Z. J. Med.,* 5:7.
18. Freyschuss, V., Sjoqvist, F., Tuck, D., et al. (1970): Circulatory effects in man of nortriptyline, a tricyclic antidepressant drug. *Pharmacol. Clin.,* 2:68.
19. Thorstrand, C., and Lindblad, L. E. (1976): The effect of amitriptyline on forearm blood flow. *Scand. J. Clin. Lab. Invest.,* 36:17.
20. Muller, O. F., Goodman, N., and Bellet, S. (1961): The hypotensive effect of imipramine hydrochloride in patients with cardiovascular disease. *Clin. Pharmacol. Ther.,* 2:300.
21. Kantor, S. J., Glassman, A. H., Bigger, J. T., et al. (1977): The cardiac effects of therapeutic plasma concentrations of imipramine. Presented at the Meetings of the American Psychiatric Association, Toronto, May, 1977.
22. Maxwell, R. A., Keenan, P. D., and Chaplin, E., et al. (1969): Molecular features affecting the potency of tricyclic antidepressants and structurally related compounds as inhibitors of the uptake of tritiated norepinephrine by rabbit aortic strips. *J. Pharmacol. Exp. Ther.,* 166:320.
23. Kaumann, A., Basso, N., and Aramendia, P. (1965): The cardiovascular effects of the N-(γ-methylaminoproply-iminodibenyzl)-HCl (desmethylimipramine) and guanethidine. *J. Pharmacol. Exp. Ther.,* 147:54.
24. Laddu, A. R., and Somani, P. (1969): Desipramine toxicity and its treatment. *Toxicol. Appl. Pharmacol.,* 15:287.
25. Van Zwieten, P. A. (1973): The central action of antihypertensive drugs, mediated via central α-receptors. *J. Pharm. Pharmacol.,* 25:89.
26. Cardiovascular complications of tricyclic antidepressants (1971): *N.Z. Med. J.,* 74:330.

27. Kristiansen, E. S. (1961): Cardiac complications during treatment with imipramine (Tofranil). *Acta Psychiatr. Neurol. Scand.,* 36:427.
28. Gaultier, M., Boissier, J. R., Gorceix, A., et al. (1965): The cardiotoxicity of imipramine in man. *Eur. Soc. Study. Drug. Toxicol.,* 6:171.
29. Buckley, J. P., Steenberg, M. L., Jandhyala, B. S., et al. (1975): Effects of imipramine, desmethylimipramine and their 2 OH metabolites on hemodynamics and myocardial contractility. *Fed. Proc.,* 34:450.
30. Baum, T., Shropshire, A. J., Rowles, G., et al. (1971): Antidepressants and cardiac conduction: Iprindole and imipramine. *Eur. J. Pharmacol.,* 13:287.
31. Cairncross, K. D., and Gershon, S. (1962): A pharmacological basis for the cardiovascular complications of imipramine medication. *Med. J. Aust.,* 2:372.
32. Häfliger, F. (1959): Chemistry of Tofranil. *Can. Psychiatr. Assoc. J.,* 4:69.
33. Cassano, G., Sjöstrand, S. E., and Hansson, E. (1965): Distribution and fate of C^{14}-amitriptyline in mice and rats. *Psychopharmacologia,* 8:11.
34. Barth, N., Manns, M., and Muscholl, E. (1975): Arrhythmias and inhibition of noradrenaline uptake caused by tricyclic antidepressants and chlorpromazine on the isolated perfused rabbit heart. *NSAP,* 288:215.
35. Weld, F. M., Bigger, J. T., Swistel, D., et al. (1978): Effects of imipramine hydrochloride on electrophysiological properties of sheep. Cardiac purkinje fibers. *Am. J. Cardiol.* 41:386 (Abstr.).
36. Rawling, B. A., and Fozzard, H. A. (1978): Electrophysiological effects of imipramine on cardiac purkinje fibers. *Am. J. Cardiol.,* 41:387 (Abstr.).
37. Barth, N., and Muscholl, E. (1974): The effect of tricyclic antidepressants desipramine, doxepin and iprindole on the isolated perfused rabbit heart. *Nauyn Schmiedebergs Arch. Pharmacol.,* 284:215.
38. Langslet, A., Johansen, W. G., Ryg, M., et al. (1971): Effects of dibenzepine and imipramine on the isolated rat heart. *Eur. J. Pharmacol.,* 14:333.
39. Matsuo, S. (1967): Comparative effects of imipramine and propranolol on the transmembrane potentials of the isolated rabbit's atria. *Jpn. J. Pharmacol.,* 12:279.
40. Kristiansen, E. S. (1961): Cardiac complications during treatment with imipramine (Tofranil). *Acta Psychiatr. Neurol.,* 36:427.
41. Moir, D. C., Cornwell, W. S., Crooks, J., et al. (1972): Cardiotoxicity of amitriptyline. *Lancet,* 2:561.
42. Freeman, J. W., Mundy, R. G., Beattie, R. R., et al. (1969): Cardiac abnormalities in poisoning with tricyclic antidepressants. *Br. Med. J.,* II:610.
43. Williams, R. B., Jr., and Sherter, C. (1971): Cardiac complications of tricyclic antidepressant therapy. *Ann. Intern. Med.,* 74:395.
44. Fletcher, G. F., and Kazamia, T. M. (1969): Cardiotoxic effects of mellaril—Conduction disturbances and supraventricular arrhythmias. *Am. Heart J.,* 78:135.
45. Giardina, E. G. V., Bigger, J. T., Kantor, S. J., et al. (1978): Electrocardiographic and antiarrhythmic effects of imipramine hydrochloride. *Clin. Res.,* 26:482A.
46. Boakes, A. J., Laurence, D. E., Teoh, P. C., et al. (1973): Interactions between sympathomimetic amines and antidepressant agents in man. *Br. Med. J.,* 1:311.
47. Moir, D. C. (1973): Tricyclic antidepressants and cardiac disease. *Am. Heart J.,* 86:841.
48. Kantor, S. J., Bigger, T., Glassman, A. H., et al. (1975): Imipramine induced heart block. *JAMA,* 231:1364.
49. Moorehead, C. N., and Knox, S. J. (1965): Imipramine induced auricular fibrillation. *Am. J. Psychiatry,* 122:216.
50. Rasmussen, E. B., and Kristjansen, P. (1963): ECG changes during amitriptyline treatment. *Am. J. Psychiatry,* 119:781.
51. Smith, R. E., and Rusbatch, B. J. (1967): Amitriptyline and heart block. *Br. Med. J.,* 3:311.
52. Burckhardt, D., Raeder, E., Muller, V., et al. (1978): Cardiovascular effects of tricyclic and tetracyclic antidepressants. *JAMA,* 239:213.
53. Vohra, J., Burrows, G. D., Hunt, D., et al. (1975): The effect of toxic and therapeutic doses of tricyclic antidepressant drugs on intracardiac conduction. *Eur. J. Cardiol.,* 3:219.
54. Burrows, G. D., Vohra, J., Dumovic, P., et al. (1977): Tricyclic antidepressant

drugs and cardiac conduction. In: *Proceedings of the 10th Congress of the College of International Neuropsychopharmacology*. Pergamon Press, London.
55. Coull, D. C. (1970): Amitriptyline and cardiac disease. *Lancet,* 2:590.
56. Boston Collaborative Drug Surveillance Program (1972): Adverse reactions to the tricyclic antidepressant drugs. *Lancet,* 1:529.
57. Biamino, G., Fenner, H., Neyes, J., et al. (1975): Comparative in vitro and in vivo studies on the effects of tricyclic antidepressants on myocardial contractility. In: *Metabolism of Contraction,* edited by P. E. Roy and G. Rona, pp. 59–69. University Park Press, Baltimore.
57a. Schwartz, P. J., and Wolf, S. (1978): QT interval prolongation as predictor of sudden death in patients with myocardial infarction. *Circulation,* 57:1974.
57b. Haynes, R. E., Hallstrom, A. P., and Cobb, L. A. (1977): Repolarization abnormalities in sudden cardiac death syndrome. *Clin. Res.* 25:143a (Abstr.).
58. Robinson, D. S., and Barker, E. (1976): Tricyclic antidepressant cardiotoxicity. *JAMA,* 236:2089.
59. Steele, C. M., O'Duffy, J., and Brown, S. S. (1967): Clinical effects and treatment of imipramine and amitriptyline poisoning in children. *Br. Med. J.,* 9:663.
60. Bain, D. J. G. (1973): A criticism of the use of tricyclic antidepressant drugs in the treatment of childhood enuresis. *J. R. Coll. Gen. Pract.,* 23:222.
61. Rhoads, J. M., and McCollum, D. E. (1969): A hypotensive episode caused by amitriptyline. *Lancet,* 2:741.
62. Smith, R. B., and Rusbatch, B. J. (1967): Amitriptyline and heart block. *Br. Heart J.,* 3:311.
63. Silverman, G. (1972): Cardiotoxicity of amitriptyline. *Lancet,* 2:710.
64. Thorstrand, C. (1976): Cardiovascular effects of poisoning by tricyclic antidepressants with special reference to the ECG. *Acta Med. Scand.,* 199:337.
65. Brackenridge, R. G., Peters, T. J., and Watson, J. M. (1968): Myocardial damage in amitriptyline and nortriptyline poisoning. *Scot. Med. J.,* 13:208.
66. Noble, J. J., and Matthew, H. (1969): Acute poisoning by tricyclic antidepressants: Clinical features and management of 100 patients. *Clin. Toxicol.,* 2:403.
67. Crocker, J., and Morton, B. (1969): Tricyclic (antidepressant) drug toxicity. *Clin. Toxicol.,* 2:397.
68. Hawthorn, J. W., Marcus, A. M., and Kaye, M. (1963): Management of massive imipramine overdose with mannitol and artificial dialysis. *N. Engl. J. Med.,* 268:33.
69. Crome, P., Dowling, S., Braitwaite, R. A., et al. (1977): Effect of activated charcoal on absorption of nortriptyline. *Lancet,* 2:1203.
70. Spiker, D. G., and Biggs, J. T. (1976): Tricyclic antidepressants. Prolonged plasma levels after overdose. *JAMA,* 236:1711.
71. Biggs, J. T., Spiker, D. G., Petit, J. M., et al. (1977): Tricyclic antidepressant overdose. Incidence of symptoms. *JAMA,* 238:135.
72. Asberg, M., Cronholm, B., Sjoquist, F., et al. (1970): Correlation of subjective side effects with plasma concentrations of nortriptyline. *Br. Med. J.,* 4:18.
73. Berger, F. M. (1976): Present status of clinical psychopharmacology. *Clin. Pharmacol. Ther.,* 19:725.
74. Braithwaite, R. A., Goulding, R., Theano, G., et al. (1972): Plasma concentration of amitriptyline and clinical response. *Lancet,* 1:1297.
75. Gram, L. F., Reisby, N., Ibsen, I., et al. (1976): Plasma levels and antidepressant effect of imipramine. *Clin. Pharmacol. Ther.,* 19:318.
76. Brown, T. C. K., Barker, G. A., Dunlop, M. E., et al. (1973): The use of sodium bicarbonate in the treatment of tricyclic antidepressant induced arrhythmias. *Anaesth. Intensive Care,* 1:203.
77. Snyder, B. D., Blonde, L., and McWhirter, W. R. (1974): Reversal of amitriptyline intoxication by physostigmine. *JAMA,* 230:1433.
78. Slovis, T. L., Ott, J. E., Teitelbaum, D. T., et al. (1971): Physostigmine therapy in acute tricyclic antidepressant poisoning. *Clin. Toxicol.,* 4:451.
79. Newton, R. W. (1975): Physostigmine salicylate in the treatment of tricyclic antidepressant dosage. *JAMA,* 231:941.
80. Tobias, J., and Das, B. N. (1976): Cardiac complications with amitriptyline poisoning—Successful treatment with physostigmine. *JAMA,* 235:1474.

81. Vessell, E. S., Passananti, G. T., and Greene, F. E. (1970): Impairment of drug metabolism in man by allopurinol and amitriptyline. *N. Engl. J. Med.*, 283:1484.
82. El Yousef, M. K. (1974): Tricyclic antidepressants and phenothiazines. *JAMA*, 229:1419.
83. Heiman, E. M. (1977): Cardiac toxicity with thioridazine-tricyclic antidepressant combination. *J. Nerv. Ment. Dis.*, 165:139.
84. Hansten, P. D. (1976): *Drug Interactions*, third edition, p. 193. Lea and Febiger, Philadelphia.
85. Persson, G., and Siwers, B. (1975): The risk of potentiating effect of local anesthesia with adrenalin in patients treated with tricyclic antidepressants. *Swed. Dent. J.*, 68:9.
86. Pettinger, W. A. (1975): Clonidine, a new antihypertensive drug. *N. Engl. J. Med.*, 293:1179.
87. Briant, R. H., Reid, J. L., and Dollery, C. T. (1973): Interaction between clonidine and desimipramine in man. *Br. Med. J.*, 1:522.
88. Mitchell, J. R., Cavanaugh, J. H., Arias, L., et al. (1970): Guanethidine and related agents: III Antagonism by drugs which inhibit the norepinephrine pump in man. *J. Clin. Invest.*, 49:1596.
89. Meyer, J. F., McAllister, C. K., and Goldberg, L. I. (1970): Insidious and prolonged antagonism of quanethidine by amitriptyline. *JAMA*, 213:1487.
90. Sjöquist, F. (1965): Psychotropic drugs (2). Interaction between monoamine oxidase (MAO) inhibitors and other substances. *Proc. R. Soc. Med.*, 58:967.
91. Page, L., Vager, H. M., and Sidd, J. J. (1976): Drugs in the management of hypertension Part II. *Am. Heart J.*, 92:114.
92. Goldberg, L. I. (1964): Monoamine oxidase inhibitors. *JAMA*, 190:456.
93. Carlson, A., and Kindquist, M. (1962): In vivo decarboxylation of methyldopa and methylmetatyrosine. *Acta Physiol. Scand.*, 54:87.
94. Rossum, J. M., and Hurkmans, J. A. (1963): Reversal of effect of methyldopa by monoamine oxidase inhibitors. *J. Pharm. Pharmacol.*, 15:493.
95. Dollery, C. T. (1965): Physiological and pharmacological interactions of antihypertensive drugs. *Proc. R. Soc. Med.*, 58:983.
96. Lemberger, L. (1974): Chemically important antihypertensive drug interactions. *Drug Ther.*, 4:49.
97. Cade, J. F. J. (1949): Lithium salts in the treatment of psychotic excitement. *Med. J. Aust.*, 36:349.
98. Schou, M., Amdisen, A., Trap-Jensen, J. (1908): Lithium poisoning. *Am. J. Psychiatry*, 125:520.
99. Federal Drug Administration Statement (1970): *Ann. Intern. Med.*, 73:291.
100. Good, C. A. (1903): An experimental study of lithium. *Am. J. Med. Sci.*, 125:273.
101. McKusic, V. A. (1954): The effect of lithium on the electrocardiogram of animals and relation of their effects to the ratio of the intracellular and extracellular concentrations of potassium. *J. Clin. Invest.*, 33:598.
102. Riciotti, M. A., Lisi, K. R., and Damato, A. N. (1971): A metabolic basis for the electrophysiological effects of lithium. *Circulation* [*Suppl.*], 44:217.
103. Polumbo, R. A., Branzi, A., Schroeder, J. S., et al. (1973): The antiarrhythmic effect of lithium chloride for experimental ouabain induced arrhythmias. *Proc. Soc. Exp. Biol. Med.*, 142:1200.
104. Horgan, J. H., Proctor, J. D., Velandia, J., et al. (1973): Antiarrhythmic effect of lithium. *Arch. Int. Pharmacodyn.*, 206:105.
105. Carmeliet, E. Z. (1964): Influence of lithium ions on the transmembrane potential and cation content of cardiac cells. *J. Gen. Physiol.*, 47:501.
106. Singer, I., and Rotenberg, D. (1973): Mechanism of lithium action. *N. Engl. J. Med.*, 289:254.
107. Horowitz, L. C., and Fisher, G. U. (1969): Acute lithium intoxication. *N. Engl. J. Med.*, 281:1369.
108. Tangedahl, T. N., and Gau, G. T. (1972): Myocardial irritability associated with lithium carbonate therapy. *N. Engl. J. Med.*, 287:867.
109. Tseng, H. L. (1972): Interstitial myocarditis probably related to lithium carbonate intoxication. *Arch. Pathol.*, 92:444.

110. Swedberg, K., and Winblap, B. (1974): Heart failure as a complication of lithium treatment. *Acta Med. Scand.,* 196:279.
111. Tilkian, A. G., Schroeder, J. S., Kao, J. J., and Hultaren, H. N. (1976): The cardiovascular effects of lithium: A review of the literature. *AMS Med.,* 61:665.
112. Wilson, J. R., Kraus, E. S., Bailas, M. M., et al. (1976): Reversible sinus node abnormalities due to lithium carbonate therapy. *N. Engl. J. Med.,* 294:1223.
113. Wellens, H. J., Cats, V. M., and Duren, D. R. (1975): Symptomatic sinus node abnormalities following lithium carbonate therapy. *Am. J. Med.,* 59:285.
114. Demers, R. G., and Heninger, G. R. (1971): Electrocardiographic T wave changes during lithium carbonate treatment. *JAMA,* 218:381.
115. Tilkian, A. G., Schroeder, J. S., and Kao, J. (1976): Effect of lithium on cardiovascular performance. Report on extended ambulatory monitoring and exercise testing before and after lithium therapy. *Am. J. Cardiol.,* 38:701.
116. Wren, J. C., and Dana, J. B. (1976): Electrocardiographic changes during lithium therapy. *J. Maine Med. Assoc.,* 67:185.
117. Peterson, V., Huidts, S., Thomsen, K., et al. (1974): Effect of prolonged thiazide treatment on renal lithium clearance. *Br. Med. J.,* 3:143.
118. Thompson, K., and Schon, M. (1968): Renal lithium excretion in man. *Am. J. Physiol.,* 215:823.
119. Byck, R. (1977): Drugs used in the treatment of psychiatric disorders. In: *Pharmacologic Basis of Therapeutics,* edited by L. Goodman and A. Gilman, p. 185. Macmillan, New York.
120. Grant, A. P. (1962): Sequential trial of isocarboxazid in angina pectoris. *Br. Med. J.,* 1:513.
121. Cole, S. L., Kaye, D., and Griffith, G. C. (1963): Assay of antianginal agents: A long acting nitrate, psychic energizers and a tranquilizer. *Am. J. Cardiol.,* 11:639.
122. Barber, J. M., Murphy, F. M., and Cheeseman, E. A. (1958): A clinical trial of isocarboxazid (Marplan) in angina pectoris. *Br. Heart J.,* 20:162.
123. Shamsie, S. J., and Barriga, C. (1971): The hazards of use of monoamine oxidase inhibitors in disturbed adolescents. *Can. Med. Assoc. J.,* 71:517.
124. Blackwell, B., Marley, E., Price, J., et al. (1967): Hypertensive interactions between monoamine oxidase inhibitors and food stuffs. *Br. J. Psychiatry,* 113:349.
125. Villiers, J. C. (1966): Intracranial hemorrhage in patients treated with monoamine oxidase inhibitors. *Br. J. Psychiatry,* 112:109.
126. Jounela, A. J., and Kiuimakis, T. (1973): Possible sensitivity to meperidine in phenylketonuria. *N. Engl. J. Med.,* 288:1411.
127. Rom, W. N., and Brenner, E. J. (1972): Toxicity by interaction of tricyclic antidepressant and monoamine oxidase inhibitor. *Calif. Med.,* 117:65.
128. Stimmel, B. (1975): The effects of mood-altering drugs on the heart. In: *Current Cardiovascular Topics. Vol. 1: Drugs in Cardiology,* edited by E. Donoso, pp. 219–221. Stratton Intercontinental, New York.

Chapter 9

Marijuana

The cannabis sativa plant has been known to humankind since the early milleniums, being capable of abundant growth in tropical and temperate climates. Many local names have been assigned to the products of this plant, depending on the portion utilized to make the consumable substance and the country where the plant is cultivated. Hashish or charas represents the resin extracted from the tops of the flowering plant and is considered to be much more potent than other preparations. Preparations of dry leaves and flowering shoots are termed bhang, kif, dugga, macohna. Ganga refers to an extract of the smaller leaves. Marijuana is the American term usually referring to any preparation of the plant consumed to produce psychic changes (1).

It is difficult to estimate with any precision the magnitude of marijuana use (Chapter 1) since the illegality of the drug prevents accurate record keeping. In 1971, the United States National Commission on Marihuana and Drug Abuse (2) estimated 24 million Americans to have used marijuana at some time. A more recent estimate by Dupont has indicated that up to 13 million Americans may now be smoking marijuana, with at least 15% of the general population age 11 and over having used this drug on at least one occasion (3). Most users tend to be in the younger age ranges, with increases in marijuana use between high school and 5 years after graduation in several studies reported as changing from 20 to 62% (4). Marijuana use decreases precipitously in adults over age 35 in whom continued use is a rarity (5).

PHARMACOLOGY

Regardless of the components of the plant that are consumed, the active principles are the cannabinoids (Table 1), with delta^9-tetrahydrocannabinol (Δ^9-THC) being primarily responsible for the psychic effects of the drug. Cannabinol (CBN) and cannabidol (CBD), the two other major cannabinoids, are essentially inactive in humans (6). In most instances, consumption of marijuana is by smoking. When used in this manner, a variable amount of Δ^9-THC is lost through exhaled air, the respiratory dead space, or elimination in the smoke. Pyrolysis may also destroy some of the drug, although it is likely that volatilization in the smoke occurs prior to the actual burning of the tobacco (7). The efficacy of delivery of marijuana through smoking has

TABLE 1. *Constituents of cannabis isolated from cannabis sativa*

Cannabinol (CBN)
Cannabidol (CBD)
Cannabinolic acid
Cannabidolic acid
Cannabigerol (CBG)
Cannabicyclol
8-Tetrahydrocannabinol (Δ^8-THC)[a]
9-Tetrahydrocannabinol (Δ^9-THC)[a]

[a] Psychoactive substances.

been reported to range from 20 to 80%, with an average efficiency of 50% (8). An American marijuana cigarette approximates 500 mg marijuana and is estimated to contain 5 to 20 mg Δ^9-THC, with 2.5 to 5 mg Δ^9-THC being absorbed.

Oral doses of Δ^9-THC are also effective, with the equivalent dosage needed reported to be 2.5- to threefold higher. This is probably related to the destruction of marijuana in the gastrointestinal tract.

Biotransformation

After smoking, Δ^9-THC, which is highly lipophilic, is absorbed rapidly by the mucous membranes, with pharmacologic effects noted within minutes. Oxidation to 11-hydroxy-Δ^9-THC, an active metabolite, occurs with subsequent metabolism to inactive products. Δ^9-THC is an avid binder to plasma proteins. Plasma concentrations reach peak values between 10 and 30 min, with an initial rapid fall reflecting a wide distribution to lipid-rich tissues (9). Plasma levels may remain elevated for more than 2 hr, although traces of Δ^9-THC can be found in the plasma for up to several days. This finding probably reflects a gradual metabolism as well as the release of Δ^9-THC from tissues. The plasma half-life of Δ^9-THC and its metabolites is 5 to 7 days (10).

When ingested, a delay in appearance of plasma levels occurs, with peak levels seen from 30 to 120 min. Subjective effects persist for 3 to 5 hr. There is little evidence to indicate that consumption of repeated doses of marijuana for several days or daily smoking for several weeks will produce permanent, clinically detectable accumulation in tissues (11). Increased dosages over more prolonged periods, however, may result in persistent deposition in fatty tissue (12).

Δ^9-THC is metabolized in the liver and excreted in the urine and feces, with urinary metabolites detected for weeks. 11-Hydroxy-Δ^9-THC is one of the major metabolites and is believed to be predominantly although not solely responsible for the clinical effects of Δ^9-THC (13). Animal studies have suggested that the metabolites produced in the biotransformation of marijuana may vary, depending on whether the liver or lung is the primary organ involved (5). The clinical relevance of these findings with respect to effects observed following smoking or ingestion remains to be clarified. Chronic marijuana smokers metabolize Δ^9-THC more rapidly than do nonsmokers (14). This might explain the considerable amount of tolerance that has been observed clinically in regular users of cannabis products.

CARDIOVASCULAR EFFECTS

There is a general consensus that marijuana can affect the cardiovascular system primarily through the actions of Δ^9-THC. The magnitude of such an effect, however, is dependent on (a) dose employed, (b) route of administration, (c) prestudy status of the subject with respect to the presence of chronic marijuana usage, and (d) whether such effects are measured acutely or on a long-term basis.

Hemodynamics

Normal Subjects

Single Dose Studies

Experimentally, Δ^9-THC administered intravenously in doses of approximately 1 mg/kg may reduce blood pressure in dogs, cats, and monkeys often associated with bradycardia (15). This effect is consistent and at times considerable. Synthetic derivatives have also been shown to produce marked hypotension in both laboratory animals and humans (16).

Studies of cardiac performance in normal subjects given intravenous infusions of Δ^9-THC at a rate equivalent to smoking one 5-mg Δ^9-THC marijuana cigarette show a significant increase in heart rate and left ventricular ejection time (LVET), with a shortened preejection period (PEP). There is no change in arterial pressure or afterload, suggesting an increased venous return associated with an increase in cardiac volume and stroke output to be responsible for these changes. Administration of propranolol prior to Δ^9-THC, although preventing a shortening in PEP, did not affect either heart rate or LVET (17).

Oral doses of 10 to 70 mg Δ^9-THC (120 to 946 μg/kg) produce a consistent early increase in pulse rate (7,18–20). It is controversial whether a linear relationship exists between dose administered and pulse rate. Kipplinger et al. (21) have reported a linear dose response with the increase in pulse rate enhanced in the presence of alcohol at a blood concentration of 0.05% and blocked by the use of propranolol. Supine blood pressure has been reported as remaining stable or slightly decreasing. At higher doses, however, several instances of orthostatic hypotension have been observed. Congestion of the conjunctival blood vessels is one of the most constant findings. The congestion persists longer than tachycardia, being apparent more than 90 min after smoking. It is dose related and considered to be secondary to a direct effect of cannabis on the conjuctival vessels rather than to an irritant effect of the cigarette smoke.

Beaconsfield et al. (22,23) studied the circulatory response to Δ^9-THC consumed in one cigarette at a dose equivalent to that used by habitual smokers in both regular smokers and nondependent subjects. An increase in pulse rate, as well as lymph blood flow, was noted. The degree of tachycardia was related to the amount of Δ^9-THC absorbed. A maximum rate was reached within 30 min of smoking and persisted for more than 40 min. This response could be produced and at times potentiated after administration of atropine but not after pretreatment with propranolol.

In a study of conditioned marijuana smokers utilizing Δ^9-THC in a dose approximating one to two marijuana cigarettes, Weiss et al. (24) found, in addition to an increased heart rate and forearm blood flow, an increase in recumbent mean arterial blood pressure and an increase in forearm conductance and urinary excretion of free epinephrine. There was a significant shortening of the ventricular PEP and attenuation of reflex venoconstriction in response to deep breathing. These changes were indicative of increased sympathoadrenal activity.

Similarly, Tashkin et al. (25) measured parameters of left ventricular performance of marijuana smoking in 21 experienced marijuana smokers. No change was noted in stroke volume or PEP/LVET. Cardiac rate, cardiac output, and circumferential fiber shortening velocity increased slightly, suggesting the absence of any adverse effect on myocardial contractility.

In summary, tachycardia is the most consistent change reported with single-dose marijuana use. Conflicting findings exist with respect to its effect on blood pressure. In one instance, syncope was reported in several intoxicated subjects (26). The discordant findings may be related to the dosage of Δ^9-THC utilized, the inability to distinguish the effects of posture, and the effects of single doses as compared to chronic marijuana administration.

Long-Term Administration

Several investigators have described the cardiovascular effects of long-term, rather than single-dose, administration of Δ^9-THC. Bernstein et al. (27) noted a lowering of systolic and diastolic blood pressure in volunteers who smoked three to six marijuana cigarettes per day for 21 days. Benowitz et al. (28) performed a double-bind study with 10 volunteers involving various dosage schedules of daily doses of 210 mg Δ^9-THC. They found that, in normal subjects, prolonged ingestion of Δ^9-THC resulted in a significant lowering of blood pressure and slowing of the heart rate. Orthostatic hypotension in the absence of hypovolemia was observed, associated with a submaximal compensatory increase in heart rate. The orthostatic changes were of sufficient intensity to result in the appearance of dizziness during the period of maximal postural hypotension. The Valsalva maneuver resulted in a delayed and diminished slowing of the heart rate post-Valsalva release.

Weight gain occurred in all subjects, with a mean increase of 3.6 kg. This increase in weight started with administration of Δ^9-THC, continued throughout day 10 of the study, and fell sharply subsequent to discontinuing the drug, reaching baseline levels by day 3 or 4. Hemoglobin concentrations were also altered, inversely proportional to weight gain. These findings suggest that an increase in plasma volume represents a compensatory response to the hypotensive effects of the drug.

On exercise, all subjects experienced a less-than-expected rise in systolic and diastolic blood pressure based on their basal state values, although the heart rate did increase. These effects were most pronounced during early administration and less with continued use.

Continued use of Δ^9-THC in this study resulted in a tolerance to the orthostatic hypotensive changes, the initial tachycardia, and the blunting of blood pressure rising during exercise. No tolerance was noted, however, with respect to the supine hypotensive effects of the drug. On discontinuing the Δ^9-THC, no effects were noted on the cardiovascular system. A return to baseline values of all measured cardiovascular parameters occurred within 1 day. These findings suggest that although tissue accumulation occurs in organs with a high adipose content, on prolonged administration cardiovascular effects are dependent on the presence of increased plasma levels of Δ^9-THC or its active metabolites.

Persons With Coronary Artery Disease

The attributes of marijuana as an antianxiety or euphoria-producing drug suggest the possibility of its use in coronary artery disease to alleviate anxiety and tension not infrequently found in the anginal or postmyocardial infarction patient.

The specific effect of marijuana in persons with known cardiac disease has been studied by Aronow and Cassidy (29), who compared marijuana and placebo marijuana in subjects with angina pectoris. These authors found a significant decrease of 48% in mean exercise performance until the onset of angina following smoking one marijuana cigarette as compared to a mean decrease in exercise performance of 8.6% with placebo. An increase in carboxyhemoglobin levels was noted with both marijuana and placebo; however, no changes were recorded in resting heart rate or blood pressure. Marijuana was also noted to increase systolic pressure heart rate product, resulting in a further increase in myocardial oxygen demand. When these effects are combined with a decrease in myocardial oxygen delivery and increased epinephrine release, angina may be induced early.

The echocardiographic effects of marijuana versus placebo in anginal patients were also studied by this group (30) in a double-blind crossover study. Both placebo and marijuana decreased the end-diastolic volume, cardiac index, and ejection fraction. In addition, marijuana caused a significant increase in heart rate and systolic and end-diastolic pressure. The hemodynamic changes induced by the placebo were attributed to the elevations in carboxyhemoglobin levels, whereas the additional effects of marijuana were related to the known actions of Δ^9-THC. The net effect of marijuana in anginal patients was a decrease in myocardial oxygen delivery, an increase in myocardial oxygen demand, and a decrease in exercise time until onset of angina. Whether these changes are caused by a Δ^9-THC-induced increase in heart rate and afterload or a direct negative inotropic effect on the myocardium remains to be determined.

It is of interest that psychologic studies in patients with angina have also demonstrated less than salutary findings. Smoking marijuana resulted in an increased cognitive impairment and a disruption in the expected relationship between affect measures and specific cardiovascular variables in five of 10 patients (31).

Although these studies involve small numbers of patients, the ability of marijuana to cause increases in pulse rate and blood pressure in normal subjects, associated with decrease in exercise capacity in patients with angina, suggests that the use of this drug in patients with hypertension or coronary heart disease may be associated with more liabilities than benefits.

Electrocardiographic Changes

In addition to sinus tachycardia, other electrocardiographic changes can occur secondary to Δ^9-THC. Miller et al. (32) studied His bundle recordings in subjects administered intravenous Δ^9-THC at a dose equivalent to smoking one 5-mg Δ^9-THC-containing marijuana cigarette. A markedly enhanced sinus automaticity was noted associated with facilitation of sinoatrial and AV nodal conduction. Nonspecific ST and T-wave changes indicative of mild alterations and repolarization may also occur. Kochar and Hosko (33) studied the electrocardiographic effects of intermediate and large doses (200 and 300 μg/kg) in seven subjects whose smoking history varied from heavy use (3 times weekly) to no use whatsoever. After the small dose of Δ^9-THC, only two of the seven subjects showed electrocardiographic changes. Administration of the larger dose, however, was followed by increased heart rate in six subjects, ST segment and T-wave changes developing in two, and premature ventricular contractions noted in one. Interestingly, these electrocardiographic abnormalities were prominent only in previous cannabis users.

Roth et al. (34) utilized continuous electrocardiographic monitoring in 10 normal subjects during marijuana administration. The dosage of marijuana administered in cigarettes was adjusted to a Δ^9-THC content of 20 mg. Although marijuana-induced tachycardia was noted, T-wave changes were slight, and only five ventricular premature contractions occurred in all sessions. These data suggest that marijuana does not ordinarily increase the incidence of ventricular premature contractions in young male subjects and that hypotensive episodes occasionally reported with the use of marijuana may be idiosyncratic rather than arrhythmia induced.

Although the clinical relevance of these findings remains to be determined, the appearance of ventricular premature contractions and ventricular bigeminy subsequent to Δ^9-THC or marijuana administration, sometimes accompanied by dizziness and syncope, have been noted by several investigators (35). Further evaluations of these alterations with the use of long-term halter monitoring is warranted, especially in populations at high risk for development of arrhythmias.

Mechanism of Action

The cardiovascular effects of Δ^9-THC appear to be biphasic, depending on dosage and mode of administration (acute or chronic) (Table 2). Acute administration of single, moderate doses results in a sympathetic stimulation, whereas prolonged administration or administration of large single doses appears to inhibit the sympathetic system.

The mechanism by which Δ^9-THC acts on the cardiovascular system has not been precisely defined, but the predominant action appears to be on the autonomic nervous system, affecting both sympathetic and parasympathetic pathways. Weiss et al. (24) have demonstrated increased urinary excretion of epinephrine after Δ^9-THC administration. Other investigators have invoked a stimulation of the beta-adrenergic system as the main mechanism of action. Although this site may be active during a single dose administration, other mechanisms appear to predominate with continued use. Most recently, Gash et al. (46) have demonstrated an enhancement of plasma norepinephrine levels which persist for as long as 2 hr.

Benowitz and Jones (28) studied the effect of sympathomimetic amines, atropine, and propranolol on volunteers chronically maintained on Δ^9-THC. In contrast to animal studies, which revealed an increased pressor response to catecholamines after Δ^9-THC, these investigators did not note an alteration in Δ^9-THC-induced hemodynamic responses with either alpha- or beta-

TABLE 2. *Hemodynamic effects of marijuana administration*

Dose	Heart rate	Blood pressure	Orthostatic changes	Plasma volume	Myocardial contractility
Acute administration, small or moderate dose	↑	V	—	—	—
Chronic administration or administration of large single dose	↓	↓	+	↑	NM
Coronary artery disease, acute administration	↑	↑	—	NM	↓

↑, Increase; ↓, decrease; V, variable responses reported; —, no change; NM, not measured.

sympathetic agonists. Parasympathetic block with atropine was found to result in a greater heart rate during Δ^9-THC ingestion, suggesting an enhancement of parasympathetic tone. After both sympathetic and parasympathetic block, however, Δ^9-THC was still able to induce an increase in heart rate. This suggests a direct cardiac action of Δ^9-THC in addition to its effect on the autonomic system. It is also possible that Δ^9-THC may have an antihistamine effect. Experimentally, it can prevent hypotensive changes normally induced by histamine and acetylcholine (23). The clinical relevance of this finding remains to be clarified.

OVERDOSE REACTIONS

Adverse physical reactions to marijuana are relatively rare when the drug is smoked or consumed orally, with nausea and vomiting being most frequently reported with large doses. In the street setting, marijuana is rarely injected intravenously, and overdose reactions are infrequent. Intravenous injection is associated with considerable toxicity (35–37). Toxic effects may be dependent on both dosage and the presence of allergic or idiosyncratic reactions to existing contaminants or other substances. Following injection, nausea, vomiting, and diarrhea are frequent. Hypotension, renal failure, and associated hematologic alterations, consisting of a leukemoid reaction, anemia, and thrombocytopenia, have also been reported.

The hypotension, which at times may be considerable, may be related to a hypovolemia secondary to copious diarrhea or may be the result of a direct central nervous system (CNS) effect of marijuana on the vasomotor receptor. The occurrence of renal failure is related to the preceding hypotension and is quite transient, responding quickly to fluid replacement. Proteinurea of 3 g/day has been reported in one patient, suggesting transient glomerular damages (37).

DRUG INTERACTIONS

Since metabolism of marijuana occurs mainly through the hepatic microsomal enzyme system, interactions with other drugs also metabolized through this pathway may occur. Metabolism of Δ^9-THC can be accelerated by pretreatment with phenobarbital and inhibited *in vitro* by acute administration of nortriptyline and desmethylimipramine metabolites, phenobarbital, amphetamine, and meprobamate (38). The clinical relevance of these reactions remains unknown. The combined use of marijuana and some tranquilizers may result in adverse effects.

The use of marijuana is frequently associated with consumption of other mood-altering drugs. In a survey of 107 marijuana users, Carlin and Post (39) found more than 74% to be simultaneously using other drugs. Alcohol and stimulants are most often used with marijuana. Since marijuana acts on the autonomic nervous system, it is possible that combined use of such drugs might have added deleterious cardiovascular effects (Table 3). Evans et al. (40) noted combined use of marijuana and dextroamphetamines to cause additive increases in tachycardia and elevations of systolic blood pressure. This was not associated with any interactive effect on psychomotor performance. Alcohol has also been shown to enhance Δ^9-THC-induced tachycardia; however, synergistic effects were observed on impairment of psychomotor performance (41). Administration of secobarbital and marijuana smoking can produce effects similar to those seen with alcohol in regard to both subjective responses and psychomotor impairment (42).

Benewitz et al. (28) demonstrated the ability of atropine to induce an increase in blood pressure in patients maintained on chronic Δ^9-THC. Whether this interaction is central or peripheral has not been clearly defined. Concomitant use of parasympathetic blocking agents and Δ^9-THC may result in a potentially dangerous drug interaction. Gregg et al. (43) noted prolonged

TABLE 3. *Interactions of other mood-altering drugs with marijuana*

Drug	Clinical effect
Alcohol	Impaired psychomotor performance; enhancement of Δ^9-THC-induced tachycardia
Amphetamines	Synergistic effect on heart rate and blood pressure
Atropine	Synergistic effect on heart rate and blood pressure
Barbiturates	Synergistic impairment of both subjective and psychomotor responses
Diazepam	Enhancement of diazepam-induced CNS depression
Oxymorphone	Enhancement of narcotic-induced CNS depression

postoperative tachycardia in a series of patients who had smoked marijuana within 72 hr before undergoing outpatient general anesthesia for oral surgery.

Intravenous administration of Δ^9-THC to healthy subjects pretreated with oxymorphone or followed by an injection of diazepam results in prominent CNS depression, marked by drowsiness and difficulty in arousal. These effects are much more pronounced with oxymorphone but are clearly detectable with diazepam (44). Clinically important potentiation of narcotic effects with concomitant use of marijuana, however, has not been consistently demonstrated (45).

SUMMARY

Marijuana has been shown to elicit an effect on the cardiovascular system in all studies reported in the literature. The particular physiologic response elicited varies with dose, duration of administration, and presence of preexisting coronary artery disease. Acute administration in essentially healthy persons is consistently associated with a tachycardia, whereas changes in blood pressure are variable and probably not of clinical importance. Myocardial contractility is unaffected. Long-term administration can result in a decrease in heart rate and blood pressure, at times associated with orthostatic changes and an expansion of plasma volume. Marijuana administered to persons with coronary artery disease is accompanied by a deleterious physiologic response, which includes an increase in myocardial oxygen demand and a decrease in myocardial oxygen delivery accompanied by signs of diminished myocardial contractility. The end result of these effects is a decrease in mean exercise performance with a more rapid onset of angina. The use of marijuana in persons with coronary disease should therefore be discouraged.

REFERENCES

1. Lieberman, C. M., and Lieberman, B. W. (1972): Marihuana: A medical review. *N. Engl. J. Med.,* 284:88.
2. National Commission on Marihuana and Drug Abuse (1972): Marihuana. A signal of misunderstanding. Vol. 1, March, 1972, U.S. Government Printing Office, Washington, D.C.
3. Marijuana and Health: The Fourth Annual Report to the U.S. Congress from the Secretary of Health, Education and Welfare (1974): NIDA, Rockville, Maryland.
4. Green, M. H., Nightingale, S., and Dupont, R. (1975): Evolving patterns of drug abuse. *Ann. Intern. Med.,* 83:402.
5. Marihuana Research Findings (1976): National Institute on Drug Abuse Research Monograph Series No. 14. U.S. Dept. HEW, No. 017–024–00622–0, Washington, D.C.
6. Hollister, L. E. (1973): Cannabidol and cannabinol in man. *Experientia,* 29:825.
7. Hollister, L. E. (1971): Marihuana in man: Three years later. *Science,* 172:21.
8. Manno, J. E., Kiplinger, G. F., Scholz, N., et al. (1971): The influence of alcohol and marihuana on motor and mental performance. *Clin. Pharmacol. Ther.,* 12:202.
9. Kreuz, D. S., and Axelrod, J. (1973): Delta 9 tetrahydrocannabinol: Localization in body fat. *Science,* 179:391.

10. Paton, W. D. M. (1975): The pharmacology of marihuana. *Ann. Rev. Pharmacol.,* 15:191.
11. Isbell, H., Gorodetzsky, G. W., Jasinski, D., et al. (1967): Effects of (−) Δ^9-trans-tetrahydrocannibinol in man. *Psychopharmacologia,* 11:184.
12. Leighty, E. G., Fentiman, A. F., and Poltz, R. L. (1976): Long retained metabolites of $^9\Delta$ and Δ^8-tetrahydrocannabinols identified as novel fatty acid conjugates. *Res. Commun. Chem. Pathol. Pharmacol.,* 14:13.
13. Perez-Reyes, M., Wagner, D., Brine, D. R., et al. (1976): Tetrahydrocannabinols: Plasma disappearance in man and rate of penetration to mouse brain. In: *Pharmacology of Marihuana,* edited by M. C. Braude and S. Szara, pp. 117–123. Raven Press, New York.
14. Lemberger, L., Tamarkin, N. R., Axelrod, J., et al. (1971): Delta 9-tetrahydrocannabinol: Metabolism and disposition in long term marihuana smokers. *Science,* 173:22.
15. Boyd, E. S., Boyd, E. H., Muchmore, J. S., et al. (1971): Effects of two tetrahydrocannabinols and of pentobarbitol on cortical evoked responses in the squirrel monkey. *J. Pharmacol. Exp. Ther.,* 170:480.
16. Hardman, H. F., Domino, E. F., and Seevers, M. H. (1971): General pharmacological actions of some synthetic tetrahydrocannabinol derivatives. *Pharmacol. Rev.,* 23:295.
17. Kanakis, C., Pouget, J. M., and Rosen, K. M. (1976): Effects of delta-9-tetrahydracannabinol (Cannabis) on cardiac performance with and without beta blockade. *Circulation,* 53:703.
18. Mechoulam, R., Shani, A., Edery, L. T., et al. (1968): Chemical basis of hashish activity. *Science,* 169:611.
19. Johnson, S., and Domino, E. F. (1971): Some cardiovascular effects of marihuana smoking in volunteers. *Clin. Pharmacol. Ther.,* 12:762.
20. Renault, P. E., Schusler, C. R., Heinrich, R., et al. (1971): Marihuana—Standardized smoke administration and dose effect curves on heart rate in humans. *Science,* 174:589.
21. Kipplinger, G. F., Manno, J. E., Rodda, B. E., et al. (1971): Dose response analysis of the effects of tetrahydrocannabinol in man. *Clin. Pharmacol. Ther.,* 12:650.
22. Beaconsfield, P., Ginsberg, J., and Rainsbury, R. (1972): Marihuana smoking—cardiovascular effects in man and possible mechanisms. *N. Engl. J. Med.,* 287:209.
23. Beaconsfield, P. (1974): Some cardiovascular effects of cannabis. *Am. Heart J.,* 87:143.
24. Weiss, J. L., Watanabe, A. M., Lemberger, L., et al. (1972): Cardiovascular effects of delta 9-tetrahydrocannabinol in man. *Clin. Pharmacol. Ther.,* 13:671.
25. Tashkin, D. P., Levisman, J. A., Abbasi, A. S., et al. (1977): Short term effects of smoked marijuana on left ventricular function in man. *Chest,* 72:20.
26. Hollister, L. T., Richards, R. K., and Gillespie, H. K. (1968): Comparison of tetrahydrocannabinol and synhexyl in man. *Clin. Pharmacol. Ther.,* 9:783.
27. Bernstein, J. G., Becker, D., Tabor, T. F., et al. (1974): Physiological assessments: Cardiovascular function. In: *The Use of Marijuana. A Psychological and Physiological Inquiry,* edited by J. Mendelson et al., pp. 147–160. Plenum Press, New York.
28. Benowitz, N. L., and Jones, R. T. (1976): Cardiovascular effects of prolonged delta-9-tetrahydrocannabinol ingestion. *Clin. Pharmacol. Ther.,* 18:287.
29. Aronow, W. S., and Cassidy, J. (1974): Effect of marihuana and placebo marihuana smoking on angina pectoris. *N. Engl. J. Med.,* 291:65.
30. Prokash, R., Aronow, W. S., Warren, M., et al. (1975): Effect of marihuana and placebo marihuana smoking on hemodynamics in coronary disease. *Clin. Pharmacol. Ther.,* 18:90.
31. Gottschalk, L. A., Aronow, W. S., and Prakash, R. (1977): Effect of marijuana and placebo marijuana smoking on psychological state and on psychophysiological cardiovascular functioning in anginal patients. *Biol. Psychiatry,* 12:255.
32. Miller, R. H., Dhingra, R. C., Kanakis, C., et al. (1977): The electrophysiologic effects of delta-9-tetrahydrocannabinol (Cannabis) on cardiac conduction in man. *Am. Heart J.,* 94:740.

33. Kochar, M., and Hosko, M. J. (1973): Electrocardiographic effects of marihuana. *JAMA,* 225:25.
34. Roth, W. T., Tinklenberg, J. R., Kopell, B. S., et al. (1972): Continuous electrocardiographic monitoring during marihuana intoxication. *Clin. Pharmacol. Ther.,* 14:533.
35. King, A. B., and Cowen, D. L. (1969): Effect of intravenous injection of marihuana. *JAMA,* 210:724.
36. Payne, R. S., and Brand, S. N. (1975): The toxicity of intravenously used marihuana. *JAMA,* 233:351.
37. Henderson, A. H., and Pugsley, D. J. (1968): Collapse after intravenous injection of hashish. *Br. Med. J.,* 3:229.
38. Siemens, A. J., deNie, L. C., Kalant, H., et al. (1975): Effects of various psychoactive drugs on the metabolism of delta 9 tetrahydrocannabinol by rats in vivo and in vitro. *Eur. J. Pharmacol.,* 31:136.
39. Carlin, A. S., and Post, R. D. (1971): Pattern of drug use among marijuana smokers. *JAMA,* 218:867.
40. Evans, M. A., Martz, R., Rodda, B. E., et al. (1976): Effects of marijuana-dextroamphetamine combination. *Clin. Pharmacol. Ther.,* 20:350.
41. MacAvoy, M. G., and Marks, D. F. (1975): Divided attention performance of cannabis users and nonusers following cannabis and alcohol. *Psychopharmacologia,* 44:147.
42. Dalton, W. S., Martz, R., Zemberger, L., et al. (1975): Effects of marijuana combined with secobarbital. *Clin. Pharmacol. Ther.,* 18:298.
43. Gregg, J. M., Campbell, R. L., Levin, K. J., et al. (1976): Cardiovascular effects of cannabinol during oral surgery. *Anesth. Anal. Curr. Res.,* 55:203.
44. Smith, T. C., and Kulp, R. A. (1976): Respiratory and cardiovascular effects of delta-9-tetrahydrocannabinol alone and in combination with oxymorphone pentobarbital and diazepam. In: *The Therapeutic Potential of Marihuana,* edited by S. Cohen and R. C. Stillman, p. 123. Plenum Press, New York.
45. Johnstone, R. E., Lief, P. L., Kulp, R. A., et al. (1975): Combination of Δ^9 tetrahydrocannabinol with oxymorphone or pentobarbital: Effects on ventilatory control and cardiovascular dynamics. *Anesthesiology,* 42:674.
46. Gash, A., Karliner, J. S., Janowsky, D., et al. (1978): Effects of smoking marihuana on left ventricular performance and plasma norepinephrine. *Ann. Intern. Med.,* 89:448.

Chapter 10

Hallucinogenic Agents

THE ALKYLAMINES AND ALKYLTRYPTAMINES

The nonprescribed use of hallucinogens (Table 1) reached a peak in the late 1960s and then started to decline. Abuse of these drugs, however, still occurs. A survey of drug abuse episodes occurring nationwide at crisis centers or emergency rooms showed lysergic acid diethylamide (LSD) consumption to rank sixth among psychedelic drugs reported. In most instances, LSD contacts involved persons under 30 years of age (1). LSD is considered the prototype for the drugs in this group, since the majority of these agents produce similar effects despite their different chemical structures (Table 2).

Pharmacology

LSD, an indole derivative, is rapidly absorbed from the gastrointestinal tract. When injected intravenously, plasma levels initially fall steeply, followed by a slow decline over an 8-hr. The plasma half-life is approximately 175 min. Distribution is widespread and rapid, with the highest concentrations found in the lung, liver, kidney, and brain (2). Symptomatic changes are perceived within 40 min after ingestion, with the severity of the psychologic effects proportionate to dose. Symptoms begin to resolve in about 12

TABLE 1. *Commonly used hallucinogenic agents*

Group	Drug	Street terminology
Indole alkylamines		
Ergot alkaloids	Lysergic acid diamide	LSD, acid
Tryptamine derivatives	Psilocybin	
	Psilocin	
	Dimethyltryptamine	DMA, DMT
	Diethyltryptamine	DET
Phenylalkylamines	Mescaline	
	2,5 Dimethoxy-4-ethyl-amphetamine	DOET
	2-5 Dimethoxy-4-methyl-amphetamine	DOM, STP
	3 Methoxy-4-5-methyl-enedioxyamphetamine	MMDA
	3,4 Methylenedioxy-amphetamine	MDA, businessman's high, love drug
Hydrocarbons	Glue, paint thinner, aerosol propellants	
Anticholinergics	Atropine	
	Scopolamine	
Miscellaneous	Phencyclidine	PCP, angel dust, mist, goon, tic and toc, crystal, hog, superweed, busy bee
	Muscimol	
	Piperidylglycolate esters	
	Nutmeg	
	Nitrous oxide	

TABLE 2. *Comparison of effects of hallucinogenic drugs to LSD*

Drug	Effects compared to LSD
Alkyltryptamines	
Psilocybin	Similar but earlier onset, shorter duration, absence of hyperactivity and salivation
DMT	Similar but more intense and of much shorter duration
DET	Similar to DMT but less severe
Phenylalkylamines	
Mescaline	Similar but much greater dose needed to produce same intensity of effects; true hallucinations infrequent, pseudohallucinations most common
DOM, STP	Similar but less potent; much more potent than mescaline; hallucinations as intense in higher doses; accompanied by uncontrollable emotions

hr, although aftereffects lasting days have been reported (3). Metabolism is in the enterohepatic system and is relatively complete with the formation of 2-oxy-LSD, which is subsequently excreted in the feces.

The precise mechanism by which LSD produces its effects has not been clearly defined, although interactions with serotonin and other neurotransmitters are considered to be responsible. *In vitro* LSD is an antagonist of the peripheral actions of 5-hydroxytryptamine (5-HT). It has been postulated that LSD blockage of 5-HT within the central nervous system (CNS) produces the psychic effects of the drug. More recent evidence suggests, however, that LSD may actually mimic 5-HT action at synapses in the brain, the decreased rate of turnover of 5-HT representing the phenomenon of negative feedback (4,5).

Cardiovascular Effects

Little work has been performed concerning the cardiovascular effects of these drugs. Intravenous administration of LSD in dogs is associated with depression of left ventricular contractility and moderate tachycardia (6); but the relevance of this finding to oral use in humans is unclear. The quality of drugs purchased on the street may vary greatly, with the frequent presence of numerous adulterants.

Ingestion of hallucinogens generally produces dilated pupils and hyperactivity. Sympathomimetic signs include tachycardia, mild hypertension, diaphoresis, and tremor. Although sympathetic effects predominate, parasympathomimetic activity, such as hypotension, bradycardia, and respiratory depression, rarely may occur. If the hallucinogen is an agent chemically related to the amphetamines, e.g., 2-5 dimethoxy-4 methylamphetamine (STP), the sympathetic response may be greatly accentuated (7). Tolerance to these effects occurs, contingent on dose and frequency of ingestion. The hemodynamic changes observed might represent reactions to the psychologic effects of the drug rather than being a primary physiologic response.

Overdose Reactions

With high doses of hallucinogenic drugs, a toxic acute brain syndrome, manifested by disorientation and clouding of consciousness, occurs. If amphetamines are mixed with the hallucinogen, a marked sympathetic reaction, manifested by tachycardia, hypertension, and increased motor activity, is frequent. Although death has been reported following the ingestion of hallucinogens, the fatal outcome was probably related to the presence of adulterants, such as belladonna alkaloids or solvents. In such instances, cardiovascular or respiratory failure is the usual mode of exodus (7,8).

In the treatment of toxic symptoms, it is important to elicit the name of the specific hallucinogen consumed. The administration of phenothiazines to one who has taken STP can result in an accentuation of excitation as well as profound hypotension and circulatory collapse (9,10). In such patients, diazepam is helpful and may be required for as long as 1 week, as the reaction to STP can be quite prolonged.

Severe agitation secondary to LSD can be managed with phenothiazines or benzodiazepines in a dosage to allow the patient to enter a sleep state from which awakening can occur easily. Since the adverse reaction lasts from 8 to 24 hr, tranquilizing medication after this period is usually unnecessary, unless a psychotic state persists.

If the offending hallucinogen cannot be identified or is considered to be a substance with anticholinergic activity, the use of phenothiazines can result in an anticholinergic reaction that may include coma, tachycardia, arrhythmia, hypotension, and, rarely, circulatory and respiratory collapse. In such instances, slow intravenous administration of 1 to 4 mg physostigmine can abolish the toxic symptoms. The short duration of action of physostigmine mandates close observation, with administration every 1 to 2 hr if needed (8).

Drug Interactions

The action of LSD on 5-HT suggests that important interactions can occur with other drugs that effect this neurotransmitter (11). Reserpine-induced depletion of 5-HT can result in an accentuation of LSD activity. Conversely, the coadministration of monoamine oxidase (MAO) inhibitors with attendant increases in 5-HT can attenuate the response to LSD. The use of chlorpromazine or phenoxybenzamine can antagonize LSD and improve adverse psychic symptoms. The use of these agents, however, may be associated with an increased risk of orthostatic hypotension. The combination of mescaline and amphetamine has been associated with a potentiation of hallucinogenic effects.

INHALANTS: GLUE, SOLVENTS, AND AEROSOL PROPELLANTS

The inhalants are among the least expensive and most easily available hallucinogenic agents. For this reason, abuse of airplane glue, solvents, and aerosol propellants is usually confined to the preadolescent and adolescent years. The prevalence of solvent abuse and the specific solvent abused varies with time and place (Table 3). During the past several years, the aerosol propellants have become increasingly more popular, as has the custom of combining inhalation with ingestion of alcohol and sedative drugs. Surveys of junior high and high school students have reported solvent use in 2.8% of all students (12,13). Although most solvent inhalation occurs in the young and healthy, the toxicity of many of these substances on the cardiovascular system in laboratory animals is well known, and the potential for clinically adverse reactions is quite real. The aliphatic nitrites (amylnitrite

TABLE 3. *Commonly available solvents*

		Vehicle abused				
	Abuse reported	Paint lacquer, thinner	Gasoline	Glue	Propellants	Cardiac toxicity[a]
Aliphatic hydrocarbons n-Hexane, n-pentane, isooctaine	+	+	+			+
Aromatic hydrocarbons Benzene, tolvene styrene, xylene, naphthalene	+	+	+			+
Halogenated hydrocarbons						+
Dichlorinated Methylene,[b] Acetylene, ethylene, propylene	−	+			+	+
Trichlorinated Chloroform, Methyl-chloroform, Trichloro-ethylene	+	+		+	+	+
Fluorinated Trichlorofluoromethane, dichlorodifluoromethane, cyroflurane, dichlorotetrafluoromethane	+				+	+
Ketones	+	+				
Alcohols	+	+				
Aliphatic nitrates	+					

[a] In laboratory animals: Reduce ventricular fibrillation threshold and/or sensitize the myocardium to ventricular fibrillation.

[b] During biotransformation in the liver, carbon monoxide is formed, which may enhance the cardiotoxicity of this agent.

and isobutylnitrite) alone or at times commercially mixed with isobutyl alcohol are abused frequently by young adults to prolong orgasm rather than to produce a specific hallucinogenic effect.

The inhalants abused most frequently are the aliphatic and aromatic hydrocarbons, trichloroethylene and the fluorinated propellants (Table 3). Although the dichlorinated hydrocarbons do not have a history of abuse, these substances are likely to replace the fluorinated hydrocarbons in propellants and, unfortunately, have been demonstrated to be cardiotoxic in laboratory animals (14).

Fatal complications associated with solvent inhalation were initially attributed to anoxia. Subsequent studies in animals, however, have challenged this concept. Many of the solvents have been shown to induce ventricular arrhythmias through the ventricular fibrillation threshold or by hypersensitizing the myocardium to the effects of epinephrine (9,14–18). Flowers and Horan (10,19) have reported cardiac arrhythmias in dogs inhaling aerosols propelled with hydrocarbons. The arrhythmias produced consisted of junctional or ventricular escape rhythms ultimately terminating in asystole or ventricular fibrillation.

Bass (20), in a review of more than 100 cases of sudden death among teenage sniffers, noted a period of hyperactivity or emotional stress to precede the terminal event. Autopsy examinations of these patients were usually unremarkable, suggesting a fatal arrhythmia to be the mode of exodus. The precise etiology of arrhythmias induced in the clinical setting remains speculative. Based on the experimental studies, one may hypothesize (a) a direct toxic effect of the solvent, (b) an increased circulation of epinephrine associated with euphoria superimposed on a conduction system sensitized to an epinephrine effect, (c) anoxia secondary to solvent-induced depression of the respiratory center, or (d) anoxia secondary to suffocation when the solvent is inhaled in a plastic bag.

Although the greatest potential for toxicity occurs in situations involving abuse, evidence for adverse cardiologic effects exists even when an unwitting association with these agents is present or when propellants are used therapeutically. Speizer et al. (21) have suggested that the use of an aerosol containing monochlorodifluoromethane by pathology residents to accelerate fixing of tissue is associated with a 3.6-fold higher risk of palpitations than in unexposed residents. A statistical association without a confirming pathologic diagnosis between sympathomimetic bronchodilators and mortality in British asthmatics was made as early as 1966. However, the asthmatic death rate in England has declined subsequent to this time, despite the continued use of inhalers (22,23).

PHENCYCLIDINE

Phencyclidine [1-(1-phenylcyclohexyl)-piperidine] hydrochloride (PCP) is a white crystalline powder developed in the late 1960s for use as a short-acting intravenous anesthetic. The dissociative anesthesia produced was accompanied by considerable adverse side-effects, including hallucinations and hypertensive reactions. As a result, PCP was abandoned for human use in 1965 but retained as a veterinary anesthetic under the trade name of Sernylan (24).

PCP appeared as a street drug in California in the mid to late 1960s, marketed as the "PeaCe pill" or "angel dust." PCP was consumed by mixing with other substances or smoking PCP sprinkled on marijuana. Soon, clandestine laboratories began producing this substance in increasing amounts containing more impurities and associated with severe toxic reactions, at times terminating fatally. Although its use initially spread to other areas in the country, the associated adverse effects made PCP less desirable than the other readily available hallucinogens. Unfortunately, its use has increased during the past several years. It is estimated that at least 7 million persons have tried PCP, with adverse reactions recorded in more than 4,000 in 1977 (25). A recent survey (26) of youthful drug abusers revealed 32% of a sample of 2,750 to have a history of past or present PCP use. Since PCP can presently be purchased in tablet, powder, leaf, or rock crystal form, it can be consumed through ingestion, smoking, snorting, or injection.

Pharmacology

PCP is readily soluble in both water and ethanol. Intravenous or intramuscular injection results in an immediate clinical response, whereas a lag time of approximately 15 min follows oral consumption. Effects may last from hours to days, with the duration of action directly related to increasing dosage. Metabolism is rapid, with the monohydroxypiperidine derivative excreted primarily in the urine. The metabolites have little or no pharmacologic activity.

Cardiovascular Effects

PCP is a sympathomimetic drug with CNS stimulant and depressant properties that vary with dosage administered (Table 4). Experimentally, cardiovascular effects may also vary, with hypertension and tachycardia reported at low doses and arrhythmia and hypotension at higher doses (27,28). Clinically, cardiovascular changes are minimal with low doses, consisting of tachycardia and increases in both systolic and diastolic blood pressure (29,30).

Overdose Reactions

Toxic reactions are associated with marked agitation or drowsiness, nystagmus, tachycardia, elevation in blood pressure (which at times may be severe), pupillary miosis, hypotonia, ventilatory disturbances, and severe cases of markedly depressed respiration associated with hypotension and coma (31). The presence of normal or constricted pupils is an especially helpful sign, as intoxication with other hallucinogens is usually associated with pupillary dilatation.

Treatment is mainly supportive. The rapid absorption of PCP from the intestinal tract makes gastric lavage relatively ineffective once symptoms occur. Hydration with subsequent diuresis may aid in clearance of drug metabolites in the urine. Seizures may be controlled with anticonvulsive medications. Diazepam, 10 to 20 mg orally or 10 mg i.m., has been considered to be satisfactory in treating spasticity, opisthotonos, and nystagmus. Hypertension, if severe, must be treated. Hypotension, if mild, can be

TABLE 4. *Clinical effects of PCP*

Effect	
Low dose	High dose
Neurologic	
Nystagmus	
Variable pupil size (miotic)	
Depressed light reflex	
Blurred vision	
Diminished pain, proprioception, temperature sensation	
Increased deep tendon reflex/clonus	Decreased deep tendon reflex
Tremors	Convulsions
Slurred speech	
Drowsiness	Coma
Psychologic	
Amnesia	Delirium
Anxiety/agitation	Hallucinations (frequent)
Body image distortion	
Euphoria	
Depersonalization	
Disordered thought process	
Hallucinations (rare)	
Cardiovascular	
Increased pulse rate	Arrhythmias
Increased blood pressure (systolic and diastolic)	Decreased blood pressure
Gastrointestinal	
Nausea and vomiting, excessive salivation	
Renal	
Increased urine output	Decreased urine output
Respiratory	
Variable changes in depth and rate	Depression with respiratory arrest
Muscular	
Ataxia, muscle weakness, purposeless limb movements	Opisthotonos

treated supportively. The use of sympathomimetic agents or belladonna alkaloids are contraindicated. Haloperidol or phenothiazines may be helpful in modifying anxiety and agitation if reassurance is ineffective.

ANTICHOLINERGIC HALLUCINOGENS

The natural anticholinergics in the alkaloids of the belladonna plants have been used through the centuries by both physicians and poisoners alike. The hallucinogenic effects of these plants were recognized in Africa, India, and in this country by the American Indians, who chewed the leaves to promote

TABLE 5. *Over-the-counter anticholinergic drugs*

Trade name	Contents
Asthmador	Stramonium, belladonna
Mr. Sleep	Scopolamine, methapyrilene
Sleep Eze	Scopolamine, methapyrilene
Sominex	Scopolamine, methapyrilene, salicylamide
Sominex II	Scopolamine, methapyrilene, salicylamide, benadryl

visions during religious ceremonies. There are several alkaloids found in these plants, notably, atropine, hyoscyamine, and scopolamine. Since the actions of the other substances differ only quantitatively from that of atropine, this drug is considered the prototype.

At present, the use of the anticholinergics is mainly through physician prescription or purchase of over-the-counter medication (Table 5). However, several reports have appeared in the literature describing the use of jimson weed seeds by teenagers for a hallucinogenic effect (32).

Pharmacology

Atropine and related alkaloids, through competition at receptor sites, inhibit the muscarinic actions of acetylcholine and actually are more antimuscarinic than anticholinergic, having little effect at nicotinic receptor sites. Their actions can be overcome by increasing the concentration of acetylcholine at receptor sites either through administering drugs with cholinergic activity or by the use of anticholinesterase (33).

Absorption from the intestinal tract following ingestion is rapid, accompanied by a prompt disappearance from the blood with wide tissue distribution. Excretion is through the urine, with the majority of the ingested dose eliminated within the first 12 hr. This is in contrast to scopolamine, which is excreted in the urine to only a minor degree (34).

Cardiovascular Effects

The prominent action of atropine on the cardiovascular system is to alter heart rate through its effect on vagal tone. Initial effects may actually result in a transient bradycardia secondary to central vagal stimulation in the absence of peripheral muscarinic receptor block. This initial effect may be more pronounced with low doses of scopolamine (33). The predominant effect, however, is an increase in heart rate secondary to its blocking the vagal effect on the S-A and A-V nodes. Conduction through the S-A and A-V node increases, with tachycardia being most prominent in those persons with a high resting degree of vagal tone. The effect of atropine on blood pressure is variable but minimal. Systemic doses have been noted to result in transient rises in both systolic and diastolic blood pressure (35).

The effectiveness of atropine on increasing conduction through the S-A and A-V node has resulted in its recommendation in cases of severe sinus bradycardia and partial A-V block, especially in the presence of acute myocardial infarction. Since the initial effects of atropine, especially when administered in low doses, may be bradycardia, should a further slowing of the heart or A-V dissociation occur following administration of atropine, a larger dose should be given (36).

Recently, the use of atropine to accelerate heart rate in acute myocardial infarction has been questioned. Criticism is centered on the demonstration of an augmented myocardial oxygen consumption, with an extension of myocardial damage accompanying the increase in heart rate (37,38). In addition, some of the more malignant forms of premature ventricular contractions have been reported to persist, despite an increase in heart rate. In the face of severe bradycardia accompanied by diminished cardiac output, however, the judicious use of atropine can be beneficial (39).

Overdose Reactions

Poisoning from belladonna overdose may occur in infants and young children who accidently ingest medications containing these substances. Infants are particularly susceptible to the toxic effects of these agents, and intoxication has been reported secondary to conjunctival instillation of atropine-like drugs or from atropine in medications used to treat enuresis (33). Overuse of nonprescription medications containing scopolamine can result in intoxication, as can deliberate misuse of these drugs to obtain euphoria.

The anticholinergic syndrome may consist of dry mouth, flushing of skin, blurred vision associated with pupillary dilatation, elevated temperature, hypertension, tachycardia, palpitations, A-V conduction defects, and delirium. Severe cases may result in coma, respiratory depression, hypotension, circulatory failure, and death. This syndrome can exist with overdose from any drug that has anticholinergic actions, such as the tricyclic antidepressants. Diagnosis can best be made by noting early signs of inhibition of the parasympathetic system. This includes dryness of mucous membranes, pupillary dilatation nonresponsive to light, and tachycardia in the presence of confusion or delirium.

Treatment, in addition to supportive measures, should include gastric lavage if the medication has been taken orally and the intramuscular administration of physostigmine (in the absence of hypotension) in doses of 1 to 2 mg (in adults) to counteract the anticholinergic effects (41).

It should be emphasized that the duration of action of physostigmine is relatively short, so that repeated doses every 30 min to 2 hr may be needed.

Careful titration of physostigmine is necessary, as excessive doses may result in poisoning, manifested by severely miotic pupils, increased secretions, and muscle fasciculation. Phenothiazines are specifically contraindicated as a general sedative, since their antimuscarinic action may intensify toxicity. If sedation is mandatory or if seizures are present, diazepam may be used in judicious doses to avoid intensification of CNS depression.

REFERENCES

1. Drug Abuse Warning Network Phase III Report April 1974–1975 (1976): BNDD No. 72–47. IMS America, National Institute of Drug Abuse, Rockville Pike, Maryland.
2. Aghajanian, G. K., and Bing, O. H. L. (1964): Persistence of lysergic acid diethylamide in the plasma of human subjects. *Clin. Pharmacol. Ther.,* 5:611.
3. Freedman, D. X. (1968): The use and abuse of LSD. *Arch. Gen. Psychiatry,* 18: 300.
4. Aghajanian, G. K., Foote, W. E., and Sheard, M. H. (1970): Action of psychotogenic drugs on single midbrain raphe neurons. *J. Pharmacol. Ther.,* 171:178.
5. Brimblecombe, R. W. (1973): Psychotomimetic drugs: Biochemistry and pharmacology. In: *Advances in Drug Research,* edited by N. J. Harper and A. B. Simmons, p. 165. Academic Press, New York.
6. Schlant, R. C., and Nutter, D. O. (1970): Effect of lysergic acid diethylamide (LSD) upon ventricular function and myocardial contractility. *Circ. Res.,* 18:72.
7. Snyder, S. H., Faillace, L., and Hollister, L. (1967): 2-5 Dimethoxy-4-methylamphetamine (STP). A new hallucinogenic drug. *Science,* 158:669.
8. Solursh, L. P., and Clement, W. R. (1968): Hallucinogenic drug abuse. Manifestations and management. *Can. Med. Assoc. J.,* 98:407.
9. Taylor, G. J., and Harris, W. S. (1970): Glue sniffing causes heart block in mice. *Science,* 170:866.
10. Flowers, N. C., and Horan, L. G. (1972): Nonanoxic aerosol arrhythmias. *JAMA,* 219:33.
11. Hollister, L. E. (1968): *Chemical Psychoses: LSD and Related Drugs.* Charles C Thomas, Springfield, Illinois.
12. Chambers, C. D. (1971): An assessment of drug use in the general population. Special Report No. 1. Drug Use in New York State. New York State Narcotic Addiction Control Commission.
13. Towfighi, J., Gonatas, N. K., Pleasure, D., et al. (1976): Glue sniffers neuropathy. *Neurology,* 26:238.
14. Aviado, D., Zakhari, S., Simaan, J., et al. (1976): *Methylchloroform and Trichlorethylene in the Environment.* CRC Press, Cleveland.
15. Taylor, G. J., Harris, W. W., and Bogdonoff, M. B. (1971): Ventricular arrhythmias induced in monkeys by inhalation of aerosol propellents. *J. Clin. Invest.,* 50:1546.
16. Chenoweth, M. (1946): Ventricular fibrillation induced by hydrocarbons. *J. Ind. Hyg. Toxicol.,* 28:151.
17. Winek, C., and Collom, W. (1971): Benzene and toluene fatalities. *J. Occup. Med.,* 13:259.
18. Clark, D., and Tinston, D. (1973): Correlation of the cardiac sensitizing potential of halogenated hydrocarbons with their physiochemical properties. *Br. J. Pharmacol.,* 49:355.
19. Flowers, N. C., and Horan, L. G. (1972): The electrical sequelae of aerosol inhalation. *Am. Heart J.,* 83:644.
20. Bass, M. (1970): Sudden sniffing death. *JAMA,* 212:2075.
21. Speizer, F. E., Wegman, D. H., and Ramirez, A. (1975): Palpitation rates associated with flurocarbon exposure in a hospital setting. *N. Engl. J. Med.,* 292:624.

22. Reinhardt, C. F., Azar, A., Maxfield, M. E., et al. (1971): Cardiac arrhythmias and aerosol sniffing. *Arch. Environ. Health,* 22:265.
23. Standing Medical Advisory Committee for the Central Health Services Council, Secretary of State for Social Services and the Secretary of State for Wales (1973): *Deaths from Asthma.* Department of Health and Social Security.
24. Eastman, J. W., and Cohen, S. N. (1975): Hypertensive crisis and death associated with phencyclidine poisoning. *JAMA,* 231:1270.
25. Clark, M., and Agrest, S. (1978): The deadly angel dust. In: *Newsweek,* March 13, p. 34.
26. Services Research Report (1978): Phencyclidine use among youths in drug abuse treatment. NIDA-USPH Alcohol Drug and Mental Health Administration. (ADM 78–635).
27. Chen, G., Ensor, C. R., Russell, D., et al. (1959): The pharmacology of 1-(1 phenylcyclohexyl)-piperidine hydrochloride. *J. Pharmacol. Exp. Ther.,* 727:241.
28. Domino, E. F. (1964): Neurobiology of phencyclidine. *Int. Rev. Neurobiol.,* 6:303.
29. Gool, R. Y., and Clarke, H. L. (1964): Anesthesia for underdoctored areas. *Anesthesia,* 18:265.
30. Munch, J. C. (1974): Phencyclidine: Pharmacology and toxicology. *Bull. Narc.,* 26:9.
31. Linden, C. B., Lovejoy, F. H., and Costello, C. E. (1975): Phencyclidine: Nine cases of poisoning. *JAMA,* 234:513.
32. Mahler, D. A. (1975): Jimson weed. *Ann. Intern. Med.,* 83:905.
33. Innes, I. R., and Nickerson, M. (1976): Atropine, scopolamine and related antimuscarinic drugs. In: *The Pharmacological Basis of Therapeutics,* edited by L. S. Goodman and A. Gilman, p. 594. Macmillan, New York.
34. Kalser, S. C. (1971): The fate of atropine in man. *Ann. N.Y. Acad. Sci.,* 179:667.
35. Cullumbine, H., McKee, W. H. E., and Creasy, N. H. (1955): The effects of atropine sulfate on healthy male subjects. *J. Exp. Physiol.,* 40:309.
36. Das, G., Talmers, F. N., and Weissler, A. M. (1975): New observations on the effects of atropine on the sinoatrial and atrioventricular nodes in man. *Am. J. Cardiol.,* 36:281.
37. Epstein, S. E., Goldstein, R. E., Redwood, D. R., Kent, K. M., et al. (1975): The early phase of acute myocardial infarction in pharmacologic aspects of therapy. *Ann. Intern. Med.,* 78:918.
38. Knoebel, S. B., McHenry, P. L., Phillips, J. F., et al. (1974): Atropine induced cardioacceleration and myocardial blood flow in subjects with and without coronary artery disease. *Am. J. Cardiol.,* 33:327.
39. Lown, B., Klein, M. D., Hershberg, P. I. (1969): Coronary and precoronary care. *Am. J. Med.,* 46:705.
40. Hurst, J. W., Logue, R. B., Walter, P. F. (1978): The clinical recognition and management of coronary athersclerotic heart disease. In: *The Heart,* edited by J. W. Hurst and R. B. Logue, p. 1272. McGraw-Hill, New York.
41. Comstock, E. (1976): Chemotherapy for drug abuse related emergencies. In: *Acute Drug Abuse Emergencies,* edited by P. G. Bourne, pp. 277–296. Academic Press, New York.

Chapter 11

Narcotic Analgesics 1: Morphine, Synthetic Opiates, and Narcotic Antagonists

The history of the poppy begins in antiquity. Although the exact date of the first systematic cultivation of this plant is unknown, seeds and capsules of poppies were found as early as the Stone Age in the area of lake dwellers. In Mesopotamia (4000–3000 B.C.), the poppy was cultivated by the Sumarians in order to extract opium. The Sumarian term *gil,* meaning happiness and joy, was applied to this flower. The Babylonian culture subsequently spread the cultivation of the poppy eastward to Persia and westward to Egypt.

The medicinal value of the poppy is first described in the works of Hippocrates (463–377 B.C.), where various types and preparations of the plant were recommended for use as a hypnotic, cathartic, styptic, and narcotic. The 18th century marked the beginning of large-scale organized trade and importation of opium, most popular in the Orient. In the early part of the 19th century, Serturner in Germany separated meconic acid from opium, producing morphine from the alkaline base. Robiquet in France isolated narcotine in 1817 and codeine in 1832. By this time, the use of opium and its products had become fashionable and widespread both in the United States and abroad. The popularity of morphine and its derivatives for medicinal as well as abusive purposes has continued unabated to present times.

Pharmacology

Currently used narcotic agents can be classified into three main groups: (a) the naturally occurring opium alkaloids, (b) the semisynthetic opiates (Table 1), and (c) the synthetic narcotic analgesics (Table 2). The opium alkaloids consist of the phenanthrenes, containing morphine, codeine, and thebaine, and the benzylisoquinolines, containing papaverine and noscapine. Derivatives of morphine are formed by substitution at the phenolic (R) or the alcoholic (R_1) hydroxy groups. In general, modification at the R position produces a decrease in both analgesic activity and side-effects.

Morphine, the prototype of narcotic analgesics, is the original derivative of the opiates and semisynthetic narcotic analgesics. Its actions are consistent and have been studied extensively. Oral administration, whether as snuff or through smoking, results in rapid absorption from the gastrointestinal tract or the nasal mucosal membranes and the lung. When morphine or its congeners are administered intravenously, a rapid onset of action occurs. Radioim-

TABLE 1. *Opium alkaloids and semisynthetic derivatives*[a]

Generic name	Trade name	Average dose[b] (mg)	Relative potency[c]	Duration of action (hr)
Morphine and derivatives				
Morphine		10	1	4–5
Heroin (diacetylmorphine)		2–5	3–4	3–4
Hydromorphone (dihydromorphinone)	Dilaudid	1–2	6	4–5
Metopon (methyldihydromorphinone)	Metopon	3	3	4–5
Oxymorphone (dihydrohydroxymorphinone)	Numorphan	1–2	5–10	4–5
	Pantopon[f]	15	1	4–5
Codeine and derivatives				
Codeine (methylmorphine)		120 (10–60)	0.08	(4–6)
Hydrocodone (dihydrocodeinone)	Hycodan[e]	(5–10)		(4–6)
Dihydrocodeine	Paracodin	60	0.16	
Oxycodone (dihydrohydroxycodeinone)	Percodan[d]	10 (3–5)	1	4–5 (4–5)

[a] Modified from Jaffe and Martin, ref. 18, and Lasagna, ref. 36.
[b] Dose is that producing the same effects equivalent to subcutaneous administration of 10 mg morphine. Figures in parentheses refer to oral dosage.
[c] In relation to morphine, equivalent of a potency of 1.
[d] Also contains homatropine, aspirin, and phenacetin.
[e] Also contains homatropine.
[f] Contains all the alkaloids of opium in approximately same proportion as occurring in nature.

TABLE 2. *Synthetic narcotic analgesics*[a]

Generic name	Trade name	Average dose[b] (mg)	Relative potency[c]	Duration of action hr
Benzomorphans				
Phenazocine	Prinadol	3	3	4–5
Morphinans				
Levorphanol	Levodromoran	2–3	4	4–5
Phenylheptylamines (diphenylpropylamines)				
Acetylmethadol	LAAM			
Methadone	Dolophine	7.5–10	1–1.5	3–5
Phenadoxone	Heptalgin	10–20	0.5–1	1–3
Propoxyphene	Darvon	(240)	0.04	(4–5)
Phenylpiperidines				
Alphaprodine	Nisentil	40	0.25	2–3
Anileridine	Loritine	40	0.25	2–3
Diphenoxylate	Lomotil[c]			
Meperidine	Demerol	75	0.1	2–4
Piminodine	Alvodine	10	1	2–4

[a] Modified from Jaffe and Martin, ref. 18, and Lasagna, ref. 36.
[b] Dose is that producing the same effects equivalent to subcutaneous administration of 10 mg of morphine. Figures in parentheses refer to oral dosage.
[c] In relation to morphine, equivalent of a potency of 1.
[d] Also contains atropine sulfate. Used only orally.

munoassay techniques have demonstrated a multiphasic decline in plasma levels, with a slow disappearance following a rather precipitous decline within the first 5 to 10 hr (1). Morphine is concentrated in free or bound form in parenchymal tissue, most prominently in the liver, kidney, lung, spleen, adrenals, and thyroid (2). Detoxication is rapid, and tissue levels are minimal 24 hr after the last injection. At 48 hr, however, very low levels of morphine may be detectable in the serum, with urinary metabolites identifiable for several days. This may be related to a slow release from tissues or absorption via the enterohepatic circulation.

Biotransformation

Excretion occurs mainly as the glucuronide (85 to 90%) free morphine (5 to 10%), in the urine (90%), or through the enterohepatic circulation in the bile with fecal elmination (8 to 10%). Excretion is rapid, with 90% occurring within the first 24 hr through glomerular filtration. Small amounts of normorphine and codeine have also been detected in the urine after administration of both heroin and morphine (3).

A discussion of the cardiovascular changes induced by these drugs can best be understood by dividing these drugs into the licit and illicit agents. The major narcotic in the latter category is heroin, which is considered separately in the following chapter.

Hemodynamics

Narcotics, administered medically in therapeutic doses, are associated with little effect on blood pressure, heart rate, or rhythm in the supine patient. Even in toxic doses resulting in respiratory depression, a significant effect on the vasomotor center is delayed; thus hypotension seen late in the course of narcotic overdose is usually secondary to hypoxia. Physiologic response to gravitational shifts, however, is altered; hypotension may occur on sitting or standing secondary to peripheral vasodilatation. Intravenous morphine causes significant arteriolar dilatation, manifested by a reduction in both forearm and systemic vascular resistance.

The mechanism producing this vasodilatation has not been clearly defined because a direct arteriolar dilating effect has not been demonstrated. Morphine-induced histamine release may be a responsible factor. The duration of hypotension exceeds that of histamine release, however, and the plasma levels of histamine in such settings are considerably less than those seen in histamine-induced hypotension (4–6). In addition, antihistamines are not completely effective in blocking morphine-induced hypotension, suggesting that other mechanisms may be operative. Intraarterial atropine has been shown to be unable to prevent morphine-induced vasodilatation, making activation of cholinergic fibers an unlikely possibility (7,8). Although propranolol is ineffective in preventing vasodilatation subsequent to morphine injection, intraarterial phentolamine has been shown to completely abolish this response, suggesting a morphine-induced reduction in sympathetic alpha-adrenergic tone to be a prominent mechanism, although the precise site of this reaction is not known (7).

In clinical studies utilizing forearm blood flow, morphine has been shown to affect venous tone. Immediately after intravenous infusion of morphine, Zelis et al. (8) recorded a significant degree of venoconstriction, which reached a peak in 1 to 2 min and subsided in 5 min. This was followed by a significant decrease in venous pressure, accompanied by venodilation. The mechanism of this action has not been determined. Morphine does not cause a block of either the alpha-adrenergic receptor or the ganglion, as had been previously reported in animals (7). The most likely operative mechanisms may be either a decrease in afferent stimuli or an inhibition of central nervous system (CNS) determinants of venous tone.

The effect of morphine on heart rate is variable, with increases, decreases, and unchanged rates being reported (9,10). Cardiac output is not significantly altered. Regional circulatory changes, with the exception of renal blood flow, which has been found to be decreased, are relatively unchanged (6).

Cerebral vasodilatation may occur, however, secondary to carbon dioxide retention in the presence of an overdose reaction.

Persons With Coronary Disease

In patients with cardiac disease, especially acute myocardial infarction, the cardiovascular response to narcotic agents may be more attenuated. Alderman et al. (11) have demonstrated a decrease in oxygen consumption, cardiac index, left ventricular end-diastolic pressure, and cardiac work in persons with coronary artery disease. Studies in patients with coronary artery disease and normal left ventricular contractility using large doses of morphine (2 mg/kg i.v.) resulted in a decrease in oxygen consumption manifested by a decrease in rate-pressure product (12). Eleven patients tolerated the analgesia without difficulty, and no episodes of hypotension were observed. Changes in coronary blood flow, coronary vascular resistance, ejection time, heart rate, blood pressure, and tension time index were all considered to be insignificant. No change was noted in pulmonary vascular resistance, although a slight increase in pulmonary arterial pressure occurred. It should be emphasized that this study was performed in persons with normal myocardial contractility with a relatively slow infusion rate of morphine (5 mg/min). Infusion rates of 10 mg/min or more have been associated with precipitous transient hypotension (13).

Scott and Orr (14), in a double-blind study evaluating the effects of intravenous heroin (diamorphine) 5 mg, methadone 10 mg, morphine 10 mg, and pentazocine 30 mg in 118 patients with pain caused by suspected acute myocardial infarction, noted that all these agents, with the exception of pentazozine, resulted in a decrease in blood pressure of up to 10 mg Hg in approximately one half the patients. Clinically significant bradycardia did not occur with any of the drugs. Despite these minor alterations in blood pressure, no adverse clinical reactions were reported. These findings were confirmed by Lee et al. (15), who also noted the absence of any deleterious hemodynamic effects in persons with acute myocardial infarctions treated with intravenous morphine and meperidine. In this study, morphine was not found to significantly lower pulmonary capillary wedge pressure even in those patients whose left ventricle filling pressure was elevated. None of these patients, however, was in respiratory distress or experiencing chest pain.

To assess the effects of morphine in persons with acute pulmonary edema, Vismara et al. (16) compared the venous response in forearm blood flow in such patients with that of normal controls following intravenous infusion of 1 mg/kg morphine sulfate. Although morphine immediately improved the clinical state of those patients in pulmonary edema and induced a significant venodilation in forearm vessels, the magnitude of the venodilation was similar to that observed in normal subjects. The ability of morphine to improve the clinical state without significantly affecting venous dilation may be explained by the finding that neurohumoral sympathetic system discharge is responsible for only about 16% of the increase in venous tone seen in congestive heart failure (17). Other mechanisms that might explain the beneficial action of morphine include: (a) increased pooling in the splanchnic circulation secondary to arteriolar dilation and passive filling of previously underperfused venous segments, (b) dilatation of resistance vessels resulting in a diminished ventricular afterload, and (c) a CNS effect resulting in a decrease in dyspnea and euphoria.

Regardless of the mechanism of action, however, the data indicate that morphine, when used appropriately, is a useful and safe drug in patients with cardiac disease, whether used as an analgesic agent or in the treatment of pulmonary edema. Alterations in the cardiovascular system are minimal and closely resemble those seen with normal adult volunteers.

Narcotic Use in Special Populations

It should be emphasized that persons with cor pulmonale and hepatic dysfunction secondary to congestive changes or primary hepatic disease may be much more sensitive to standard doses of narcotic agents. Similarly, these agents must be used cautiously in the presence of diminished respiratory reserve. Respiratory depressant effects may be heightened with concomitant use of phenothiazines, monoamine oxidase (MAO) inhibitors, and tricyclic antidepressants through mechanisms that have not yet been clearly defined (18). Treatment of narcotic overdose, a subject of considerable importance, is discussed in the following chapter.

METHADONE CONGENERS

Methadone and L-Acetylmethadol

Although significant alterations in the cardiovascular system have not been reported in persons receiving narcotic agents in the therapeutic setting, these drugs are administered for a relatively short period of time, in most instances, relating to the need for transient analgesia. The establishment of methadone maintenance as a therapeutic modality in the rehabilitation of heroin addicts has resulted in a great number of persons being placed on methadone for prolonged periods. In New York city alone, there are more than 30,000 persons currently maintained on this drug. The long-term effects of methadone and its congeners on the myocardium are a matter of concern. The most prominent congeners are propoxyphene (Darvon®) and L-acetylmethadol (LAAM). LAAM is presently being extensively studied as a possible replacement for methadone in maintenance therapy for chronic heroin dependency. Methadone is a 6-dimethylamino-4-4-diphenyl-3-heptanone first synthesized as an analgesic in Germany during World War II. Its structure is markedly different from morphine, but its actions are qualitatively similar; it is, however, much more effective orally and, on a milligram-for-milligram basis, when administered parenterally, it is slightly more potent. The *l*-isomer is much more potent than *d*-methadone by a range of eight- to 50-fold.

Cardiovascular Effects

The effects of methadone on cardiovascular hemodynamics are minimal and similar to those of other narcotics. There is no clinical evidence of adverse effects of methadone on the electrocardiogram (ECG) with either acute or chronic administration. Experimentally, however, Beagle dogs given daily doses of 20 mg/kg body weight methadone developed tachycardia and T-wave changes as early as 3 months after commencement of therapy (19). Similarly, in animals given 4 to 8 mg/kg LAAM daily, considerable electrocardiographic changes developed consisting of tachycardia (31%), ST segment of T-wave changes (69%), and alterations in the QRS complex (16%). These changes reverted toward normal within 4 weeks of discontinuing LAAM therapy. The doses of both methadone and LAAM used in these experiments, however, far exceed those used clinically in maintenance therapy (19).

To assess these effects in a clinical setting, Towery and Rios (20) reviewed ECGs of 430 patients without evidence of previous cardiovascular disease maintained on either methadone or LAAM for a 4-month period. Baseline ECGs were normal in 84 and 88% of patients prior to maintenance therapy on LAAM or methadone, respectively. Although 12 to 16% of these patients initially had abnormal ECGs, it should be emphasized that 15 to 20% of the entire group of patients were also using tranquilizers and/or antidepressants at the time of the study. Information was not available as to whether the use of these agents correlated with those individuals noted to have abnormal baseline ECGs. After 4 months of drug therapy, a review of the ECGs revealed the absence of any significant changes observed in patients maintained on either LAAM or methadone.

Propoxyphene

Propoxyphene, an ester of methadone, is a commonly prescribed analgesic medication. Indeed, in its various proprietary forms alone or in combination with aspirin, phenacetin, or caffeine, produced by 35 companies, it may be among the most commonly prescribed analgesics. It is used most frequently to bridge the gap between aspirin and the more potent narcotics. Dextropropoxyphene is the active isomer with effects similar to those of codeine, although its potency is approximately one-third as great. In the usual therapeutic doses, few effects are seen on the cardiovascular system. Ingestion of large doses, however, has been associated with ventricular bigeminy (21). Overdose reactions result in respiratory and/or cardiac arrest, convulsions, cardiovascular collapse, and pulmonary edema. Finkle et al. (22), in a national assessment of propoxyphene-related deaths, noted cardiac arrest as the mode of demise to be almost as frequent as respiratory depression (45 versus 50%) in 180 cases where an adequate medical history was obtained. Treatment of overdose reactions is similar to that seen with the other narcotic drugs, with naloxone being the antagonist of choice.

NARCOTIC ANTAGONISTS

The substitution of the methyl group attached to the tertiary nitrogen of the opiates or synthetic narcotics results in formation of a narcotic antagonist (Table 3). These drugs may be grouped as those with solely antagonist activity and those which, in addition to their antagonistic actions, also produce effects similar to those seen with morphine (agonist-antagonist). In general, all these drugs can reverse the antidepressant effetcs of morphine and related compounds.

Absorption from the gastrointestinal tract following oral administration of all the commonly used naroctic antagonists is good. Nalorphine and naloxone, however, are so rapidly metabolized in the liver subsequent to absorp-

TABLE 3. *Narcotic antagonists*

Generic name	Trade name	Derivative	N-group substitution	Antagonist activity[a,b]	Physical dependence liability
Nalorphine	Nalline	Morphine	$CH_2CH{=}CH_2$	1.0	Present
Levallorphan	Lorfan	Levorphanol	$CH_2CH{=}CH_2$	3.7	
Pentazocine	Talwin	Phenazocine	$CH_2{-}CH{=}C(CH_2)(CH_2)$	0.025	Present
Cyclazocine		Phenazocine	$CH_2{-}CH(CH_2)(CH_2)$ (ring)	3.5	Present
Naloxone	Narcan	Oxymorphone	$CH_2CH{=}CH_2$	7.0	None
Naltrexone[c]		Oxymorphone	$CH_2CH(CH_2)(CH_2)$ (ring)	17	None

[a] Ability to precipitate abstinence syndrome in morphine-dependent monkeys utilizing nalorphine as a standard of one.

[b] From Eddy and Jacobson, ref. 37.

[c] Naltrexone is the N-cyclopropylmethyl congener of naloxone.

tion to make oral use of these two agents ineffective. Duration of action of naloxone and nalorphine following parenteral administration is 30 min to 4 hr, pentazocine 4 to 6 hr, and naltrexone and cyclazocine up to 24 hr.

The mechanism of action of these agents is presumed to be competitive with the narcotic for a position at the narcotic receptor site. Clinically, these agents have been used for (a) analgesia, (b) detection of narcotic use, (c) treatment of acute narcotic overdose, and (d) prevention of heroin-induced euphoria.

Pentazocine

The narcotic antagonist used clinically most frequently as an analgesic drug is pentazocine (Talwin®). Although the major effects of pentazocine on the CNS, smooth muscle, and gastrointestinal tract are similar to those of the opiates, the cardiovascular response differs considerably (14,15). Pentazocine produces elevations in plasma epinephrine and norepinephrine, with associated increases in blood pressure and heart rate.

In normal subjects, renal plasma flow is decreased with a change noted in glomerular filtration rate. When used as an analgesic in patients with acute myocardial infarction, pentazocine induces significant increases in systemic arterial pressure, pulmonary artery pressure, pulmonary capillary wedge pressure, and systemic vascular resistance. These adverse effects are particularly evident in those patients whose left ventricular filling pressures were increased prior to receiving pentazocine (11,14,15). The increase in pulmonary capillary wedge pressure is of such a degree that, in one study, the use of this agent was discontinued in any other than Killip class 1 patients. Pentazocine administration is also associated with significant increases in left ventricular systolic and diastolic dimension, with decreases in ejection fraction and mean velocity of left ventricular fiber shortening noted on echocardiography. Significant decreases of systemic arterial PO_2 have also been noted following use of this drug. The mechanism of action of pentazocine appears to be related to peripheral vasoconstriction and a negative inotropic action.

Although pentazocine is reported to be a nonnarcotic analgesic and particularly suitable as an alternative for the relief of pain in acute myocardial infarction, the findings described above suggest that its use is contraindicated or, at best, should be undertaken with extreme caution. In addition, contrary to the proposed benefits of pentazocine with respect to drug dependence, experience has shown this agent to be dependency producing, with many cases of pentazocine addiction being reported in the literature (23,24). Intravenous injection of pentazocine by the addict is associated with complications similar to those seen with illicit heroin use (Chapter 12).

Morphine and its derivatives continue to be the agents of choice for the treatment of ischemic myocardial pain. It should be emphasized, however, that if pentazocine is administered to patients who have been receiving narcotics on a regular basis, withdrawal symptoms may occur. An opiate-free interval of several days is recommended prior to the use of this agent.

Naloxone and Naltrexone

Naloxone hydrochloride (Narcan®), the N-allyl derivative of oxymorphone, is currently the antagonist of choice in the treatment of narcotic overdose (25). It is one of the few antagonists to be devoid of all agonist activity. It has a relatively short duration of action, with a serum half-life of approximately 20 min. Metabolism occurs rapidly in the liver through conjugation to an inactive glucoronide. Naloxone has not been associated with any changes in the cardiovascular system. It is a relatively safe, extremely efficient drug to use in narcotic-induced depression, regardless of the presence of cardiovascular disease.

Naltrexone is the N-cyclopropylmethyl derivative of naloxone. It is more effective orally and has a much longer duration of action than naloxone. This is related to its metabolite β-naltrexol, which also has opiate agonist activity. Naltrexone has been associated with some small changes in diastolic blood pressure, but these changes have not been found to be of clinical importance (26–29).

DRUG INTERACTIONS

Simultaneous use of narcotic agents and cardiac medications has not been clinically associated with adverse effects. Combinations of narcotic agents and other mood-altering drugs, however, may result in untoward reactions (Table 4). Clinically, alcohol and barbiturate ingestion, most frequently associated with injection of heroin, can intensify the depressant action of heroin, often with fatal results, although the concentration of each individual agent may be sublethal. A prolongation of morphine-induced respiratory depression has also been reported with phenothiazines, MAO inhibitors, and tricyclic antidepressants (18,30).

Concomitant administration of dextroamphetamine and morphine can potentiate morphine analgesia without enhancing the undesirable side-effects of morphine analgesia. Forrest et al. (31) found this combination to enhance the analgesic potency of morphine by 50 to 100%, depending on the dose of dextroamphetamine.

The amount of narcotic required to produce a given level of analgesia can be reduced by administration of some of the phenothiazines. The respiratory depressant effect of these drugs may be enhanced; although the degree of sedation is increased, an antianalgesic effect may sometimes occur, requiring an increased amount of narcotics to produce satisfactory analgesia. The basal depressor activity of the phenothiazines may result in an accentuation of the mild hypotension of that seen in morphinized subjects. Concomitant

TABLE 4. *Interactions of narcotics with other drugs*

Drug	Effect
Alcohol	Enhanced narcotic depressant effect[a]
Amphetamines	Potentiation of morphine analgesia without increasing toxic effects
Diazepam	Enhanced depressant effect of methadone;[b] prolongation and potentiation of methadone analgesia[b]
MAO inhibitors	Enhanced narcotic depressant effect; with meperidine can produce excitation syndrome, hyperpyrexia, and convulsions
Phenothiazines	Enhanced narcotic depressant effect; reduction in amount of narcotic required for analgesia;[c] potentiation of hypotension
Sedatives	Enhanced narcotic depressant effect[a]
Tricyclic antidepressants	Enhanced narcotic depressant effect; potentiation of heroin toxicity and intensification of naloxone-induced morphine withdrawal;[b] potentiation and prolongation of methadone analgesia[b]

[a] Respiratory depressant effects prominent with acute administration.
[b] Effects documented only in laboratory animals.
[c] Effects variable. Antianalgesic effect may sometimes occur.

use of meperidine and MAO inhibitors has been associated with respiratory depression, excitation, delirium, hyperpyrexia, and even convulsions (31).

Several interactions between the tricyclic antidepressants and narcotic drugs have been reported in the laboratory setting (32,33). An increase in morphine analgesia has been shown to occur in the imipramine-treated rabbit. Imipramine can also enhance meperidine-induced respiratory depression, potentiate heroin toxicity, and intensify morphine withdrawal precipitated by naloxone. Desipramine has been shown to potentiate and prolong methadone analgesia by increasing the brain concentration of methadone as well as by inhibiting metabolism of methadone in the liver (34). Diazepam has also been observed to inhibit methadone metabolism, resulting in increased methadone levels (35).

Although the mechanism of these interactions has not been fully elucidated, it is more than likely that these drugs cause alterations in the metabolic pathways of the narcotic agents or in the concentration of neurotransmitters involved in producing opiate effects.

REFERENCES

1. Spector, S., and Vesell, E. (1971): Disposition of morphine in man. *Science,* 174: 421.
2. Robinson, A. E., and Williams, F. M. (1971): Postmortem distribution of morphine in heroin addicts. *Med. Sci. Law,* 11:135.

3. Roe, B., Boerner, V., Abbott, S., et al. (1972): Morphine metabolism in man: A clinical marker of tolerance. *Clin. Res.,* 21:245.
4. Eckenhoff, J., and Oech, S. (1960): The effects of narcotics and antagonists upon respiration and circulation in man. *Clin. Pharmacol. Ther.,* 1:483.
5. Pur-Shahriari, A. A., Mills, R. A., and Hoppin, F. G. (1967): Comparison of chronic and acute effects of morphine sulfate on cardiovascular function. *Am. J. Cardiol.,* 20:654.
6. Ryan, T. J., Brand, E., and Ramaswamy, K. (1966): The effect of morphine on ventricular function of man. *Clin. Res.,* 14:260.
7. Ward, J. M., McGrath, R. L., and Weil, J. V. (1972): Effects of morphine on peripheral vascular response to sympathetic stimulation. *Am. J. Cardiol.,* 29:659.
8. Zelis, R., Mansour, J., Capone, R. J., et al. (1974): The cardiovascular effects of morphine. *J. Clin. Invest.,* 54:1249.
9. Pettus, W. W., Geiger, A. J., and Grezebien, S. T. (1942): Effects of morphine on the electrocardiogram of men. *Yale J. Biol. Med.,* 14:493.
10. Drew, J. M., Dripps, R. D., and Comroe, J. H. (1946): Clinical studies of morphine II. The effect of morphine upon the circulation of man and upon the circulatory and respiratory responses to tilting. *Anesthesiology,* 7:44.
11. Alderman, E. L., Barry, W. H., Graham, A. F., et al. (1972): Hemodynamic effects of morphine and pentazocine differ in cardiac patients. *N. Engl. J. Med.,* 287:623.
12. Lappas, D. G., Geha, D., and Fischer, J. E. (1975): Filling pressures of the heart and pulmonary circulation of the patient with coronary artery disease after large intravenous doses of morphine. *Anesthesiology,* 42:153.
13. Stoelting, R. K., and Gibbs, P. S. (1973): Hemodynamic effects of morphine and morphine-nitrous oxide in vascular heart disease and coronary artery disease. *Anesthesiology,* 38:45.
14. Scott, M. E., and Orr, R. (1969): Effects of diamorphine, methadone, morphine and pentazocine in patients with suspected acute myocardial infarction. *Lancet,* 1:1065.
15. Lee, G., DeMaria, A. N., Amsterdam, E. A., et al. (1976): Comparative effects of morphine, meperidine and pentazocine on circulatory dynamics in patients with acute myocardial infarction. *Am. J. Med.,* 60:949.
16. Vismara, L., Leaman, D. M., and Zelis, R. (1978): The effects of morphine on venous tone in patients with acute pulmonary edema. *Circulation,* 54:335.
17. Zelis, R. (1974): The contribution of local factors to the elevated venous tone of congestive heart failure. *J. Clin. Invest.,* 54:219.
18. Jaffe, J. H., and Martin, W. K. (1975): Narcotic analgesics and antagonists. In: *The Pharmacological Basis of Therapeutics,* edited by L. S. Goodman and A. Gilman, pp. 245–283. Macmillan, New York.
19. Ettinger, S. J. (1975): Report to the National Institute on Drug Abuse: One year chronic oral toxicity with methadone in beagle dogs. Industrial Biotest Laboratories, HSM 42–73–178.
20. Towery, O. B., and Rios, J. (1975): The effect of LAAM on the electrocardiogram. Report to the National Institute of Drug Abuse.
21. McCarthy, W. H., and Kennan, R. L. (1964): Propoxyphene hydrochloride poisoning. *JAMA,* 187:460.
22. Finkle, B. S., McCloskey, K. L., Kiplinger, G. F., et al. (1976): A national assessment of propoxyphene in postmortem medical legal investigation 1972–1975. *J. Forensic Sci.,* 21:706.
23. Inciardi, J. A., and Chambers, C. D. (1971): Patterns of pentazocine abuse and addiction. *N.Y. State J. Med.,* 71:1727.
24. Swanson, D. W., Weddige, R. L., and Morse, R. M. (1973): Hospitalized pentazocine abusers. *Mayo Clin. Proc.,* 48:93.
25. Martin, W. R. (1976): Naloxone. *Ann. Intern. Med.,* 85:765.
26. Gritz, E. R., Shiffman, S. M., and Jarvik, M. E. (1976): Naltrexone: Physiological and psychological effects of single doses. *Clin. Pharmacol. Ther.,* 19:773.
27. National Institute on Drug Abuse Research Monograph Series No. 9 (1977): Narcotic antagonists: Naltrexone progress report, p. 171. DHEW Publ. no. ADM 77–387, Washington, D.C.

28. Evans, J. M., Hogg, M. I. J., Lunn, J. N., et al. (1974): A comparative study of the narcotic agonist activity of naloxone and levallorphan. *Anaesthesia,* 29:721.
29. Resnick, R., Volavka, J., and Freedman, A. M. (1974): Studies of EN 1639A (Naltrexone): A new narcotic antagonist. *Am. J. Psychiatry,* 131:646.
30. Evans-Prosser, C. D. G. (1968): The use of pethidine and morphine in the presence of monoamine oxidase inhibitors. *Br. J. Anaesthiol.,* 40:279.
31. Forrest, W. H., Jr., Brown, B. W., Jr., Brown, C. R., et al. (1977): Dextroamphetamine with morphine for the treatment of postoperative pain. *N. Engl. J. Med.,* 296:712.
32. Hansten, P. D. (1969): Tricyclic antidepressants. Drug interactions. *Hosp. Management,* 4:25.
33. Saarnivaara, L. (1969): Analgesic activity of some sympathetic drugs and their effect on morphine analgesia in rabbits. *Ann. Med. Exp. Biol. Fenn.,* 47:180.
34. Liu, S. J., and Wang, R. I. H. (1975): Increased analgesia and alterations in distribution and metabolism of methadone by desipramine in the rat. *J. Pharmacol. Exp. Ther.,* 195:94.
35. Spaulding, T. C., Minium, L., Kotake, A. N., et al. (1974): The effect of diazepam on the metabolism of methadone by the liver of methadone dependent rats. *Drug Metab. Dispos.,* 2:458.
36. Lasagna, L. (1964): The clinical evaluation of morphine and its substitutes as analgesics. *Pharmacol. Rev.,* 16:47.
37. Eddy, N., and Jacobson, A. E. (1971): In: *Current Medical Digest,* pp. 329–338.

Chapter 12

Narcotic Analgesics 2: Heroin Addiction

Although pharmacologically pure narcotics are associated with minimal alterations in the cardiovascular system, the effects of illicit preparations are far more serious. Heroin is the predominant narcotic used in street addiction. The number of persons dependent on heroin is extremely difficult to determine with any precision. As discussed in Chapter 1, however, national estimates of heroin users have ranged as high as 724,000.

Complications relating to illicit use of heroin, with the exception of pharmacologic overdose, are unrelated to its narcotic properties. Within minutes of injection, heroin starts to be converted into monoacetylmorphine and subsequently to morphine, with the latter drug being responsible for the majority of narcotic effects. The cardiovascular complications associated with heroin addiction are therefore related to the adulterants with which the heroin mixtures are "cut" (Table 1) and to the unsterile methods of injection.

The most common adulterants seen on the streets are maltose, lactose, and quinine. These substances are called "fillers" and are readily soluble in the blood stream. Other substances, however, such as talc, may be mixed with the heroin; or tablets designed for oral consumption containing talc (Table 2) may be frequently injected with the heroin mixture in an attempt to obtain a heightened euphoric state. In addition to the adulterants and other drugs that may be combined with the heroin for synergistic effects, the method of injecting these drugs also provides for additional contamination. Prior to injection, the contents of the heroin mixture are dissolved in water, heated in a bottle cap or other small container (cooker), and drawn up in an eyedropper or syringe through a small amount of cotton. This filtration

TABLE 1. *Adulterants reported in heroin mixtures*

Arsenic	Lactose
Baking soda (sodium bicarbonate)	Magnesium trisilicate
Barbiturates	Mannite (mannitol)
Battery acid	Methapyrilene
Butacaine	Nicotine
Caffeine	Parathion
Cocaine	Procaine
Cotton fibers	Quinine
Cyanide	Starch
Gum resin	Strychnine

TABLE 2. *Tablets containing talc that are frequently injected with heroin mixtures intravenously*

Generic name	Trade name
Amphetamines	
Methadone	
Methylphenidate	Ritalin
Phenmetrazine	Preludin
Propoxyphene	Darvon
Tripelennamine	Pyribenzamine

process is thought to remove "impurities" but, in reality, provides an additional source for injection of particulate matter in the form of cotton strands.

CARDIOMYOPATHY

Since most cases of heroin-induced acute respiratory failure experience pulmonary edema attributable to hypersensitivity or anoxia, cardiac size is usually normal. Cardiotonic drugs are not required, and, providing therapy is promptly instituted, most persons respond to the administration of a narcotic antagonist, oxygen, and assisted ventilation (see section on overdose reactions). Several reports have recently appeared in the literature describing cardiac dilatation and acute left ventricular failure (1,2). The clinical course in these patients resembles an acute cardiomyopathy. In such instances, appropriate treatment of left ventricular failure is necessary.

ELECTROCARDIOGRAPHIC CHANGES

Electrocardiographic alterations in illicit heroin users have been described. Bradycardia and repolarization abnormalities may occur, consisting of QT prolongation and T-wave changes in more than 50% of asymptomatic heroin addicts and multiple drug abusers (3) (Figs. 1 and 2). Duberstein and Kaufman (4), in a review of 149 symptomatic patients with heroin intoxication, found 25% to exhibit atrial arrhythmias or conduction disturbances. Paroxysmal atrial fibrillation with a slow ventricular response has been seen following heroin injection, with a reversion to regular sinus rhythm after administration of a narcotic antagonist (5) (Fig. 3).

Etiologic Mechanisms

The etiology of these alterations has not been well defined. The rapid deacetylation of heroin to morphine in the body makes it unlikely that heroin per se is the responsible agent, although bradycardia may be a manifestation

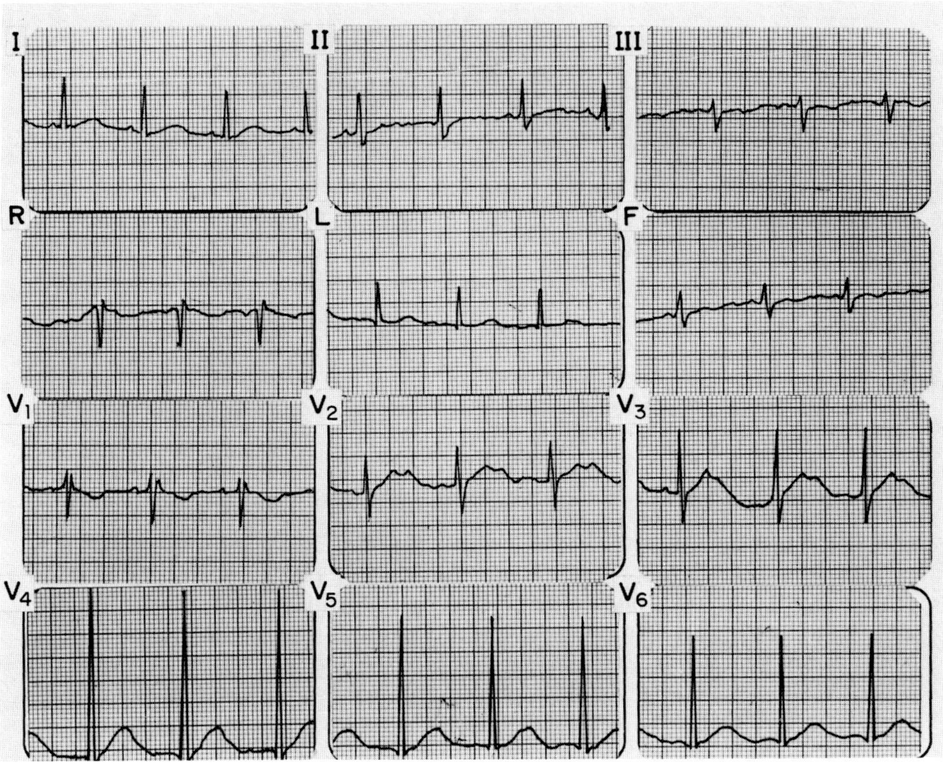

FIG. 1. Tracing of an ECG of an asymptomatic 35-year-old woman addicted to heroin with no history of cardiac disease. Serum electrolytes were within normal limits. Prolongation of QTc interval (0.48 sec) and dimpling of T-wave in precordial leads are prominent.

of a narcotic effect. It is more likely that the adulterants in the injected mixture play a prominent role. Quinine, frequently found in heroin packets, alters the electrocardiogram (ECG) in the same manner as quinidine, with a greater dose required to produce a similar effect. Although low doses may increase the sinus rate, at increasing concentrations bradycardia may be produced. The effects of other heroin combinations containing cocaine and amphetamine may also contribute to the abnormalities seen.

Hypoxemia, associated with hypercapnia and/or respiratory acidosis, has been postulated as a major cause of heroin-induced arrhythmias, especially in a setting where a pharmacologic overdose has occurred. Duberstein and Kaufman (4) considered hypoxemia and acidosis to be the major cause of atrial fibrillation in their series of patients. Reversion to sinus rhythm, however, did not occur until both nalorphine and oxygen were administered. Glauser et al. (6) compared electrocardiographic changes in 25 patients with heroin overdose with those seen in 25 individuals with oral barbiturate poisoning. There was no significant difference between PaO_2, $PaCO_2$, pH, or

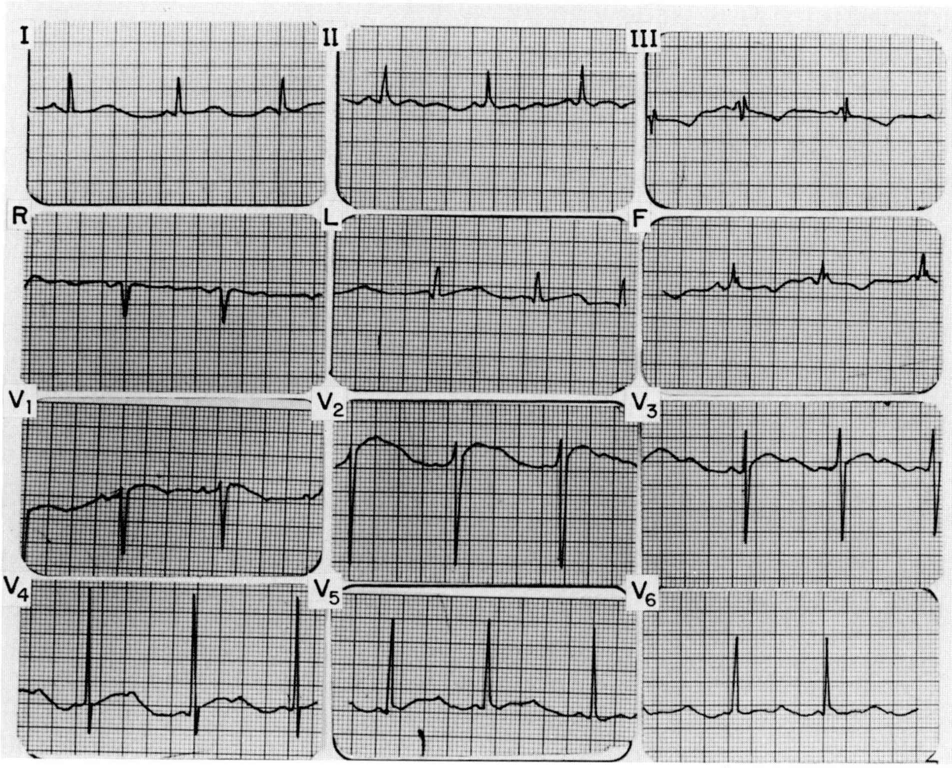

FIG. 2. Tracing of an ECG obtained on screening physical of an asymptomatic 31-year-old man addicted to heroin with no history of cardiac disease. Serum electrolytes were within normal limits. Marked prolongation of QT interval is present with prominant U-waves. The patient refused observation and expired several hours later when walking on the street. Postmortem examination was essentially negative except for pulmonary congestion and the presence of morphine on toxicologic examination. (Reprinted from Stimmel, ref. 88.)

serum potassium, with supplemental oxygen required in both groups. A PaO_2 of 74.8 and a pH of 7.31 was achieved in the heroin overdose group with administration of oxygen. The percentage of patients in each group experiencing minor electrocardiographic alterations was also similar, with only 16% of heroin overdose patients and 20% of barbiturate overdose patients having normal ECGs. Serious arrhythmias, however, were noted only in the heroin overdose group. Five patients (20%) experienced arrhythmias, consisting either of atrial fibrillation or ventricular tachycardia. Arterial blood gases in these patients were no different than in those patients not experiencing the arrhythmias. Guenter (7) has demonstrated that hypoxemia alone in persons with a normal myocardium subjected to exercise does not induce arrhythmias. These findings suggest that hypoxemia does not play the sole role in the serious electrocardiographic changes recorded in heroin users.

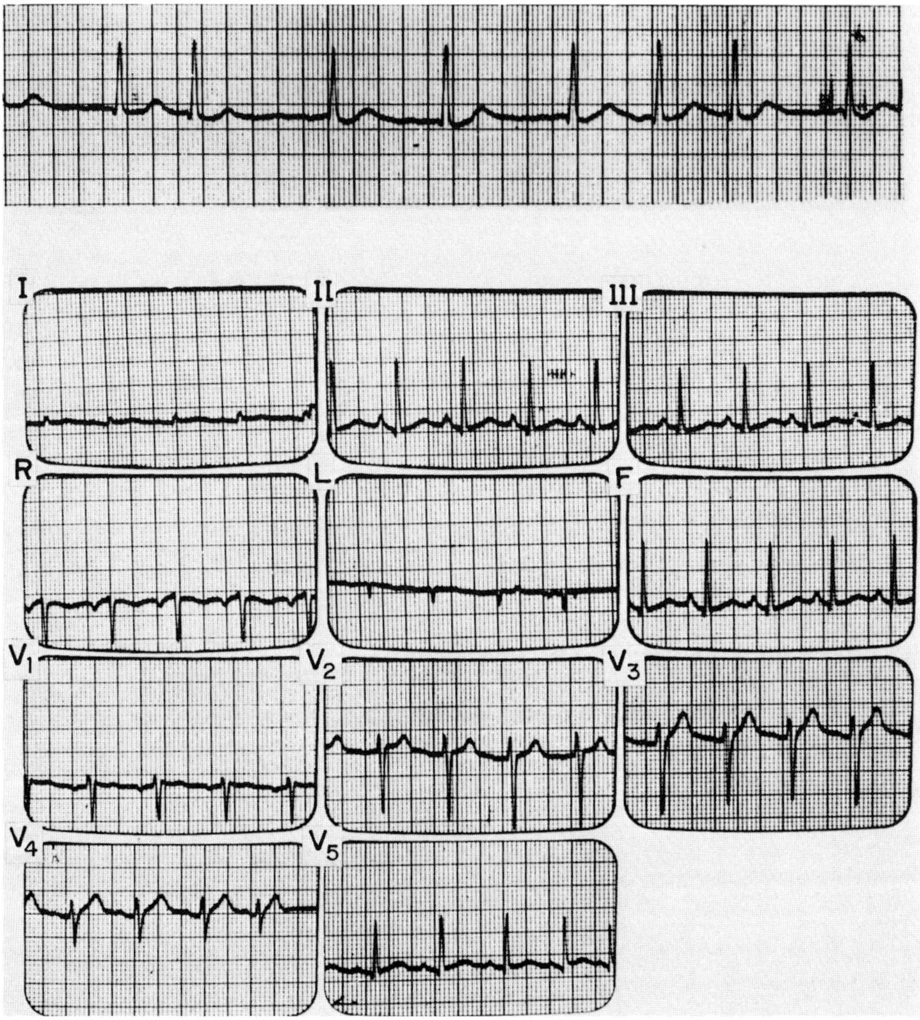

FIG. 3. ECGs from a 22-year-old heroin addict admitted in coma. Upper panel: Rhythm strip on admission showing rapid atrial fibrillation with a slow ventricular response of 70 beats/min. Lower panel: 11-lead ECG after treatment with oxygen and a narcotic antagonist revealing sinus rhythm at 100/min. (Reprinted from Labi, ref. 89.)

Clinical Relevance

The importance of these electrocardiographic alterations is only now becoming apparent. QT prolongation and other repolarization abnormalities may give rise to ectopic or reentrant rhythms with resultant ventricular arrhythmias. Excitement or fright has been shown to cause further prolongation of the QT interval (8). When stress is superimposed on abnormal repolarization and accompanied by injection of illicit materials, a fatal ventricular arrhythmia might occur. Lupovich et al. (9) reported cardiac arrest and atroventricular block in two young persons who were subsequently found to have injected heroin with quinine. These repolarization abnormalities may play a role in the acute fatal reaction and sudden death noted to occur after heroin injection.

ENDOCARDITIS[1]

Infective endocarditis represents one of the most serious cardiovascular complications of parenteral drug abuse, being second only to tetanus in morbidity and mortality (10,11). It is difficult to estimate the prevalence of endocarditis among narcotic addicts; however, it has been reported to be present in 20% of admissions for infectious complications of heroin dependency and in 9% of all general hospital admissions in heroin users (12–15). Local pyogenic infections and endocarditis were responsible for 2 to 8% of all deaths in narcotic addicts in New York city over a 19-year period (11).

Kearns (16) reported the first case of endocarditis in a heroin user in 1936. Since that time, over 250 cases of narcotic addiction associated with infective endocarditis have appeared in the literature (17–25). This disease in the addict tends to be an acute process, caused by virulent invasive organisms resistant to commonly used antibiotics, occurring most frequently on a valve free from preexisting disease and running a fulminating course mandating early diagnosis and aggressive therapy.

Pathologic Determinants

The description given earlier of the conditions under which illicit heroin is injected allows for an understanding of the prevalence of infectious complications in narcotic addicts. Hussey and Katz (15), in a series of infections resulting from narcotic addiction between 1931 and 1947, found that severe infections were almost entirely restricted to the use of heroin as compared to morphine (38 versus 3%), concluding that this association was due primarily to the method of adulteration and also to the common technique of group administration. Since that time, it has been commonly believed that bacterial and/or fungal contamination of the injection paraphernalia or the heroin mixtures has provided the primary focus for the initiation of the endocarditis process (11,13).

---

[1] Portions of this section have been published in Stimmel, B., and Dack, S. (1978): Infective endocarditis in narcotic addicts. In: *Infective Endocarditis,* edited by S. H. Rahimtoola, p. 195. Grune and Stratton, New York.

Contaminated Injection Paraphernalia

Recent studies involving culturing of samples of street heroin and paraphernalia used for injection have cast doubt on this theory. Tuazon et al. (26), in an analysis of 100 samples of heroin and 100 paraphernalia used for injection confiscated by the Bureau of Narcotics and Dangerous Drugs over a 7-month period, found an absence of bacterial growth in 32% of heroin samples and 11% of cultures of syringes and needles. The most common organism found was the bacillus species. Diphtheroids were grown in 17% of paraphernalia cultures and in 9% of heroin samples. Other bacteria frequently isolated included coagulase negative staphylococcus, aspergillus, and clostridium species. Fungi represented 15% of organisms cultured. Candida species other than candida albicains, however, were not found. Aspergillus was the most common fungus cultured from heroin, with saccharomyces, rhodotorula, and aspergillus cultured from the paraphernalia.

The distinct absence of the coagulase-positive *Staphylococcus aureus* was quite surprising, as *S. aureus* is considered to be responsible for 90% of acute endocarditis in narcotic addicts. It is possible that *S. aureus* was present either in the diluent (which was not available for analysis) used to dissolve the heroin or on the skin of narcotic addicts. In a subsequent study, Tuazon and Sheagren (27) demonstrated the carrier rate of *S. aureus* among recent drug users to be increased by more than 300% when compared to a control population (35 versus 11%). Abstinence from drug injection for a period of more than 2 weeks was associated with a decline of the carrier rate to that of control levels. In a comparable study of nonaddicts and diabetics, almost identical carrier rates to heroin addicts were found in those diabetics using insulin (34%). Diabetics on oral hypoglycemic therapy had a carrier rate similar to that of a control group (28). The findings suggest that daily parenteral self-medication may predispose to an increased carrier rate of *S. aureus,* which may result in septicemia when these organisms are introduced into the blood stream subsequent to heroin injection.

Gram negative organisms were found in 22 of 148 (15%) cultures of the injection equipment and 3 of 109 (3%) isolates of heroin samples. *Escherichia coli* was the predominant organism isolated in 17% of paraphernalia samples. This finding also differs from series of gram negative organisms causing endocarditis in narcotic addicts where pseudomonas species predominate. That this organism is rarely a contaminant of heroin mixtures was also confirmed by Reyes et al. (21), who also cultured heroin mixtures from 23 addicts in whom pseudomonas endocarditis developed. Only one specimen was found to contain pseudomonas.

Valve Damage Caused by Adulterants

Exposure to an infective organism, although necessary, is not a sufficient cause for the development of endocarditis in the presence of a normal valve. Weinstein and Schlesinger (29) related the pathologic process terminating in infective endocarditis to be dependent on the presence of one or more factors: (a) a jet of blood flowing from a high pressure area to one of low pressure on a previously damaged valve, (b) a sterile platelet-fibrin thrombus, and (c) bacteremia with a high titer of agglutinating antibody for the infective organism.

Although it must be emphasized that endocarditis secondary to narcotic addiction can develop in narcotic addicts with preexisting heart disease, in most instances such infections are found to occur on essentially normal valves. The valve structure of the heroin addict can be damaged through repeated injection of street heroin containing numerous contaminants, including cotton strands. These materials may cause subsequent subendothelial injury and serve as a nidus for a platelet-fibrin thrombus and bacterial growth. Experimental pathologic findings tend to support this hypothesis (30).

Immunologic Defects

The possibility of a narcotic-induced defect in the defense mechanism of the addict must also be considered. Administration of morphine has been associated with a decreased phagocytic activity in both animals and humans (31). Nickerson et al. (32), however, have found the serum of heroin addicts to have an increased opsonin capacity, with a normal response of phagocytic cells to ingest and kill test bacteria.

Clinical Presentation

Fever is the most frequent symptom experienced in persons with endocarditis. The association of fever, new murmur or one different from that previously known to exist in a narcotic addict, must result in a primary diagnosis of infective endocarditis until proven otherwise. Endocarditis among drug users does differ from that in the drug-free population. Heroin addicts are usually younger, have no previous history of cardiac disease, and are admitted to the hospital in a more serious condition than persons who are drug free. In addition, heroin addicts characteristically neglect their physical condition. A study comparing addicts who have endocarditis with endocarditic nondrug users, however, found that 94% of addicts report their symptoms to a physician as being 1 week in duration, as compared to 86% of the control group, whose symptoms were present for more than 2 weeks prior to hospitalization (12). This early presentation among narcotic addicts may be related to the frequent prevalence of respiratory complaints associated with hypoxia and dyspnea secondary to septic pulmonary emboli in the presence of tricuspid value endocarditis.

Tricuspid Valve Lesions

The right side of the heart is more frequently affected in narcotic addicts than in nonaddicts (Table 3), although left-sided lesions of the aortic and/or

TABLE 3. *Site of involvement in infective endocarditis in drug addicts*[a]

Site	No.	%	
Pure left sided	134		48
Aortic	63	23	
Mitral	40	14	
Aortic and mitral	31	11	
Pure right sided	118		43
Tricuspid	111	40	
Tricuspid and pulmonary	7	3	
Right and left sided	23		9
Aortic and tricuspid	8	3	
Aortic, mitral, tricuspid	5	2	
Mitral, tricuspid, pulmonic	2	1	
Mitral and tricuspid	8	3	
Total	275		100

[a] Data obtained from ref. 37–48, 56, 59, 61, 62. Cases where data needed for the table were incomplete were deleted.

mitral valve still predominate. The tricuspid valve, however, is the single valve most frequently involved in aggregate series reported in the literature (33–36). This is probably attributable to selection of cases for publication rather than to the true prevalence of tricuspid value lesions. The presence of fever and cough in a narcotic addict, however, should suggest the existence of tricuspid endocarditis with associated pneumonia or pulmonary emboli. This diagnosis must be considered even in the absence of a tricuspid valve murmur, which has been noted in only 64% of addicts with this lesion (20,37, 38). Septic-pulmonary emboli (Fig. 4) can be seen in approximately 50%

TABLE 4. *Complications of infective endocarditis in addicts*[a]

			PE		Syst emb		Mortality	
Infective organism	No.	%	No.	%	No.	%	No.	%
Staphylococcus aureus	102	43	70	68.6	23	22.6	19	18.6
Staphylococcus epidermidis	1	0.4	1	100			1	100
Streprococcus viridans	16	6.8	3	18.7	2	12.5	7	43.7
Serratia marcescens	23	9.7	3	13	9	39.1	13	56.5
Enterococcus	19	8	3	15.7	6	31.6	11	57.8
Candida	8	3.4	3	37.5	5	62.5	6	75
Gram negative rods	6	2.5	1	16.6			2	33.3
Pseudomonas	40	16.9	21	52.5	9	22.5	22	55
Diplococcus pneumoniae	1	0.4					1	100
No growth	21	8.9	4	19	1	4.8	10	47.6
Total	237	100	109	45.9	55	23.2	92	38.8

[a] Data obtained from ref. 37–48, 56, 59, 61, 62. Cases where data needed for the table were incomplete were deleted.

PE, pulmonary embolus; Syst emb, systemic emboli.

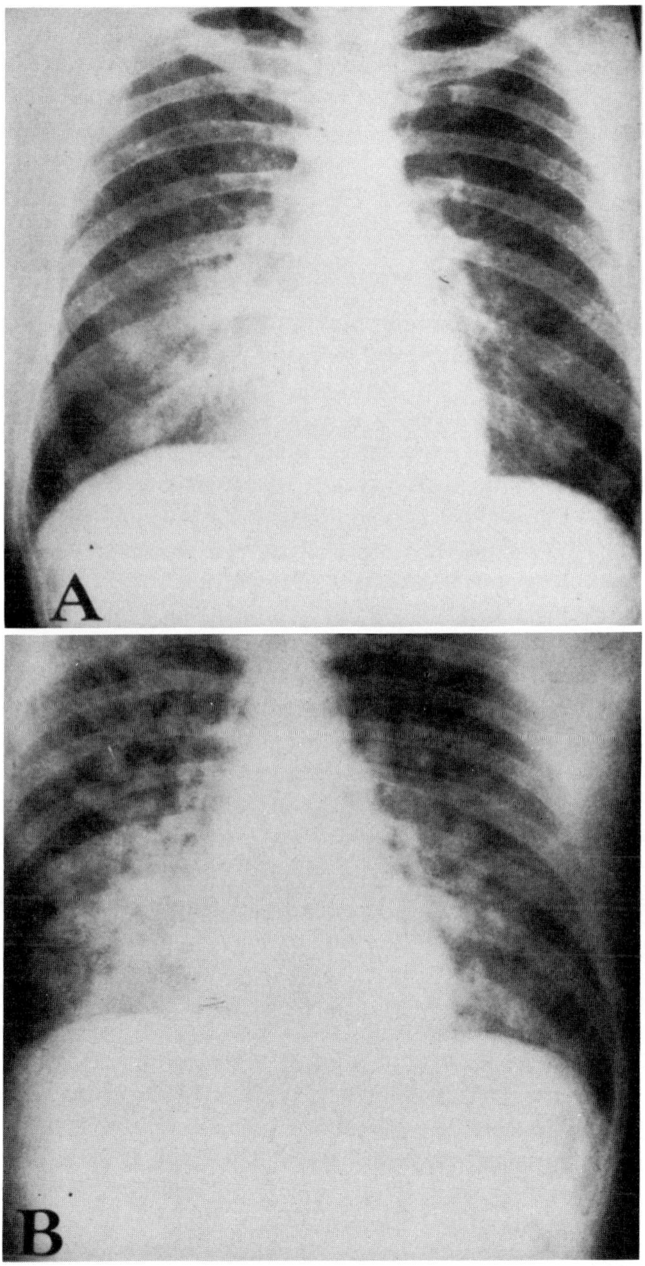

FIG. 4. Tricuspid endocarditis and septic pulmonary emboli in a 28-year-old heroin addict. A: Chest X-ray on admission revealing multiple septic pulmonary emboli. B: Chest X-ray 14 days after antibiotic therapy.

of all cases of endocarditis (Table 4) in almost all instances associated with tricuspid insufficiency. The presence of a characteristic regurgitant murmur changing with respiration allows for a diagnosis of tricuspid valve endocarditis. Other evidence suggests this condition in the absence of characteristic hemodynamic findings and includes: (a) an atrial diastolic gallop, heard best over the left sternal border and external jugular vein, (b) a short ejection murmur increasing with inspiration and lengthening in duration over several days to months, (c) early systolic clicks and gallops, which may be a forerunner of tricuspid insufficiency, and (d) the presence of midsystolic clicks secondary to scarring of the tricuspid valve.

The atrial diastolic gallop has been attributed to increased right atrial volume without compensatory right atrial dilatation, resulting in a forceful atrial contraction. The tricuspid regurgitation murmur may also be short rather than holosystolic secondary to either minimal regurgitation or a rapid ventricularization of the right atrial pressure curve secondary to severe tricuspid valve destruction.

The diagnosis of tricuspid valve endocarditis with associated tricuspid insufficiency should be considered in any heroin addict presenting with fever, bacteremia, and pulmonary emboli who, on physical examination, is noted to have a regurgitant murmur increasing with inspiration, associated with early systolic clicks or atrial gallops.

Aortic and Mitral Valve Lesions

Left-sided endocarditis alone or in combination with involvement of the tricuspid valve is reported in approximately 57% of all cases with endocarditis, usually associated with murmurs of aortic or mitral insufficiency. Cardiomegaly, with or without congestive heart failure, is frequent. The clinical presentation of left-sided endocarditis, however, can be quite variable. Murmurs of aortic or mitral stenosis may be found in the presence of large obstructive vegetations. Orlando et al. (39), in a study of 16 addicts with endocarditis, found eight presenting with musculoskeletal complaints and four with nonspecific arthralgias. In addition, the presenting symptoms may be secondary to systemic emboli. This phenomenon has been noted in 23% of cases reported in the literature.

Approximately 10 to 18% of addicts presenting with endocarditis have had some preexisting cardiac disease (12,17). In these instances, left-sided involvement with *Streptococcus viridans* is usually prominent. If the onset of endocarditis is not acute, splenomegaly and peripheral signs of subacute endocarditis, such as petechiae, Roth spots, and hematuria, may be present. It must also be emphasized that the presence of fever or a heart murmur does not invariably indicate endocarditis in a narcotic addict. Infections and pyogenic reactions are not infrequent and may be secondary to extravascular infection. The presence of a cardiac murmur of a functional nature or secondary to preexisting heart disease or pulmonary hypertension in the absence of fever and endocarditis may also be present. Respiratory distress accompanied at times by pulmonary edema may represent an acute reaction to intravenous injection of street heroin rather than the presence of septic pulmonary emboli. It is important to carefully evaluate all symptoms and signs in order to detect the presence of an acute infective endocarditis.

Laboratory Diagnosis

Although the presence of a heart murmur and a positive blood culture usually confirm the bacteriologic diagnosis of infective endocarditis, in up

TABLE 5. *Laboratory aids in diagnosis of endocarditis*

Aid	Initial diagnosis	Effectiveness of therapy
Blood cultures	+	+
Antibodies to staphylococcal[a] teichoic acids	+	+
Immune complexes in serum	+	+
Intraleukocytic bacteria in venous blood concentrates	±	
Echocardiographic demonstration[b] of vegetations	+	+

[a] Only in endocarditis caused by *S. aureus*. May not be detectable until several days after onset of endocarditis.

[b] Only if vegetations demonstrated. Endocarditis may frequently exist in absence of positive echocardiographic findings.

to 10% of reported cases no organism can be isolated, despite frequent culture attempts. Associated laboratory findings may therefore be quite helpful in suggesting the presence of this disease (Table 5).

Staphylococcal Teichoic Acid Antibodies

Nagel et al. (40) have demonstrated the presence of antibodies to staphylococcal teichoic acids in 18 of 22 (82%) patients with *S. aureus* coagulase-positive endocarditis. These antibodies were not found in 21 asymptomatic addicts who were *S. aureus* coagulase-positive carriers. The antibodies appear promptly enough to be of diagnostic value on admission to the hospital and may be helpful in diagnosing staphylococcus infections in persons with negative blood cultures (41,42). In a series of 28 cases of *S. aureus* endocarditis, the presence of antibodies was used to make the diagnosis in 64% of cases before blood cultures had become positive. The absence of teichoic acid antibodies, however, does not rule out the diagnosis of *S. aureus* endocarditis, as the titers may not become detectable until 7 days after the onset of the disease. Persistence of these antibodies in the presence of adequate antibiotic therapy suggests metastatic complications caused by systemic emboli.

The ability to culture fungi from blood specimens of patients with endocarditis varies with the specific fungal agent. Candida can be cultured relatively easily, being successfully isolated in up to 87% of cases of candida endocarditis. Aspergillus seldom can be isolated from routine culture, being detected in only 11% (43).

Other laboratory tests may be valuable in suggesting the diagnosis of endocarditis in the absence of positive blood cultures. Intraleukocytic bacteria can be demonstrated in venous blood concentrates in almost 50% of patients with endocarditis (44). Addition of different culture media, such as enriched hypertonic solutions or special media for thiol requiring streptococcal variants, may also be helpful (45). Serologic tests may be of value in diagnosing fungi infections in the absence of positive blood cultures. Wiseman et al. (46) have suggested the use of gallium-67 myocardial imaging in detecting culture negative bacterial endocarditis.

Immune Complex Deposition

Extravalvular manifestations of endocarditis are not infrequent and are commonly attributable to septic embolization from an infected valve (Table 4). Metastatic abscesses have been demonstrated, however, and light microscopy in many cases has failed to document the presence of organisms (47). In such cases, the nonseptic nature of the lesions has been attributed to the presence of a necrotizing vasculitis (48,49). In 1972, Gutman et al. (50) demonstrated the presence of immune complex on the glomerular basement membrane in nine patients with endocarditis and associated renal insufficiency. Distribution of these deposits were noted to be in a "lumpy bumpy" rather than a linear distribution.

Bayer et al. (51) found 97% of 29 patients with infective endocarditis to have elevated serum levels of immune complexes as detected by Raji cell, with significantly higher levels being seen in patients with extravalvular lesions, endocarditis of longer duration, infection of the right side of the heart, and/or the presence of mild valvulitis. The rate of decline of these levels was dependent on clinical recovery, usually being complete within 6 weeks of initiation of chemotherapy. In those cases caused by organisms more resistant to antibiotics, the decline rate was considerably slower. In several patients requiring surgical intervention for valve replacement, the immune complex levels fell only after removal of the infective valve. Serial measurement of serum immune complex levels, similar to teichoic acid antibodies in *S. aureus* infections, may provide a useful guide to effectiveness of therapy.

Echocardiography

In the past several years, echocardiography has been found to be extremely helpful in the diagnosis of valvular vegetations, with a diagnosis being made in some patients with vegetations no larger than 0.2 cm in size (52–56). In general, however, the echocardiographic features of valvular vegetation tend to be most prominent in the sickest patients and have been used to identify lesions of both the right and left side of the heart and to follow the course of endocarditis in medically treated patients. On echocardiographic examination, vegetations appear as uneven and irregular valvular shadows (Figs. 5 and 6). Motion of the valve is usually unrestricted, although masses of shaggy or fuzzy echos attached to the valves may be noted in both systole and diastole. In instances of restricted valvular movement, the echocardiogram is quite helpful in distinguishing the presence of vegetations from other causes of abnormal valve motion, such as aortic fibrosis and calcification.

Echocardiographic diagnosis of vegetations appears to be less accurate for the tricuspid valve than for the mitral or aortic valves. Andy et al. (56) noted that among 20 clinically recognized incompetent tricuspid valves, only 12 of 18 (67%) patients whose valves were adequately visualized had echocardiographic abnormalities. This was compared to detection of echocardiographic abnormalities in 11 of 12 (92%) patients with incompetent mitral valves and all of three (100%) patients with aortic incompetency.

Differential diagnosis of valvular vegetations on echocardiographic examination includes: (a) left atrial myxoma, (b) mitral valve fluttering secondary to aortic regurgitation, (c) flail leaflets without vegetations, and (d) recordings with unusually high gains. In general, left atrial myxomas present a motion on the echocardiogram independent of the valve and not continuous with it. Mitral valve fluttering secondary to aortic regurgitation is usually manifested as a fast, regular, diastolic oscillation on a normal valve. A flail leaflet in the absence of vegetations frequently demonstrates prominent systolic echos, with a marked change in motion noted during diastole.

The echocardiogram, therefore, may be helpful in diagnosing the presence of valvular vegetations in acute endocarditis. Recently, Pratt et al. (57) have presented data to suggest that the echocardiographic demonstration of vegetations indicates extensive valve destruction predicting the development of congestive failure. Serial echocardiography may also be of value in following the course of the disease once medical therapy has been instituted.

In addition to detecting vegetations, the echocardiogram is also useful in detecting ruptured chordae of the mitral valve and torn or perforated cusps of the aortic valve (55,58).

Blood Culture

The organism cultured most frequently from the blood of addicts with endocarditis is *S. aureus* (Table 6). Although this organism predominates,

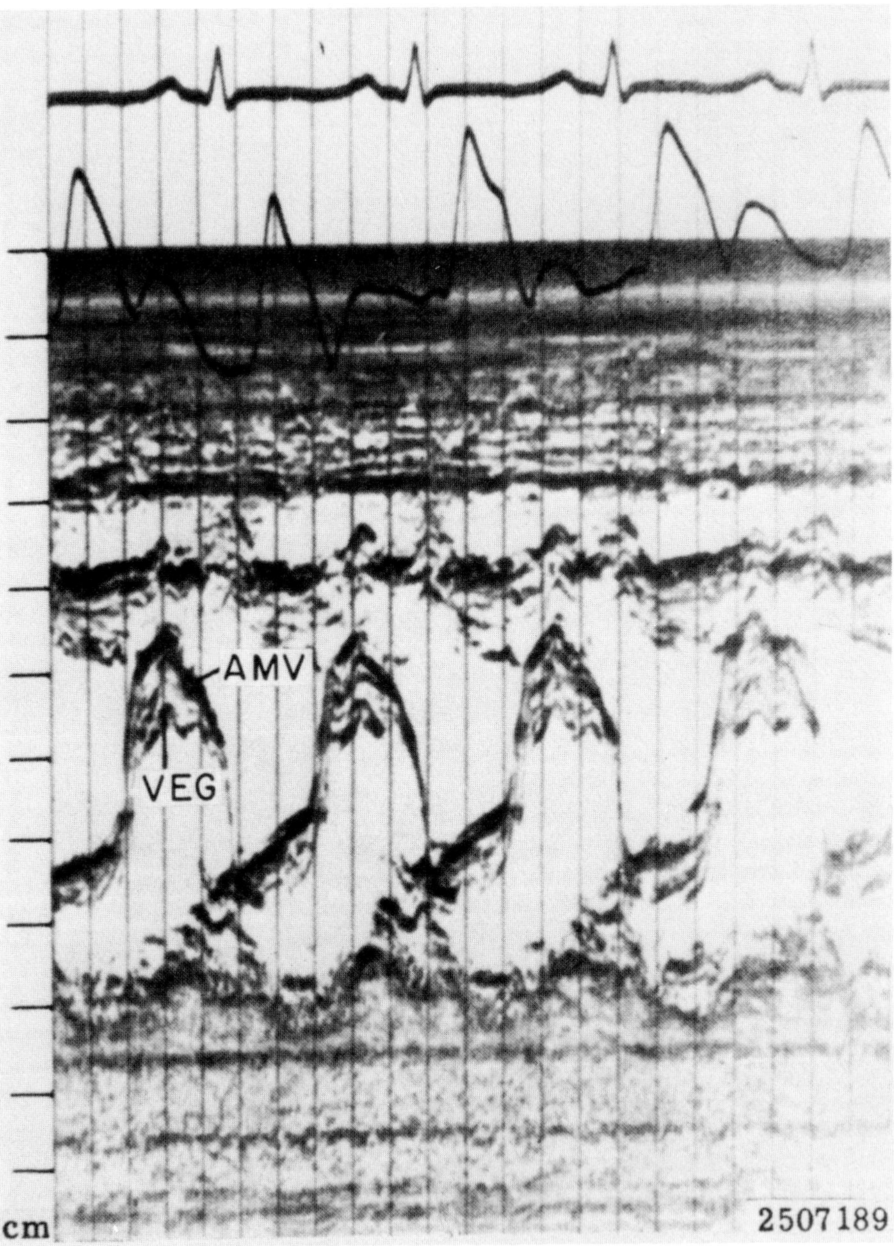

FIG. 5. Mitral valve echograms from a patient with vegetations on the anterior leaflet. There are echos (VEG) on the anterior leaflet (AMV) originating from the vegetations. Despite the leaflet thickening, the valve remains unrestricted, and an actual coarse fluttering of the valve occurs during diastole. (Reprinted from Dillion et al., ref. 90.)

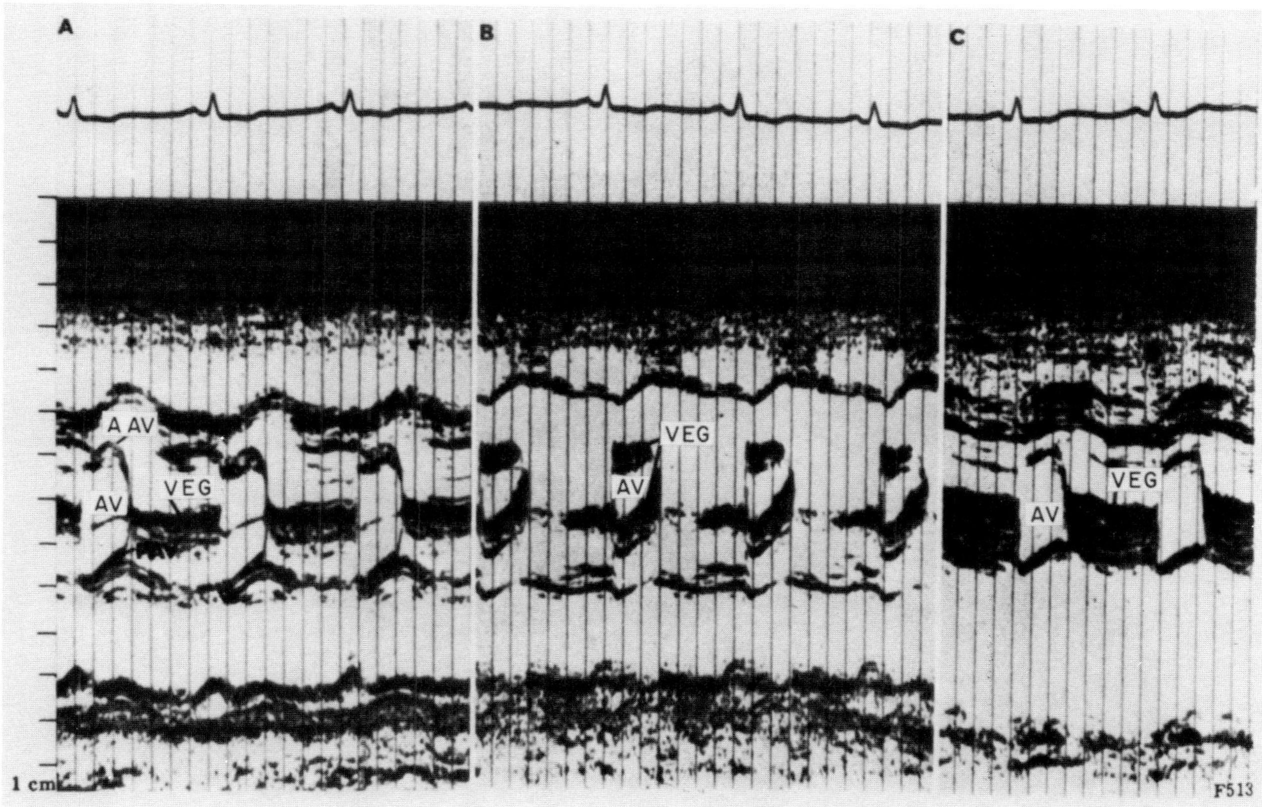

FIG. 6. Aortic valve echograms from a patient with vegetations or the aortic valve. Despite apparent valvular thickening, the motion of the leaflets remains unrestricted. AAV, anterior aortic valve leaflet; AV, aortic valve; PAV, posterior aortic valve leaflet; VEG, vegetation. (Reprinted from Dillon et al., ref. 90.)

TABLE 6. *Isolation of infective organisms in infective endocarditis in addicts*[a]

Infective organism	No.	%
Staphylococcus aureus	123	44.2
Pseudomonas species	45	16.2
Streptococcus viridans	15	5.4
Candida	10	3.6
Enterococci	42	15.1
Gram negative rods	6	2.2
Serratia marcescens	17	6.1
Staphylococcus albus	3	1.1
Staphylococcus epidermides	2	0.7
Diplococcus pneumoniae	1	0.4
No growth on repeated cultures	14	5.0
Total	278	100

[a] From refs. 37–48, 56, 59, 61, 62. Cases where data needed for the table were incomplete were deleted.

it is, fortunately, responsible for one of the lowest mortality rates (19%). This is more related to the affinity of the organism for the tricuspid valve than its invasive capacity.

Pseudomonas Species

The pseudomonas species is responsible for 16% of cases of endocarditis reported in the literature. Although in many series this organism has been rarely identified, three recent articles have stressed the prevalence of these organisms, with *P. aeruginosa* and *P. cepacia* being most frequently isolated (21–23). Similar to infection with *S. aureus,* tricuspid valve involvement predominates (60%), although left-sided lesions are not uncommon. Arterial emboli may occur when associated left atrial or mural thrombi exist. Mixed infections are not uncommon. In such cases, the pseudomonas organism is identified only after antibiotic therapy has been instituted, lowering the innoculum of the other organisms. Pseudomonas has a propensity to concentrate about arteries and veins with an invasion of the aterial media, which may result in focal vessel destruction (20). Mortality in these patients is high (55%) but varies with site of lesion, with those patients having only tricuspid or pulmonary valve involvement having mortality rates of 30% compared to 89% if left-sided lesions are present (22).

Streptococcus Viridans

Streptococcus viridans are present in approximately 5% of cases. In almost all instances, infection occurs in patients with preexisting cardiac disease. The majority of these patients presents a clinical picture similar to subacute bacterial endocarditis in nonaddicted populations, with involvement of aortic and mitral valve predominating.

Group D Streptococcus

Group D streptococcal endocarditis (enterococci) is found in varying frequency (0 to 5%), usually representing less than 2% of most series (24, 35,36). In the aggregate series, reported enterococci were present in 15% of infective organisms. The aortic or mitral valve is usually affected, with tricuspid involvement rarely noted.

Serratia Species

Serratia marcescens is a rare cause of bacterial endocarditis. A recent report by Mills and Drew (25), however, documented 19 cases of endocarditis caused by nonpigmented serratia strains. The aortic and mitral valves were the most frequently involved, with embolic episodes noted in 13 (68%) patients. The mortality rate was exceedingly high (68%), despite adequate antibiotic therapy. Twelve patients with left-sided valvulitis treated medically succumbed to this disease, suggesting the need for early surgical intervention.

Candida Species

Candida is known to be a prominent cause of endocarditis in narcotic addicts (59,60). McLeod and Remington (43), in a review of 59 cases of fungal endocarditis in narcotic addicts, found candida species to be responsible for 54 of 59 cases. Although Andriole (61) found a 20% incidence of candida endocarditis in a review of 100 cases of intravenous narcotic users, when a review of a larger number of cases is made, this rate drops to approximately 4% (Table 5). The prominence of fungal endocarditis in narcotic addicts is still impressive. When compared to all cases of fungal endocarditis, 59 of 259 (23%) were found to occur in addicts (43). All valves may be affected; but involvement of aortic and mitral valves predominates. Although the average vegetation size is 2 cm^3, vegetations larger than 8 cm^3 have been reported. Systemic large vessel emboli are not infrequent, with common sites of entrapment being kidney, brain, spleen, and lower extremities. Aspergillus, with its predilection for small size arteries and veins, may lead to necrosis and thrombosis of the peripheral vasculature (43).

Polymicrobial Cultures

During the past several years, there has been a noticeable increase in the frequency of polymicrobial endocarditis. The majority (81%) of cases reported in the literature occurs in heroin addicts (62,63). Although the clinical presentation of "mixed" infective endocarditis is usually no different than the endocarditis caused by a single organism, the prognosis is usually worse and surgical intervention more frequently needed. This may be related to the frequent occurrence of candida species and *P. aeruginosa* as causative agents.

Management

Antibiotic Therapy

Treatment of addicts strongly suspected or diagnosed as having endocarditis should be instituted promptly with appropriate antibiotic therapy. Complications of this disease are frequent. In addition to septic pulmonary emboli, other complications can include pneumonia with empyema, gastrointestinal bleeding, septic arthritis, arterial emboli to the systemic circulation, focal destruction of blood vessels, destruction of valve cusps or chordae tendineae, and progressive cardiac failure. It should be emphasized that although systemic emboli are most common in candida infections, they have also been reported in infections due to *S. aureus, S. fecalis,* enterococcus, and pseudomonas.

If after institution of appropriate antibiotic therapy, persistent fever suggests the possibility of a second infecting organism, the presence of a gram negative rod must be considered. Multiple cultures should be performed and an alteration of antibiotic coverage accomplished, as appropriate. In such cases where gram negative bacillary infection exists, serum bactericidal titers might be helpful in determining the efficacy of an antibiotic regimen.

Specific antibiotic regimens for therapy of endocarditis will not be reviewed here, as appropriate antibiotic usage is discussed extensively in the literature. In general, the specific antibiotic should be selected on the basis of both microbiologic identification and existing antibiotic sensitivity tests and administered for 4 to 6 weeks. Efficacy of therapy can be monitored by bactericidal assay techniques. With appropriate antibiotic therapy, it is anticipated that the infective locus in the valve can be eradicated with a clearing of the bacteremia and, in the case of right-sided endocarditis, a satisfactory recovery from the disease. Even with optimal therapy, however, the bacteriologically cured addict may succumb as a result of valve destruction in left-sided endocarditis, especially in the presence of severe aortic regurgitation. In such cases, surgical intervention with valve replacement is usually necessary, preferably on an elective basis.

Surgery

Not infrequently, expectant surgery is prohibited, and the necessity of acute valve replacement arises. Early surgical intervention before eradication of infection has always been a matter of concern. This relates to the difficulty in placing sutures in inflamed and easily friable tissue, as well as the dangers of prosthetic valve infection and the dissemination of systemic emboli. In the presence of clinical deterioration manifested by progressive hemodynamic failure or intractable heart failure and persistence of systemic emboli, however, surgical intervention may be lifesaving (Table 7) (64–67). In addition, in the face of persistent infection refractory to antibiotic therapy, surgical excision of the infected valve may allow for an eradication of the bacteremia.

Emergency surgical therapy usually does not allow an attempt at plastic repair of the valve. Replacement of the aortic or mitral valve is accomplished through the use of a prosthetic valve or homograft, each of these valves having its own hazards. The use of a homograft enables the patient to be free of anticoagulant therapy, which is important in individuals who cannot be relied on to take medication. These valves are quite susceptible to repeated infection however, and, when used acutely, may be associated with valve perforation and its attendant severe effects. Prosthetic valve insertion, especially with some of the newer models, may eliminate the need for anticoagulant therapy postoperatively. Although the hazard of recurrent infection is not as severe, valvular leaks through suture lines have been reported to be a major problem.

In a review of 100 reported cases, Hancock et al. (68) found that neither the species of infective organism nor the presence of these organisms in the blood or the resected valve affected the results of surgery. Extension of the infection into adjacent tissues, especially with respect to the valve ring and aortic wall, however, may adversely affect the surgical result.

The timing of surgical intervention depends on the clinical state of the patient. Although delayed intervention for 5 to 6 days allows for an optimal period of antibiotic sterilization, in the face of clinical deterioration, immediate surgical intervention is mandatory, regardless of duration of therapy.

In cases of persistent infection of the tricuspid valve, valve resection without prosthetic replacement has been attempted at several centers (69–71). The rationale behind this is to allow further medical therapy after removal of the infective source without insertion of a prothesis that might once again become a locus of infection. Early follow-up had indicated that this procedure was tolerated, with the patients experiencing mild limitation of activity but

TABLE 7. *Indications for surgical intervention in endocarditis*

Progressive hemodynamic deterioration
Progressive intractable heart failure
Persistent infection refractory to antibiotic therapy
Associated pericarditis with valve ring abscess and annular erosion
Myocardial abscesses associated with serious conduction disturbances of intracardiac fistulae
Mycotic aneurysm

not heart failure. This applies particularly to pseudomonas infection of the tricuspid valve; the cure rate with medical treatment in one series of 33 cases was only 39% (72). Two patients subjected to valve replacement died of persistent infection. Of the remaining 17 cases, tricuspid valvulectomy provided bacteriologic cure in 15. Hemodynamic studies in 10 of these cases demonstrated no evidence of right heart failure 36 months postoperatively in seven, and right heart failure 19 months postoperatively in three. This procedure is far from being fully evaluated on a long-term basis, however, and cannot be routinely recommended; the hazards of eventual intractable right-sided congestive heart failure and massive hepatic congestive and resulting hepatic failure remain a real possibility. Nevertheless, tricuspid valvulectomy may be a lifesaving measure; following bacteriologic cure, prosthetic valve insertion can be carried out at a later date if right heart failure supervenes.

Following expectant surgery, antibiotic treatment should be continued for 4 to 6 weeks or longer until the bacteremia has been eliminated. Prolonged antibiotic therapy, however, carries with it the risk of superinfection, with organisms resistant to multiple antibiotics. Braimbridge (67), in a review of 40 patients with active endocarditis undergoing surgery, found six to have reinfection of the prosthetic valve, with the infecting organism different from that originally seen in five of the six cases.

Prognosis

Complications

Septic pulmonary emboli, systemic emboli, and progressive cardiac failure represent the most frequent complications of endocarditis (Table 4) (Fig. 7). Seeding of emboli from the aortic valve may result in chordae rupture, and actual myocardial invasion is not an unknown phenomenon (Figure 8). The presence of myocardial invasion may be suggested by the appearance of a new conduction defect. Pericarditis may also be associated with the endocarditis, usually consisting of fibrinous pericardial adhesions. Aortic valve rupture and a dissection along the aortic wall may also occur. Other complications include pneumonia with empyema and septic arteritis.

Mortality

In the early or preantibiotic era, survival of addicts affected by endocarditis was extremely poor. Luttgrens (33), reporting on endocarditis in mainline opium addicts in 1949, found only one of 13 to recover, even with the use of penicillin. With new antibiotics, mortality has improved considerably; thus the mortality rate in the 184 cases listed in Table 3 is 38%. However, this is still considerably higher than that seen in nonaddicts with infective endocarditis. Buchbinder and Roberts (72) have suggested that acute endo-

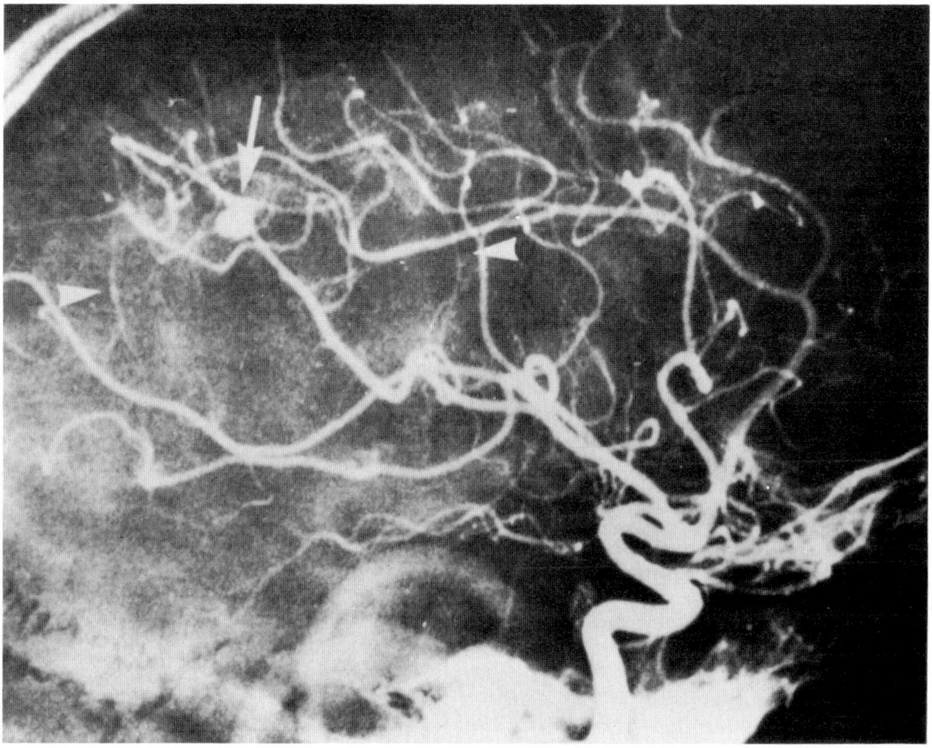

FIG. 7. Left common carotid angiogram of a 35-year-old woman with an 8-year history of heroin addiction, endocarditis, and cerebral embolus. Note mycotic aneurysm (*arrow*) with surface vessels displaced by an associated cerebral abscess (*arrowheads*). (Reprinted from Rumbaugh and Fana, ref. 91.)

carditis involving previously anatomically normal valves generally tends to be caused by a more virulent organism and is associated with a higher mortality than in those persons with previous cardiac disease. In their series, however, predisposing factors (mainly drug addiction and alcoholism) were seen in 71% of cases.

Although the decrease in mortality may reflect prompt recognition of the diagnosis with aggressive antibiotic therapy and prompt surgical intervention, other factors may be operative. The increased incidence of tricuspid endocarditis reported in the literature may favorably influence mortality. Reyes et al. (21) found mortality with pseudomonas endocarditis to be 89% if the left side of the heart was affected, as compared to 29% when only the tricuspid or pulmonary valve was involved.

Relationship to Infective Organism

The relationship between mortality and infective organism is seen in Table 4. Not unexpectedly, in the cases caused by entercoccus, candida, and

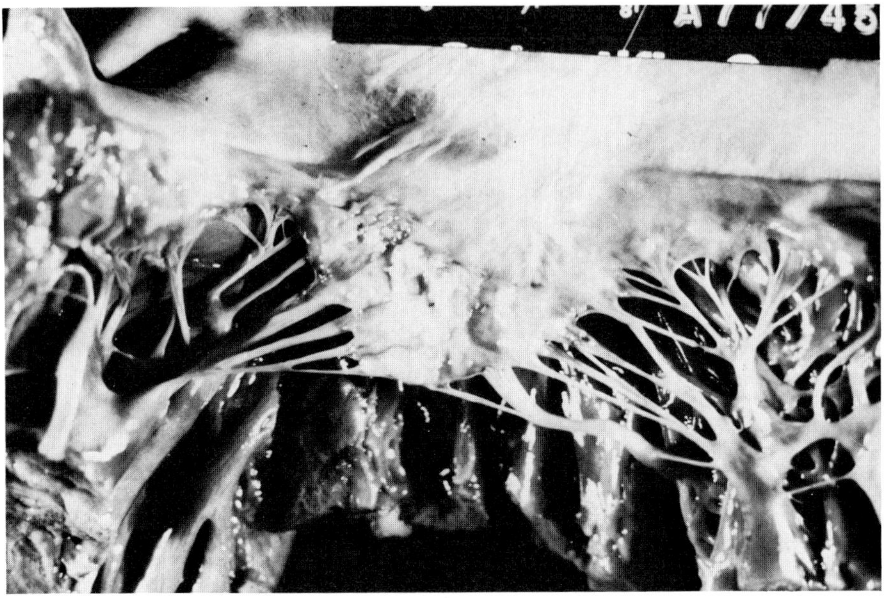

FIG. 8. Perforating endocarditis of the mitral valve. (Courtesy of Dr. Steven Geller.)

pseudomonas, mortality rates of 56, 75, and 55%, respectively, were noted. Staphylococcus, although the predominant organism in reported cases, was associated with a mortality of only 19%. This difference is probably related to predilection of this organism for the tricuspid valve, which carries a more benign prognosis.

Mortality of medical versus surgical therapy varies with reported series. Tricuspid valve replacement has been associated with a success rate of 75%, whereas in replacement of aortic and mitral valves, mortality has varied from 35 to 100% (20,21,64,72). As more experience is gained with early surgical intervention, postoperative mortality rates will, hopefully, continue to decline.

Prevention of Reinfection

Unfortunately, even though the addict with endocarditis may be successfully treated with eradication of the bacteremia and subsequent stabilization of his/her medical condition, in the face of continuing drug use, the ultimate prognosis is poor. Reinfection of the prosthetic valve will undoubtedly occur, with repeated courses of antibiotic therapy and/or valve replacement being necessary. It is therefore essential that the physician not only treat the endocarditis but also make an attempt to provide a therapeutic rationale with respect to the individual's heroin addiction. Subsequent to successful rehabilitation, instruction should be given concerning the need for prophylaxis with antimicrobial agents prior to operative procedures or manipulative dental work.

VASCULAR LESIONS

Arterial Occulsion

Inadvertent intraarterial injection of street drugs (Table 8), most specifically amphetamine, methylphenidate, and barbiturates, alone or in combination with heroin, has been known to result in mycotic aneurysm formation and arterial occulsion, with attendant vascular insufficiency and gangrene (73–76).

Complications secondary to intraarterial injection are attributed to mechanical occulsion secondary to vascular spasm. Alix et al. (77), however, in a canine model utilizing doses of drugs comparable to those available in the street setting, found that most drugs, with the exception of amphetamines, actually increase arterial flow. Amphetamines did cause arterial spasm with flow reduction. These findings were consistent, independent of the presence or absence of adulterants or in section of oral or parenteral forms of the drug. Neither *in vitro* crystalization nor increased platelet aggregation was observed. The reasons for the changes observed clinically remain unclear. It is likely, however, that vascular damage may relate to perivascular injection with hematoma formation, intimal destruction, and an actual adverse effect from prolonged use of tourniquets when injecting these medications.

TABLE 8. *Substances injected intraarterially*

Drugs	Adulterants
Barbiturates	Talc
Amphetamines	Lactate
Analgesic agents	Corn starch
Morphine sulfate	Sodium carbonate
Methadone hydrochloride	
Propoxyphene (Darvon®)	

Necrotizing Angitis

During the past several years, necrotizing angitis has been reported in parenteral drug abusers (78,79). Presenting symptoms have varied greatly, ranging from rather mild complaints to renal failure, pulmonary edema, and cerebrovascular accidents. Pathologically and angiographically, the lesions are quite similar to polyarteritis nodosa. Although the etiology of this disorder remains unknown, it is possible that immune complex formation, secondary to morphine binding antibodies or antibodies developing in response to the adulterants or other injected drugs, may play an important role. Although many persons injected heroin, coexisting amphetamine abuse or abuse of other nonnarcotic drugs was uniformly present. No specific treatment has been reported. The causal relationship of this entity to illicit drug use has been questioned (80).

Pulmonary Hypertension

When talc is injected into the blood vessels, foreign body granuloma reactions occur, most frequently in the pulmonary interstitum but also in the lumens of the small pulmonary arteries. Depositions of granulomas in the lung tissue may lead to interstitial pulmonary fibrosis with ultimate clinical manifestations of restrictive lung disease. Formation of the talc granulomas in the pulmonary vasculature can result in pulmonary arterial hypertension (Fig. 9). Pathologic studies in these patients have revealed the presence of right ventricular hypertrophy, medial hypertrophy of the muscular pulmonary arteries, and fibrous intimal proliferation with plexiform vascular lesions

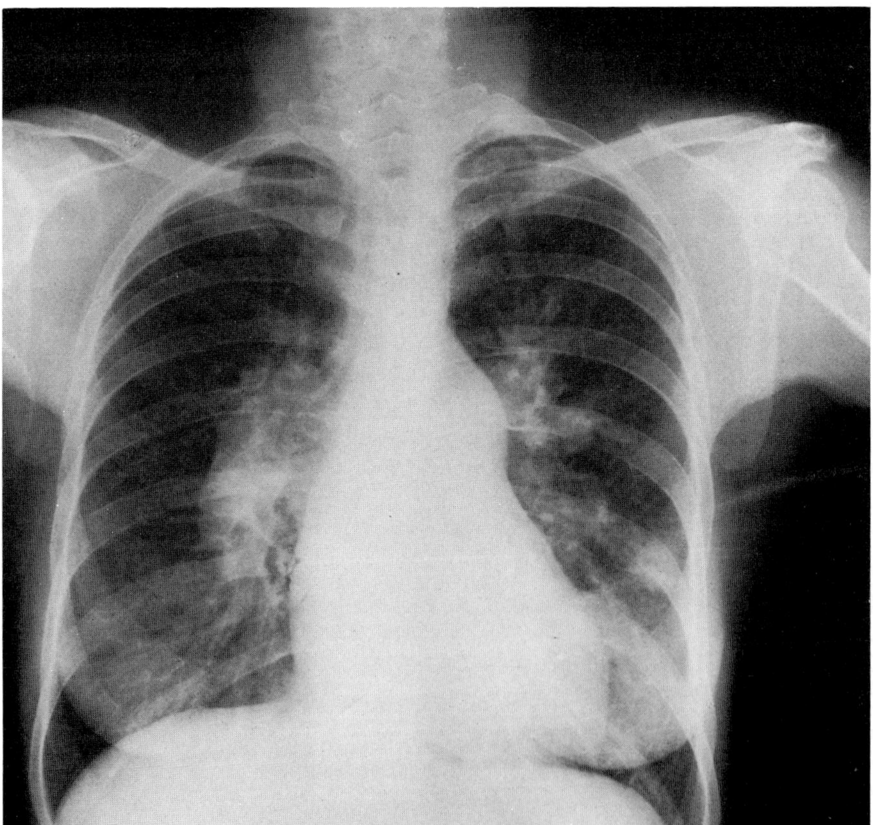

FIG. 9. Chest X-ray of a 40-year-old woman with a 20-year history of heroin addiction and pulmonary hypertension. Pulmonary conus and right and left pulmonary arteries are markedly enlarged. (Reprinted from Stimmel, ref. 92.)

(81,82). Arnett et al. (83), in a review of 21 patients with pulmonary talc granulomas, found 13 to have morphologic evidence of pulmonary hypertension and four to have changes indicative of severe pulmonary hypertension. The degree of severity of these lesions relates to individual sensitivity to talc or other materials and total dose of injected contaminants.

Pulmonary hypertension with cor pulmonale was not an infrequent phenomenon in the 1960s when paregoric was sold as an over-the-counter item in Detroit. At that time, a number of persons became dependent on a mixture of paregoric and tripelennamine (blue velvet) (84). This solution was so viscous that only the large superficial veins could be used for injections. Repeated use resulted in sclerosis of these veins, as well as obliteration of pulmonary arterioles.

Intravenous injection of foreign bodies may induce pathologic, roentgenographic, clinical, and hemodynamic changes of pulmonary hypertension. Pulmonary function tests may show a marked decrease in diffusing capacity as measured by the single breath carbon monoxide method. In a study of four patients, Robertson et al. (85) found the magnitude of decrease in diffusing capacity to be correlated with mean pulmonary artery pressure as well as pulmonary vascular resistance. This suggests that diffusing capacity may be a valuable test in screening for pulmonary hypertension in intravenous drug users.

The clinical relevance of pulmonary hypertension with respect to the high incidence of sudden deaths noted in drug addicts may be considerable. Reduction of right ventricular filling pressure, induced by contaminants having considerable vasodilatory properties in the setting of a high pulmonary vascular resistance, could be catastrophic secondary to severe hypotension. Indirect evidence of this relationship has been demonstrated by Hopkins (81), who noted extensive pulmonary granuloma in 15% of autopsy patients in whom sudden death occurred.

Thrombophlebitis

Acute suppurative thrombophlebitis may occur in both the upper and lower extremities secondary to illicit drug injection. Acute inflammation with edema is noted along the course of venous distribution. Detection may be difficult if an associated cellulitis exists. The presence of septic pulmonary emboli may be the first sign of phlebitis. Treatment with appropriate antibiotics, anticoagulants, and supportive therapy should be instituted as soon as the diagnosis is made.

OVERDOSE REACTIONS

Sudden death following illicit heroin injection is the most serious acute complication of heroin use, at one time accounting for 80% of addict deaths in New York city (86). The magnitude of this problem can be appreciated by the somber statistic that during 1970 and 1971 in New York city, heroin was the single leading cause of death in young men between the ages of 15 and 35 (87). Death is usually so rapid that in the majority of cases the person may be found with the needle still in position in the vein. The acute reaction, however, may also occur at a rate sufficiently slow to allow medical aid to be sought and appropriate therapy instituted.

Etiology

Until recently, it had been commonly assumed that all such deaths resulted from a pharmacologic overdose. Review of the evidence surrounding "overdose" deaths and the results of toxicologic examinations have suggested the possibility of multiple etiologic factors (Table 9). The term acute fatal reaction is therefore more appropriate than overdose deaths.

TABLE 9. *Etiologic mechanisms in an acute fatal reaction to heroin injection*

Allergic reactions
Aspiration of gastric contents
Cardiac arrhythmias
Pharmacologic overdose
Synergistic respiratory depressant effect of polydrug abuse
Vasodilatation in the presence of pulmonary hypertension

Cardiovascular changes during an acute fatal reaction are quite frequent. As discussed earlier, electrocardiographic abnormalities can be recorded and may be severe enough to end in death. Such arrhythmias may be the result of either hypoxia caused by a pharmacologic overdose or an allergic reaction to contaminants in the heroin mixture, or be related to a synergistic action of multiple drugs. Prompt diagnosis and treatment is essential if mortality is to be avoided.

Diagnosis

A precise history is always the best method of confirming a diagnosis of an acute fatal reaction. Unfortunately, a history may not be obtainable from the patient because of an altered level of consciousness; and, not infrequently, the patient will be "deposited" in the emergency room. For this reason, a careful physical examination is essential. In an acute fatal reaction, all vital signs may be depressed, with respiration absent or only minimally effective. In up to one-third of persons, however, an actual increase in respiratory rate may occur. The pulse can be rapid and irregular due to either hypoxia, concomitant administration of stimulant drugs, or arrhythmias. Fevers as high as 104° F may be seen. The pupils are usually miotic, unless severe hypoxia or multiple drug abuse is present; in such instances, they may be widely dilated and often nonreactive to light. In the presence of acute pulmonary edema, frothy sputum completely filling the pharynx is not uncommon. Even in the absence of increased pharyngeal secretions, bilateral rales can be heard on auscultation of the chest, and diffuse infiltrates compatible with pulmonary edema may be noted on roentgenographic examination.

Treatment

Initial treatment of narcotic overdose is similar to that of other respiratory depressant drugs. Of immediate concern is the assurance of an open airway and provision of ventilation. Intubation or tracheotomy may be necessary. Since there is no way of determining whether an actual pharmacologic overdose is present, treatment with a narcotic antagonist should be promptly instituted. The narcotic antagonist of choice is naloxone hydrochloride (Narcan®). Naloxone is an antagonist that is practically devoid of all agonist activity, having neither respiratory nor cardiovascular depressant actions when administered in the absence of a narcotic overdose. Given intravenously in doses ranging from 0.4 to 1.0 mg in the presence of a narcotic-induced reaction, a response is usually obtained within 30 to 50 sec. This response consists of lightening of the comatose state, dilatation of the pupils, and a marked increase in respiratory rate and volume. If a response is not obtained within several minutes after naloxone administration of two doses of increasing strength, it is more than likely that the comatose state is not primarily due to a pharmacologic overdose.

It should be noted that the duration of action of naloxone is 2 to 3 hr, whereas the depressant action of heroin lasts for 6 to 8 hr and that of methadone for 24 to 72 hr. Periodic administration and careful observation is therefore necessary to maintain consciousness, with continual administration of naloxone as indicated. Institution of appropriate therapy in the absence of prolonged hypoxia should result in a favorable outcome.

REFERENCES

1. Paranthaman, S. K., and Khan, F. (1976): Acute cardiomyopathy with recurrent pulmonary edema and hypotension following heroin overdose. *Chest,* 69:117.
2. Addington, W. W., Cugell, D. W., Bazley, E. S., et al. (1972): The pulmonary edema of heroin toxicity: An example of the stiff lung syndrome. *Chest,* 62:199.
3. Lipski, J., Stimmel, B., and Donoso, E. (1973): The effect of heroin and multiple drug abuse on the electrocardiogram. *Am. Heart J.,* 86:663.
4. Duberstein, J. L., and Kaufman, D. M. (1971): A clinical study of an epidemic of heroin intoxication and heroin induced pulmonary edema. *Am. J. Med.,* 51:704.
5. Labi, M. (1969): Paroxysmal atrial fibrillation in heroin intoxication. *Ann. Intern. Med.,* 71:951.

6. Glauser, F. L., Downie, R. L., and Smith, W. R. (1977): Electrocardiographic abnormalities in acute heroin overdose. *Bull. Narc.*, XXIX:85.
7. Guenter, C. A. (1975): The effects of acute severe arterial hypoxemia on the electrocardiogram during exercise. *Chest,* 68:149.
8. James, T. N. (1969): QT prolongation and sudden death. *Mod. Concepts Cardiovasc. Dis.,* 38:35.
9. Lupovich, P., Pilewski, R., and Sapira, J. D. (1970): Cardiotoxicity of quinine as an adulterant in drugs. *JAMA,* 212:1216.
10. Halpern, M., and Rho, Y. (1966): Death from narcotics in New York city. Incidence, circumstances and postmortem findings. *N.Y. State J. Med.,* 66:2391.
11. Rho, Y. M. (1972): Infections as fatal complications of narcotism. *N.Y. State J. Med.,* 72:823.
12. Stimmel, B., Donoso, E., and Dack, S. (1973): Comparison of infective endocarditis in drug addicts and nondrug users. *Am. J. Cardiol.,* 32:924.
13. Ouria, D., Hensle, T., and Rose, J. (1967): The major complications of heroin addiction. *Ann. Intern. Med.,* 67:1.
14. Curtis, J., Richman, B. L., and Feinstein, M. A. (1974): Infective endocarditis in drug addicts. *South. Med. J.,* 67:4.
15. Hussey, H. H., and Katz, S. (1950): Infections resulting from narcotic addiction. Report of 102 cases. *Am. J. Med.,* 9:186.
16. Kearns, J. J. (1936): Malignant endocarditis due to bacillus pyocyaneus. *Arch. Pathol.,* 21:839.
17. Ramsey, R. G., Gunnar, R. M., and Tobin, J. R. (1970): Endocarditis in the drug addict. *Am. J. Cardiol.,* 25:608.
18. Menda, K. B., and Gorbach, S. L. (1973): Favorable experience with bacterial endocarditis in heroin addicts. *Ann. Intern. Med.,* 78:25.
19. Dreyer, N. P., and Fields, B. N. (1973): Heroin associated endocarditis: A report of 28 cases. *Ann. Intern. Med.,* 78:699.
20. Banks, T., Fletcher, R., and Ali, N. (1973): Infective endocarditis in heroin addicts. *Am. J. Med.,* 55:444.
21. Reyes, M. P., Palutke, W. A., Wylin, R. F., and Learner, A. M. (1973): Pseudomonas endocarditis in the Detroit Medical Center. *Medicine,* 52:173.
22. Archer, G., Fekety, F. R., and Supena, R. (1974): Pseudomonas aeruginosa endocarditis in drug addicts. *Am. Heart J.,* 88:570.
23. Noriega, E. R., Rubinstein, E., Simberkoff, M. S., et al. (1975): Subacute and acute endocarditis due to pseudomonas cepacia in heroin addicts. *Am. J. Med.,* 59:29.
24. Reiner, N. E., Gopalakrishma, K. V., and Lerner, P. L. (1976): Enterococcal endocarditis in heroin addicts. *JAMA,* 235:1861.
25. Mills, J., and Drew, D. (1976): Serratia marcescens endocarditis: A regional illness associated with intravenous drug abuse. *Ann. Intern. Med.,* 84:29.
26. Tuazon, C. U., Hill, R., and Sheagren, J. N. (1974): Microbiologic study of street heroin and injection paraphernalia. *J. Infect. Dis.,* 129:327.
27. Tuazon, C. U., and Sheagren, J. N. (1974): Increased staphylococcal carrier rate among narcotic addicts. *J. Infect. Dis.,* 129:725.
28. Tuazon, C. U., Perez, A., Kishaba, T., and Sheagren, J. N. (1975): Staphylococcus aureus among insulin-injecting diabetic patients. An increased carrier rate. *JAMA,* 231:1272.
29. Weinstein, L., and Schlesinger, J. J. (1974): Pathoanatomic, pathophysiologic and clinical correlation in endocarditis. *N. Engl. J. Med.,* 291:832.
30. Durack, D. T., and Beeson, P. B. (1972): Experimental bacterial endocarditis I. Colonization of a sterile vegetation. *Br. J. Exp. Pathol.,* 53:44.
31. Krueger, H., Eddy, N. B., and Sumwalt, M. (1941): The pharmacology of the opium alkaloids. Part 1. U.S. Government Printing Office, Washington, D.C.
32. Nickerson, D. S., Williams, R. C., Jr., and Boxmeyer, M. (1970): Increased opsonic capacity of serum in chronic heroin addiction. *Ann. Intern. Med.,* 72:671.
33. Luttgrens, W. F. (1949): Endocarditis in mainline opium addicts. *Arch. Intern. Med.,* 83:653.

34. Bain, R. C., Edwards, J. E., Schiefley, C. H., and Geraci, J. E. (1958): Right-sided bacterial endocarditis and endarteritis. *Am. J. Med.,* 24:98.
35. Sapira, J. D. (1968): The narcotic addict as a medical patient. *Am. J. Med.,* 45:555.
36. Dreyer, N. P., and Fields, B. N. (1973): Associated infective endocarditis. A report of 28 cases. *Ann. Intern. Med.,* 78:699.
37. Rios, J. C., Massumi, R. A., Bressman, T. T., and Sarin, R. K. (1969): Auscultatory features of acute tricuspid regurgitation. *Am. J. Cardiol.,* 23:4.
38. Olsson, R. A., and Romansky, M. J. (1962): Staphylococcal tricuspid endocarditis in heroin addicts. *Ann. Intern. Med.,* 57:755.
39. Orlando, J., Francis, C. K., and Thadepalli, H. (1974): Variable presentation of infective endocarditis in intravenous drug abusers. *Circulation* [*Suppl. III*], 50:238.
40. Nagel, J., Tuazon, C. U., Cardella, T., and Sheagren, J. N. (1974): Serologic diagnosis of staphylococcal endocarditis: Studies in parenteral drug abusers. *Clin. Res.,* 22(3):451A.
41. Tuazon, C. U., and Sheagren, J. N. (1976): Teichoic acid antibodies in the diagnosis of serious infections with staphylococcus aureus. *Ann. Intern. Med.,* 84:543.
42. Crowder, J. G., and White, A. (1972): Teichoic acid antibodies in staphylococcal and non-staphylococcal endocarditis. *Ann. Intern. Med.,* 77:87.
43. McLeod, R., and Remington, J. S. (1978): Fungal endocarditis. In: *Infective Endocarditis,* edited by S. H. Rahimtoola, pp. 211–290. Grune & Stratton, New York.
44. Powers, D. L., and Mandell, G. I. (1974): Intraleukocytic bacteria in endocarditis patients. *JAMA,* 227:312.
45. Harache, P. (1976): Atypical bacterial forms in human disease. In: *Microbial Protoplasts Spheroplasts and L Forms,* edited by L. B. Guze, p. 484. Williams & Wilkins, Philadelphia.
46. Wiseman, J., Rovleau, J., Rigo, P., et al. (1976): Gallium-67 myocardial imaging for the detection of bacterial endocarditis. *Radiology,* 120:135.
47. Kennedy, J. E., and Wise, G. N. (1965): Clinicopathological correlation of retinal lesions: SVL acute bacterial endocarditis. *Arch. Ophthalmol.,* 74:658.
48. Levy, R. L., and Hong, R. (1973): The immune nature of subacute bacterial endocarditis (SBE) nephritis. *Am. J. Med.,* 54:645.
49. Von Gemmingen, G. R., and Winkelmann, R. K. (1967): Osler's node of subacute bacterial endocarditis. *Arch. Dermatol.,* 95:91.
50. Gutman, R. A., Striker, G. E., Gilliland, B. C., et al. (1972): The immune complex glomerulonephritis of bacterial endocarditis. *Medicine* (*Baltimore*), 51:1.
51. Bayer, A. S., Theofilopoulos, A. N., Eisenberg, R., et al. (1976): Circulating immune complexes in infective endocarditis. *N. Engl. J. Med.,* 295:1500.
52. Spangler, R. D., Johnson, M. L., Holmes, J. H., et al. (1973): Echocardiographic demonstrations of bacterial vegetations in active infective endocarditis. *J. Clin. Ultrasound,* 1:126.
53. Dillon, J. C., Feigenbaum, H., Konecke, L. L., et al. (1973): Echocardiographic manifestations of valvular vegetations. *Am. Heart J.,* 86:698.
54. DeMaria, A. N., King, J. F., Salel, A. F., et al. (1975): Echocardiography and phonocardiography of acute aortic regurgitation in bacterial endocarditis. *Ann. Intern. Med.,* 82:329.
55. Roy, P., Tajik, A. J., and Guilianc, E. R. (1976): Spectrum of echocardiographic findings in bacterial endocarditis. *Circulation,* 53:474.
56. Andy, J. J., Sheikh, M. U., Ali, N., et al. (1977): Echocardiographic observations in opiate addicts with active infective endocarditis. *Am. J. Cardiol.,* 40:17.
57. Pratt, C., Witcomb, C., Neumann, A., et al. (1978): Relationship of vegetations on echogram to the clinical course and systemic emboli in bacterial endocarditis. *Am. J. Cardiol.,* 41:384 (Abstr.).
58. Kisslo, J., Von Ramm, O. T., and Haney, R. (1976): Echocardiographic evaluation of tricuspid valve endocarditis. *Am. J. Cardiol.,* 38:502.
59. Andriole, V. T., Kravetz, H. M., Roberts, W. C., and Utz, J. P. (1962): Candida endocarditis. Clinical and pathologic studies. *Am. J. Med.,* 32:251.

60. Zimmerman, L. E. (1950): Candida and aspergillus endocarditis due to pseudomonas auruginosa. *Arch. Pathol.,* 50:591.
61. Andriole, V. T. (1970): Endocarditis in the drug user. *Conn. Med.,* 34:327.
62. Hermans, P. E., and Washington, J. A., II (1970): Polymicrobial bacteremia. *Ann. Intern. Med.,* 73:387.
63. Saravoloutz, L. D. (1978): Polymicrobial infective endocarditis: An increasing clinical entity. *Am. Heart J.,* 95:163.
64. Manhas, D. R., Hessel, E. A., Winterscheid, L. C., Dillard, D. H., and Merendino, K. A. (1970): Open heart surgery in infective endocarditis. *Circulation,* XLI:841.
65. Krishnaswami V., Reddy, S., O'Toole, J., Curtiss, E., Shaver, J., and Bahnson, H. (1974): Expectant surgical treatment of acute aortic regurgitation in infective endocarditis. *Circulation* [*Suppl. III*], 49–50:42 (Abstr.).
66. Stason, W. B., DeSanctis, R. W., Weinberg, A. N., and Austen, W. G. (1968): Cardiac surgery in bacterial endocarditis. *Circulation,* 38:514.
67. Braimbridge, M. V. (1969): Cardiac surgery and bacterial endocarditis. *Lancet,* 1:1307.
68. Hancock, E. W., Shumway, N. E., and Remington, J. S. (1971): Valve replacement in active bacterial endocarditis. *J. Infect. Dis.,* 123:106.
69. Arbulu, A., Thomas, N. W., and Wilson, R. F. (1971): Complete valvulectomy without prosthetic replacement in the treatment of tricuspid pseudomonas endocarditis. *Circulation* [*Suppl. 2*], 64:108.
70. Ganguly, S., Robin, E., Laurent, D., and Arbulu, A. (1972): Acute and chronic hemodynamic changes in dogs and man following removal of the tricuspid valve. *Clin. Res.,* 20:717 (Abstr.).
71. Robin, E., Thoms, N. W., Arbulu, A., Ganguly, S. N., and Magnisalis, K. (1975): Hemodynamic consequences of total removal of the tricuspid valve without prosthetic replacement. *Am. J. Cardiol.,* 35:481.
72. Buchbinder, N., and Roberts, W. C. (1972): Left sided valvular active infective endocarditis. A study of forty-five necropsy patients. *Am. J. Med.,* 53:20.
73. Jaffee, R. B., and Koschemann, E. B. (1970): Intravenous drug abuse—pulmonary cardiac and vascular complications. *Am. J. Roentgenol.,* 109:107.
74. Perlman, H. S., Wollowick, B. S., and Alvarez, E. V. (1970): Intra-arterial injection of propoxyphene into brachial artery. *JAMA,* 214:2055.
75. Cohen, S. M. (1948): Accidental intral arterial injection of drugs. *Lancet,* 2:361.
76. Joseph, W. L., Fletcher, H. S., Giordano, J. M., et al. (1973): Pulmonary and cardiovascular implications of drug addiction. *Ann. Thorac. Surg.,* 15:263.
77. Alix, E. C., Bogumill, G. P., and Wright, C. B. (1975): Intra arterial injection of abused drugs. *Cardiovasc. Res.,* 9:266.
78. Citron, B. P., Halpern, M., and McCarron, M. (1970): Necrotizing angitis associated with drug abuse. *N. Engl. J. Med.,* 283:1003.
79. Rumbaugh, C. L., Bergeron, R. T., and Fan, H. C. H. (1971): Cerebral angiographic changes in the drug abuse patient. *Radiology,* 101:335.
80. Baden, M. (1971): Angitis in drug abusers. *N. Engl. J. Med.,* 289:111.
81. Hopkins, C. B. (1972): Pulmonary angiothrombotic granulomatosis in drug offenders. *JAMA,* 221:909.
82. Siegel, H. (1971): Human pulmonary pathology associated with narcotics and other addictive drugs. *Hum. Pathol.,* 3:55.
83. Arnett, E. N., Battle, W. E., and Roberts, W. C. (1976): Intravenous injection of talc containing drugs intended for oral use. *Am. J. Med.,* 60:711.
84. Wendt, V. E., Puro, H. E., Shapiro, J., et al. (1964): Angiothrombotic pulmonary hypertension in addicts, "Blue Velvet" addiction. *JAMA,* 188:755.
85. Robertson, C. H., Reynolds, R. C., and Wilson, J. E. (1966): Pulmonary hypertension and foreign body granulomas in intravenous drug abusers. *Am. J. Med.,* 61:657.
86. Cherubin, C., McCusker, J., and Baden, M. (1972): The epidemiology of death in narcotic addicts. *Am. J. Epidemiol.,* 96:11.
87. Halpern, M. (1971): Fatalities from narcotic addiction in New York City. Incidence, circumstance and pathologic findings. *Hum. Pathol.,* 3:13.

88. Stimmel, B. (1975): The effects of mood-altering drugs on the heart. In: *Current Cardiovascular Topics, Vol. 1: Drugs in Cardiology,* edited by E. Donoso, p. 218. Stratton Intercontinental, New York.
89. Labi, M. (1969): Paroxysmal atrial fibrillation in heroin intoxication. *Ann. Intern. Med.,* 71:955.
90. Dillon, J. C., Feigenbaum, H., Konecke, L. L., et al., (1973): Echocardiographic manifestations of valvular vegetations. *Am. Heart J.,* 86:700.
91. Rumbaugh, C. L., and Fana, H. C. H. (1978): The effects of drug abuse on the brain. *Resident Staff Physician,* April:49.
92. Stimmel, B. (1975): In: *Heroin Dependency: Medical, Economic and Social Aspects,* p. 145. Stratton Intercontinental, New York.

Pharmacology

The amphetamines comprise a group of noncatecholamine phenylisopropylamines having potent sympathomimetic activity. They differ from sympathetic amines, such as epinephrine, by having (a) a greater stimulating effect on the CNS, (b) greater effectiveness after oral administration, and (c) duration of action measured in hours rather than minutes. Phenmetrazine (Preludin®) and diethylpropion (Tenuate®), although not phenylisopropylamines, are considered to be amphetamine-like substances because of a marked similarity in action.

Following oral ingestion, the amphetamines are readily absorbed from the intestinal tract and are distributed to the tissues, including the CNS. Inactivation occurs in the liver with excretion in bile and urine. Urinary excretion is considerably affected by pH, with acidification of urine resulting in an 80% excretion, as compared to 2 to 3% excretion in an alkaline urine (8).

Several mechanisms have been postulated to explain the actions of amphetamine. These include (a) direct and indirect release of norepinephrine or dopamine from nerve terminals, (b) inhibition of monoamine oxidase (MAO), (c) direct action on sympathetic receptors, and (d) prevention of reuptake of norepinephrine and dopamine by the nerve terminals. Although the predominant mechanism of action has not yet been clarified, amphetamine is a potent CNS stimulator and peripheral sympathomimetic activator.

Hemodynamic Effects

Ingested amphetamine in humans results in an increase in systolic and diastolic blood pressure, as well as pulse pressure secondary to the action of amphetamine on both alpha and beta receptor sites. The blood pressure elevation is directly related to the dose of amphetamine administered (9). Morselli et al. (10) have demonstrated that arterial pressures start to rise at much higher plasma levels than seen with the appearance of electrocardiographic changes (20 versus 5 ng/ml), suggesting a predominant peripheral action of amphetamine. Systolic pressures increase proportionately greater than diastolic pressures. Cerebral blood flow and cerebral oxygen consumption in laboratory animals have been shown to increase after amphetamine infusion (11).

Clinically, amphetamine ingestion or injection is followed by tachycardia, palpitations, flushing, sweating, and headache. Continued administration results in a degree of tolerance so that tachycardia and hypertension may not be prominent in chronic users (12). With increasing doses, cardiac arrhythmias may occur. Even in tolerant persons, however, intravenous use may result in flushing, palpitations, anginal pain, severe hypertension, and headache. Extremely large doses may cause arrhythmias, hyperpyrexia, hypotension, circulatory collapse, coma, and convulsions (13). Intracranial hemorrhages, secondary to severe hypertension, have also been reported (14). Zalis and co-workers (15,16) have produced subendocardial hemorrhages in dogs by intravenously administering lethal doses of pharmacologically pure amphetamines. The clinical significance of this finding is unclear.

Experimentally, when administered in relatively large doses, catecholamines can produce myocardial ischemia and necrosis in animals (17,18). These changes may be prevented by the use of reserpine and MAO inhibitors (18). Clinically, there have been few reports of amphetamine-induced myocardial disease. This may relate more to the young age of most amphetamine users than to a low potential of amphetamine to produce myocardial damage. Smith et al. (19) reported the appearance of cardiomyopathy in a 45-year-old man, without evidence of coronary disease, valve disease, or other preexisting cardiac disease, maintained on high-dose dextroamphetamine for 7 years. At postmortem examination, lesions similar to the myocarditis associated with pheochromocytoma were found, leading the authors to hypothesize a cardiomyopathy either directly related to excessive sympathetic activity or secondary to end-stage amphetamine-induced chronic myocardial hypertrophy. Although the effect of amphetamines in persons with clinical cardiac disease may be quite deleterious, the precise relationship of amphetamines to cardiac decompensation in an individual without underlying myocardial disease remains unclear.

Illicit Use

Chronic use of intravenous amphetamines is attendant with all the complications discussed in association with parenteral heroin abuse (Chapter 12), including hepatitis, bacterial or fungal endocarditis, pulmonary angiothrombotic granulomatosis, microangiopathic hemolytic anemia, and anaphylactic reactions. Some of these disorders, notably, necrotizing angitis and mycotic aneurysm formation, are specifically related to the amphetamine rather than heroin or other adulterants.

Cerebrovascular Disease

Rumbaugh et al. (20) have observed cerebral angiographic changes in young drug abusers admitted for a variety of neurologic complaints. Angiography in these patients, most of whom misused amphetamines, revealed the presence of small vessel occlusive disease (Fig. 1). Although such individuals may tend toward polysubstance abuse, with parenteral as well as oral consumption of drugs, additional experiments by these authors suggest that amphetamine, medically administered by itself, can affect the cerebral vasculature (21). Monkeys receiving daily methamphetamine (1.5 mg/kg body weight i.v.) for periods ranging from 1 week to 1 year demonstrated signifi-

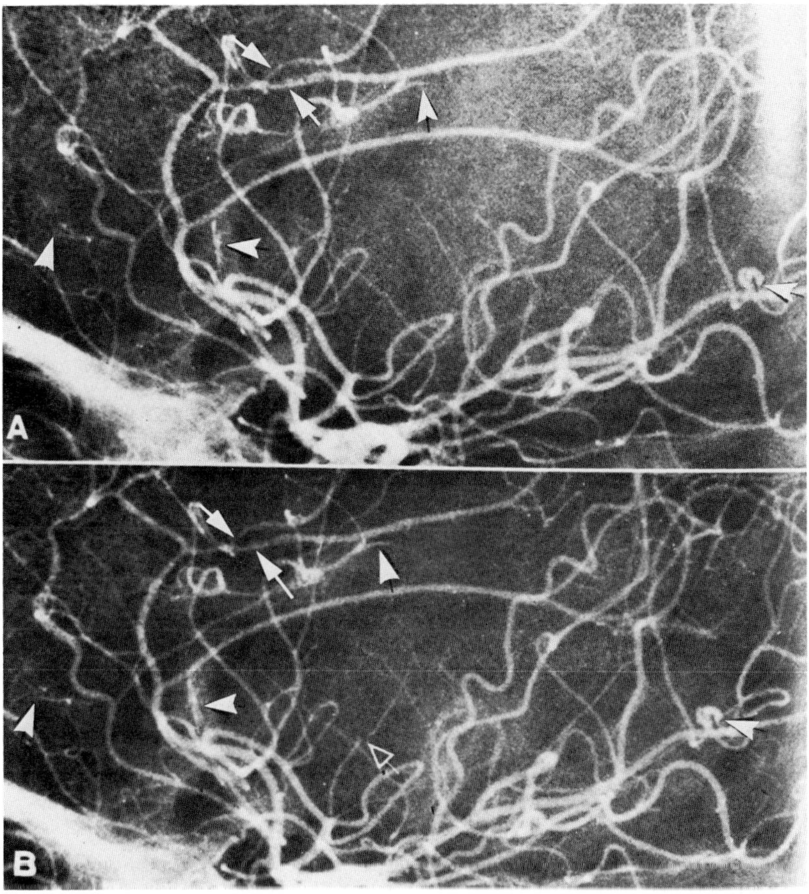

FIG. 1. Serial magnification view of carotid angiogram of a 38-year-old woman with a history of amphetamine abuse. Note moderate beading of the right callosomarginal branches (*solid arrows*) with extensive small artery branch occlusions (*open white arrows* with white tails). *Open white arrow*, small arterial filling defect. (Reprinted from Rumbaugh et al., ref. 20.)

cant vascular lesions. In the short-term study, two of three animals demonstrated a diffuse decrease in the caliber of cortical arteries, with disruption of connecting channels and perforations in the frontal cortex. Animals administered methamphetamine for 1 month showed similar changes associated with subacute neuronal cell damage. In the animals treated with methamphetamine for 1 year, occlusions and slow blood flow were seen in three of five. All animals, however, showed extensive vascular changes on histologic section, most prominent in the cortical areas of the frontal, temporal, and occipital lobes. These findings indicate the ability of long-term parenteral amphetamine use to cause central vascular damage. Whether or not such changes are attributable to the actions of amphetamine in producing vasospasm, however, is still unclear. The methamphetamine administered was prepared by dissolving 5 mg Desoxyn® tablets in sterile saline. Since talc crystals were occasionally seen in histologic section in all groups, it is possible that the filler substance plays more than a small role in producing these changes.

Intraarterial Thrombosis

Intraarterial injection of amphetamine can have a direct effect on arterial spasm and reduction in flow. Clinically, arterial insufficiency and gangrene may ensue (see Chapter 12).

Rhabdomyolysis

Kendrick et al. (22) have described the appearance of rhabdomyolysis and shock after illicit intravenous amphetamines in four patients. These patients were chronic intravenous amphetamine users and felt well before their last injection. Within 15 min to 1 hr postinjection, fevers, chills, vomiting, myalgias, and myoedema developed with increased serum creatine phosphokinase and aldolase. Myoglobinurea was also present, as was evidence of disseminated intravascular coagulation. Elevated serum and urine sodium concentrations suggested associated renal injury. Therapy with aggressive extracellular volume repletion and prevention of hyperkalemia resulted in successful outcomes.

Overdose Reactions

Acute pharmacologic overdose with amphetamines is not an infrequent phenomenon. Individual tolerance to these agents varies, with extraordinarily large doses being tolerated in chronic amphetamine users. A toxic dose may therefore vary from 30 to 125 mg in nontolerant individuals and from 300 to 1,500 mg in chronic abusers. The presence of a toxic reaction also varies with respect to environmental factors and degree of physical exertion. The tendency of large doses of amphetamines to increase oxygen consumption as well as to affect the thermoregulation center in the hypothalamus, with resulting hyperthermia, places amphetamine users performing strenuous exercises in hot weather at particular risk. Severe toxic reactions are manifested by hypertension and hyperpyrexia, followed by convulsions, cerebrovascular accidents, such as subarachnoid and subdural hemorrhage, and, ultimately, cardiovascular collapse and death.

Treatment should involve restoring the temperature toward normal and the use of sedatives (diazepam) to control seizures. The patient should be placed in a quiet environment so that agitation and environmental stimulation are minimal. In the presence of a marked psychotic reaction, appropriate use of the major tranquilizers, such as chlorpromazine (25 to 50 mg i.m. or i.v.), may be effective. The use of chlorpromazine, however, should be accompanied by careful monitoring of blood pressure; it is preferable only when severe hypertension is present because of its activity as an alpha blocker. However, degradation of amphetamine has been reported to be delayed by chlorpromazine, and the potential presence of anticholinergic contaminants in the amphetamine consumed may result in a cholinergic crisis (23). If only psychotic manifestations are present, another drug, such as haloperidol, might be preferable.

It should be emphasized that alkalinization of urine will result in an increased tubular resorption of amphetamine and a marked decrease in urinary excretion of free amphetamine (24). For this, alkalinizing solutions should not be used in fluid replacement for amphetamine overdose or in treatment of toxic psychotic reactions.

COCAINE

Cocaine is a naturally occurring alkaloid obtained from the leaves of erythroxylon coca, comprising 0.5 to 1% of the dry weight of the plant. Chemically, it consists of an ester, benzoic acid, and methylecgonine, a nitrogen-containing base. Cocaine (benzoylmethylecgonine) is a unique drug in that it is not only a local anesthetic but is also a potent sympathomimetic and CNS stimulant. Unlike the amphetamines, little or no tolerance appears to develop to its effects; some evidence has even been presented to suggest that chronic users may become hypersensitive to several of its actions (25–27).

At present, with the exception of its use as a local anesthetic, cocaine is mainly used illicitly, either by snorting or intravenous injection. Although street cocaine is relatively pure (80 to 90%) as compared to preparations of heroin, it is adulterated with a variety of substances, the most common being mannitol, glucose, and lactose. In impure preparations, other stimulants, such as caffeine and amphetamine, may be added to disguise the amount of cocaine present. Parenteral use, either in combination with other illicit drugs or as the sole agent, is associated with all the previously mentioned complications accompanying intravenous heroin and amphetamine injection.

Pharmacology

When administered locally, cocaine is rapidly absorbed, with an onset of action within minutes and a duration of action of up to 2 hr. Intravenous administration results in the appearance of cardiovascular effects within 2 min, with a peak effect seen in 5 to 10 min. Absorption through the intranasal route has a similar time of onset of effects, with a peak effect being seen at 15 to 30 min, depending on the dose administered. Intramuscular or subcutaneous administration is associated with a somewhat limited absorption rate due to the vasoconstrictive action of the drug. Although cocaine is absorbed rapidly through mucous membranes, if ingested, hydrolysis occurs with a marked decrease in absorption. The ineffectiveness of oral cocaine has recently been challenged with evidence presented to demonstrate effective plasma levels within 30 min (28).

Detoxification occurs predominantly in the liver at a rate less than absorption through mucous membranes. The main metabolic products are benzoylecgonine and ecgonine. This phenomenon may lead to toxic reactions when cocaine is absorbed in excessive doses. Elimination occurs in the urine within 24 to 36 hr as the metabolite benzoylecgonine. Less than 20% of the total absorbed dose may be eliminated unchanged in the urine. This proportion increases, however, with increasing doses of cocaine and with decreasing alkalinity in the urine. Excretion of the cocaine base is greatest in acidic urine and less in urine with a more alkaline pH (29).

The mechanism of action of cocaine is complex. It is a potent stimulator of sympathomimetic amines and, in addition, may have some sympathomimetic action of its own. Cocaine can block the uptake of amines into sympathetic nerve terminals, resulting in higher concentrations of circulating catecholamines to interact with the receptor sites. In addition, cocaine may also cause a release of norepinephrine from sympathetic nerve terminals (30). However, this effect has not been as convincingly demonstrated as its ability to block norepinephrine uptake.

Hemodynamic Effects

The experimental effects of cocaine on the heart have been well described. Small doses may actually result in a bradycardia secondary to vagal stimulation. With moderate or large amounts, however, a tachycardia accompanied by systemic hypertension commonly occurs secondary to centrally mediated tachycardia and vasoconstriction. Extremely large doses may result in sudden death due to a direct toxic effect on the myocardium or depression of the medullary centers with hypotension and respiratory arrest (31,32).

Fennel et al. (25), in a study of physiologic and behavioral effects of intravenous cocaine in 12 volunteers with a history of previous illicit drug abuse, found a dose-related increase in heart rate and systolic blood pressure after 8, 16, and 32 mg cocaine. A peak mean heart rate after the maximum dose was found to be 114 beats/min. No major cardiovascular effects were noted at lower doses. Analysis of electrocardiograms did not reveal any significant change in QRS duration, R-R interval, or frequency of atrial or ventricular premature beats. A return to control levels of heart rate and blood pressure was noted within 45 min. Similar findings were noted by Resnick et al. (31), who administered placebo and 10 or 25 mg cocaine by intravenous or intranasal routes under single- and double-blind conditions. Both doses given intravenously produced the expected elevations in heart rate and blood pressure within 2 min, with a peak effect noted within 10 min, although a correlation with plasma cocaine levels was not documented. Intranasal instillation of 10 mg cocaine, however, produced no changes different from placebo administration.

Fischman et al. (33), administering both intravenous amphetamine and cocaine to normal volunteers, found 10 mg dextroamphetamine to produce comparable heart rate and blood pressure effects as 8 to 16 mg cocaine. Disturbances in rhythm, with the exception of an increase in pulse rate, did not occur.

More profound effects of cocaine have been reported in reactions occurring at rock concerts where hypotension and tachycardia, at times reaching 100% above the expected norm, have been observed (34). In such settings, however, it is difficult to ascertain if these reactions were secondary to cocaine or to the presence of one or more unknown drugs. In addition, as described in Chapter 3, psychologic factors might have also accounted for the changes observed. Amphetamines can produce a similar but potent sympathetic response and, not infrequently, are found in substances sold on the street as cocaine. Instances of cardiac arrhythmias, other than sinus tachycardia, in patients receiving topical anesthesia with 3 ml of a 5% (150 mg) aqueous cocaine solution have been reported. These arrhythmias include multiple premature ventricular contractions and bigeminal rhythms (35). Arrhythmias have not been produced, however, when pure cocaine in doses as high as 32 mg i.v. is administered to volunteers in the laboratory setting.

Overdose Reactions

There is considerable variation with respect to the dose of cocaine considered to be toxic in humans. Fatal doses have ranged from 800 to 1,430 mg orally and from 700 to 2,500 mg subcutaneously. Up to 300 mg cocaine have been injected intravenously without adverse effects, whereas doses as low as 22 mg administered subcutaneously have resulted in severe toxic reactions (32). The toxic symptoms developing after cocaine are quite similar to those produced by amphetamines.

Pharmacologic overdose reactions are characterized by a marked stimulation of the CNS. Headache, mydriasis, tachycardia, palpitations, hypertension, hyperpyrexia, and rapid and irregular respiration are early signs. In severe cases, a progesssion to delirium, nausea, vomiting, Cheyne-Stokes respiration, hyperthermia, convulsions, and even death may occur. In instances of overdose from street cocaine, death may be extremely rapid secondary to an anaphylactic reaction to contaminants.

Treatment of acute cocaine reactions is mainly supportive. Treatment of severe CNS excitation is best handled by the use of intravenous diazepam.

Artificial respiration may be necessary in severe cases. Rappolt et al. (34) have advocated the use of propranolol to counteract the clinical sympathomimetic effects. If CNS excitation predominates, use of a sedative or tranquilizing agent, such as diazepam, by intravenous or intramuscular route may be of value. The short duration of action of cocaine, combined with a relative lack of development of tolerance, suggests that, except in circumstances secondary to consumption of large doses, pharmacologic treatment may not be necessary.

METHYLPHENIDATE

Methylphenidate (Ritalin®) is a sympathomimetic drug structurally related to amphetamine currently being used for treatment of the hyperactive child with minimal brain dysfunction. Although the precise prevalence of use of this drug is unknown, several services have revealed that 1 to 2% of school children are being treated for hyperactivity, with methylphenidate hydrocholoride the drug most frequently prescribed (35,36).

Methylphenidate is the drug of choice in the hyperkinetic syndrome since, unlike amphetamine, it is considered to be relatively free of amphetamine-related adverse side-effects, affecting primarily mental rather than motor activities. Methylphenidate, when used in the experimental setting in laboratory animals, has been shown to affect smooth muscle at receptor sites as well as the heart through augmentation of norepinephrine stimulation. This is attributable to either an alteration in the affinity of the receptor site for norepinephrine or a delay in uptake of norepinephrine by adrenergic nerve terminals. Conversely, methylphenidate has also been demonstrated to suppress the positive inotropy and vasoconstriction caused by amphetamine (37).

Clinically, in a prospective matched control study of hyperactive children, methylphenidate can significantly increase both heart rate ($p = 0.001$) and blood pressure ($p = 0.003$) in a dose-related manner (37). Although the mean difference in changes in heart rate and blood pressure was not clinically impressive, there was considerable individual variation. Differences in heart rate as great as 40 beats/min and increases in blood pressure as high as 22 mm systolic and 14 mm diastolic were recorded. Conflicting evidence exists as to whether tolerance to these effects develops with chronic use (38,39). Although the clinical relevance of these findings remains to be clarified, the large range of variation of individual response warrants careful monitoring. Physicians should closely watch for hemodynamic changes associated with increasing dosage of methylphenidate and alter therapy where appropriate.

DRUG INTERACTIONS

Amphetamine and cocaine both exert potent sympathomimetic effects. Concomitant use of either of these medications with antihypertensive drugs acting on the autonomic nervous system can be associated with interference of their antihypertensive action as well as an acute hypertensive crisis. In some instances, a specific competitive action may exist at the receptor site of the neuron between cocaine and the antihypertensive agent. Amphetamines in small doses have been shown to antagonize the antihypertensive effect of guanethidine by blocking its entry into the nerve ending and by affecting a release of norepinephrine and quanethidine from storage granules (40). These adverse reactions may occur with a combination of amphetamines or cocaine and reserpine, alpha-methyldopa, and MAO inhibitors.

Diazoxide, a benzothiadazine derivative, exerts a direct action on arterial muscle to produce vasodilatation. Since diazoxide has little effect on the cardiovascular autonomic reflexes, an increased sympathetic discharge usually occurs. A synergistic reaction may therefore occur with concomitant use of amphetamine or cocaine.

Propranolol is a beta blocker and would therefore be the agent of choice in a person with hypertension who also is using either amphetamine or cocaine. The use of propranolol has even been suggested for treatment of acute cocaine toxicity, but little evidence exists for this.

The use of cocaine in local anesthesia, associated with other local anesthetics containing epinephrine, may cause a marked tachycardia and hypertension. Although younger individuals can tolerate such effects fairly well, in the elderly patient with or without cardiac disease, such a response may be quite detrimental. Epinephrine-containing anesthetic solutions in patients also receiving cocaine for topical anesthesia should be used cautiously with careful monitoring (41).

Although cocaine is rapidly hydrolyzed subsequent to absorption, some of the drug may also undergo hepatic microsomal oxidation. Experimentally, Evans et al. (42) have demonstrated increased lethality of cocaine in laboratory mice simultaneously administered cocaine and phenobarbital. The reason for this was hypothesized to be related to a shift of cocaine metabolism to the hepatic microsomal system with the production of a toxic metabolite. Although these findings are preliminary and confined to the laboratory model, they do suggest that stimulation of microsomal metabolism can produce enhanced toxicity to the formation of a N-oxide metabolic product. The simultaneous use of cocaine with agents having a marked effect on the hepatic microsomal system, such as phenobarbital, coumarin derivatives, and diphenylhydantoin, should therefore be avoided whenever possible.

Interaction between the stimulants and other mood-altering drugs may also be attributable to synergistic reactions with those drugs exerting either an autonomic or central nervous system effect. There is little published, however, concurring the clinical relevance of such interactions.

The postulated mechanism of action of methylphenidate makes its use with guanethidine, MAO inhibitors, and tricyclic antidepressant pressor agents contraindicated (42,43). The metabolism of drugs detoxified by the liver may also be inhibited, so that a downward adjustment of their dosage may be required with concomitant administration. These agents include coumarin derivatives, diphenylhydantoin, and tricyclic antidepressants.

REFERENCES

1. American Medical Association Committee on Alcoholism and Addiction and Mental Health: Dependence on amphetamine and other stimulant drugs. *JAMA,* 197:1023.
2. National Institute of Mental Health, U.S. Dept. of Health, Education and Welfare (1909): The up and down drugs. PHS Publ. no. 1830, U.S. Government Printing Office, Washington, D.C.
3. Walsh, J. (1964): Psychotoxic drugs. *Science,* 145:1418.
4. Parry, H. S., Baeter, M. B., Mellinger, G. D., et al. (1973): National patterns of psychotherapeutic drug use. *Arch. Gen. Psychiatry,* 28:769.
5. Green, S., Nightingale, S. L., and Dupont, R. L. (1975): Evolving patterns of drug abuse. *Ann. Intern. Med.,* 83:402.
6. Student Drug Use Surveys in San Mateo, California 1968–1974 (1974): San Mateo County Dept. of Public Health and Welfare, San Mateo, California.
7. Project DAWN III Drug Enforcement Administration and National Institute of Drug Abuse (1975): BND no. 72–47.
8. Becket, A. H., and Rowland, M. (1965): Urinary excretion and kinetics of amphetamine in man. *J. Pharm. Pharmacol.,* 17:628.
9. Evans, M. A., Martz, R., Lemberger, L., et al. (1976): Effects of dextroamphetamine on psychomotor skills. *Clin. Pharmacol. Ther.,* 19:777.
10. Morselli, P. L., Placidi, G. F., Maggini, C., et al. (1976): An integrated approach for the evaluation of psychotropic drugs in man. *Psychopharmacologia,* 46:211.
11. Carlsson, C., Hagerdal, M., and Siesjo, B. K. (1975): Influence of amphetamine sulfate on cerebral blood flow and metabolism. *Acta Physiol. Scand.,* 94:128.
12. Connell, P. H. (1960): Clinical manifestations and treatment of amphetamine type dependence. *JAMA,* 196:718.
13. Committee on Alcoholism and Addiction and Council on Mental Health (1966) Dependence on amphetamines and other stimulant drugs. *JAMA,* 197:1023.
14. Goodman, S. J., and Becker, D. P. (1970): Intracranial hemorrhage associated with amphetamine abuse. *JAMA,* 212.
15. Zalis, E. G., Lundberg, G. D., and Knutson, R. A. (1967): The pathophysiology of acute amphetamine poisoning with pathologic correlation. *J. Pharmacol. Exp. Ther.,* 158:115.
16. Zalis, E. G., and Parmley, L. F. (1968): Fatal amphetamine poisoning. *Ann. Intern. Med.,* 112:822.
17. Reichenbach, D. D., and Benditt, E. P. (1970): Catecholamines and cardiomyopathy. The pathogenesis and potential importance of myofibrillar degeneration. *Hum. Pathol.,* 1:125.
18. Halpern, B. N., Morard, J. C., and Drudi-Baracco, C. (1962): Action protetrice de la reserpine sur les lesions de degenerescence myocardique alque provoquees par la DL—amphetamine et suppression de cette action par los inhibiteurs de la monoamine oxydase. *C.R. Soc. Biol.,* 156:773.
19. Smith, H. J., Roche, A. H. G., Jaqusch, M. F., et al. (1976): Cardiomyopathy associated with amphetamine administration. *Am. Heart J.,* 91:792.
20. Rumbaugh, C. L., Bergeron, R. T., Fang, H. C. H., et al. (1971): Cerebral angiographic changes in the drug abuse patient. *Radiology,* 101:335, 338.
21. Rumbaugh, C. L. (1977): Small vessel cerebral vascular disease following chronic amphetamine intoxication. In: *Cocaine and Other Stimulants,* edited by E. H. Ellinwood and M. Kilbey, pp. 241–251. Plenun Press, New York.
22. Kendrick, W. C., Hull, A. R., and Knochel, J. P. (1977): Rhabdomyolysis and shock after intravenous amphetamine administration. *Ann. Intern. Med.,* 86:381.
23. Davis, J. (1970): The effects of haloperidol and chlorpromazine on amphetamine metabolism and amphetamine stereotype behavior in the rat. *J. Pharmacol. Exp. Ther.,* 174:428.

24. Beckett, A. H., Roland, M., and Turner, P. (1965): Influence of urinary pH on excretion of amphetamines. *Lancet,* 1:303.
25. Fennel, W. H., Fischman, M. W., Schuster, C. R., et al. (1976): Cardiovascular effects of cocaine. *N. Engl. J. Med.,* 265:960.
26. Sutherland, E. W., Robism, G. A., and Butcher, R. W. (1968): Some aspects of the biological role of adenosine 3′ 5′ monophosphate (cyclic AMP). *Circulation,* 37:279.
27. Gay, G. R., Sheppard, C. W. Snaba, D. S., et al. (1973): An old girl: Flying low, dying slow, blinded by snow: Cocaine in perspective. Presented at National Research Council Committee on Problems of Drug Dependence, North Carolina.
28. Van Dyke, C., Jatlow, P., Ungorer, J., et al. (1978): Oral cocaine: Plasma concentrations and central effects. *Science,* 200:211.
29. Fish, F., and Wilson, W. D. C. (1969): Excretion of cocaine and its metabolites in man. *J. Pharm. Pharmacol.,* 21:1358.
30. Maengwyn Davies, G. D., and Kippanyi, T. (1966): Cocaine tachyphylaxis and effects on indirectly acting sympathomimetic drugs in the rabbit aortic strip and in splenic tissue. *J. Pharmacol. Exp. Ther.,* 154:481.
31. Resnick, R., Kestenbaum, R. S., and Schwartz, L. K. (1976): Acute systemic effects of cocaine in man: A controlled study by intranasal and intravenous routes. *Science,* 195:696.
32. Van Dyke, C., and Byck, R. (1977): Cocaine 1884–1974. In: *Cocaine and Other Stimulants,* edited by E. M. Ellinwood and M. Kilbey, pp. 1–30. Plenum Press, New York.
33. Fischman, M. W., Schusler, C. R., Resnekov, L., et al. (1976): Cardiovascular and subjective effects of intravenous cocaine administration in humans. *Arch. Gen. Psychiatry,* 33:983.
34. Rappolt, R. T., Gay, G. R., and Inba, D. S. (1976): Propranolol in the treatment of cardiopressor effects of cocaine. *N. Engl. J. Med.,* 295:448.
35. Krager, J. M., and Safer, D. J. (1974): Types and prevalence of medication used in the treatment of hyperactive children. *N. Engl. J. Med.,* 291:1118.
36. Sprague, R. L., and Sleator, E. K. (1973): Effects of psychopharmacological agents on learning disabilities. *Pediatr. Clin. North Am.,* 20:719.
37. Maxwell, R. A., Sylivestroiviez, H. D., Holland, R., et al. (1966): Some actions of methylphenidate on the vascular system arterial tissue and the nictitating membrane. *J. Pharmacol. Exp. Ther.,* 131:355.
38. Ballard, J. E., Boileau, R. A., Sleator, E. K., et al. (1976): Cardiovascular responses of hyperactive children to methylphenidate. *JAMA,* 236:2870.
39. Safer, D. J., and Allen, R. P. (1975): Side effects from long term use of stimulants in children. *Int. J. Ment Health,* 4:105.
40. Matsuzaki, M., Mesra, A. L., and Mule, S. J. (1975): Development of acute tolerance to cardiorespiratory function and EEG activity of cocaine and pseudococaine in the monkey. *Pharmacologist,* 17:190.
41. Brodsky, J. B., and Goldwyn, R. M. (1977): Hemodynamic effects of intranasal and I.V. cocaine. *N. Engl. J. Med.,* 295:1008.
42. Evans, M. A., Dwivedi, C., and Harbison, R. D. (1977): Enhancement of cocaine induced lethality by phenobarbital. In: *Cocaine and Other Stimulants,* edited by E. M. Ellinwood and M. Kilbey, p. 253. Plenum Press, New York.
43. Deshmankar, B. S., and Lewis, J. A. (1967): Ventricular tachycardia associated with administration of methylphenidate during guanethidine therapy. *Can. Med. Assoc. J.,* 97:1166.

Chapter 14

The Stimulants 2: Caffeine and Nicotine

CAFFEINE

Caffeine-containing beverages have been consumed for centuries. Although currently considered fairly innocuous and utilized by over 90% of the population, this was not always so. In the early 20th century, dependence on

TABLE 1. *Estimates of caffeine contents of beverages*[a]

Beverage	Cup size (ml)	Caffeine content (mg/cup)	Caffeine concentrations (ng/ml)	Sodium[b] (mg/cup)	Potassium[b] (mEq/cup)
Coffee					
Ground	140–250	88–190	352–893	0.6	2.6
Instant	140–250	30–80	194–571	1.4	1.7
Decaffeinated	140–250	2–75	7–536		
Sanka-Freeze Dried		3–5		0.3	2.3
Sanka-Ground Roast		3–5		2.0	4.0
Tea	140–250	19–150	133–500	0	2.5
Colas	140–335	19–55	40–164	15–30	0

[a] Data from refs. 1–3.
[b] 6-oz cup.

caffeine was considered equal in severity to that of morphine or alcohol. At present, the most popular caffeine-containing drinks are coffee, tea, and cola. Cocoa, another frequently consumed beverage, contains theobromine rather than caffeine.

The annual world consumption of coffee is believed to exceed 4 million tons. In the United States in 1974, the per capita daily consumption of coffee was 2.25 cups, which approximates annual per capita ingestion of 70 to 150 g caffeine (1). It must be emphasized that these figures are estimates, since references in the literature pertaining to caffeine content report conflicting and variable data. Coffee beans contain 0.7 to 2% caffeine, as well as numerous other constituents, including carbohydrates, oils, proteins, ash, nonvolatile acids, and trigonelline. Roasting alters the constituents of more than 90% of the water-soluble substances and volatizes other products. Although minute amounts of vitamins are present in coffee, with the possible exception of niacin, they are not of dietary importance (1–3). Tea contains approximately 2% caffeine, theophylline, and tannic acid.

The amount of caffeine actually consumed in coffee and tea is variable, depending on potency of brew (Table 1). Gilbert et al. (1), in a randomized survey of caffeine beverages consumed at home, found a lower caffeine content with even a greater variability than previously realized. The mean caffeine content of coffee was 74 mg/cup (range, 29 to 176 mg) and for tea 27 mg/cup (range, 8 to 91 mg).

Pharmacology

Caffeine is one of the methylated xanthines. Other drugs in this group include theophylline and theobromine. All these agents have similar properties with respect to central nervous system (CNS) stimulation, cardiac stimulation, diuretic action, and smooth muscle relaxation. Caffeine is the most

TABLE 2. *Common caffeine-containing medications*

Medication	mg/Tablet
Prescription medications	
APCs	32
Cafergot®	100
Darvon Compound®	32
Fiorinal®	40
Migral®	50
Over-the-counter drugs	
Aspirin compounds	32
Vanquish®	32
Excedrin®	60
PreMens®	60
Stimulants	100
Cold preparations	~30

potent CNS stimulant, whereas theophylline has a greater effect on the cardiovascular system and as a diuretic. These drugs are consumed as prescribed medications, as over-the-counter agents (Table 2), and, most frequently, in popular drinks.

Regardless of route of administration, caffeine is readily absorbed, but the rate of absorption from the intestinal tract may vary because of its low solubility in aqueous media. After oral administration, peak levels are reached in 1 hr, with an average half-life of 3.5 hr. Metabolism is through demethylation and oxidation to 1-methyluric acid and 1-methylxanthine. Approximately 10% of absorbed caffeine is excreted unchanged.

Xanthines are competitive inhibitors of phosphodiesterase and are believed to act by affecting the metabolism of cyclic nucleotides as well as by altering ionic flux, especially calcium (4). Administration of xanthines is associated with an accumulation of cyclic adenosine monophosphate (AMP), which in turn increases phosphorylase activity, glycogenolysis, and production of glucose (5). This is associated with an activation of triglyceride lipases with an increase in triglyceride hydrolysis and elevation of plasma free fatty acids (FFA) (6,7).

Noncardiovascular effects of xanthines include a marked stimulation of all parts of the cortex, medulla, and spinal cord, although cordal stimulation occurs only after large amounts are administered. The basal metabolic rate may increase slightly, and there is relaxation of smooth muscle, most prominently of bronchial tissue. Caffeine can increase the capacity for muscular work but does so at doses that also can cause CNS stimulation. Urine production is increased, and augmentation of gastric secretion is quite frequent, even with moderate caffeine doses. The effect on glucose metabolism may result in a disproportionate rise in blood glucose level, which may occur in response to glucose loading in diabetics.

Hemodynamics

The physiologic effects of caffeine on the heart and circulation are complex, relating to direct myocardial and vascular actions and the actions on the vasomotor centers in the medulla. In the isolated myocardium, caffeine causes an increase in contractal force and cardiac output. This positive inotropic effect may be related to the ability of caffeine to inhibit phosphodiesterase, increasing the level of cyclic AMP (8).

In the intact organism, stimulation of medullary centers with caffeine may have an opposite effect, depending on the dose employed. When stimulation occurs, it is accompanied by centrally induced vasoconstriction and cardiac irregularities. Opposite effects consist of vasodilation secondary to a direct action on the coronary, pulmonary, and systemic vasculature. These direct effects in turn are counteracted by a discharge of the vasomotor center, resulting in vasoconstriction. Cerebral vascular resistance is usually increased secondary to a direct action on cerebral arterioles.

Healthy Persons

Medical studies in humans must be divided into those using pharmacologically pure caffeine and those in which coffee is consumed, as some cardiac effects of caffeine can be duplicated only by consuming large quantities of coffee. For example, the dose of caffeine required to accelerate conduction time in animals can only be obtained in humans through the consumption of 10 to 15 cups of coffee at one time (9). In addition, the effects of caffeine on caffeine-naive subjects may be quite different from those seen in coffee drinkers, who may have become tolerant to these effects (10). Unfortunately, the literature describing the cardiovascular effects of caffeine includes few double-blind trials with placebos and even fewer studies that truly separate coffee drinkers from the caffeine naive. As a result, the administration of caffeine has been associated with ectopic beats, bradycardia, tachycardia, mild elevations of systolic and diastolic blood pressure, increased cardiac output, an increase or decrease in arterial venous oxygen difference, and an elevation of oxygen consumption (11–13). In general, the observed changes tended to decrease with repeated testing. Elevation in blood pressure, when recorded, was found to be greater in older than in younger men.

Since almost all these studies suffer from lack of randomization, the work of Robertson et al. (14) is particularly relevant. These investigators, utilizing a double-blind, randomized, crossover protocol, studied the effects of a single dose of oral caffeine in nine healthy young noncoffee drinkers maintained in appropriate sodium balance throughout the study. Caffeine (250 mg) (approximately two to three cups of coffee) was administered orally in a methylxanthine-free beverage. Subsequent to drinking this beverage, detectable hemodynamic and biochemical alterations occurred. Urinary epinephrine, norepinephrine, and vanillylmandelic acid significantly increased. The excretion of metanephrine was more affected by caffeine than was that of normetanephrine, suggesting a prominent effect of caffeine at the adrenal medullary level rather than through a generalized stimulation of the sympathetic system. Plasma renin activity was found to increase by 57% at 3 hr of observation. The magnitude of this change was such that the authors noted that the subjects would have been classified as having high renin rather than normal renin secretion if they were being evaluated for hypertension.

Hemodynamic changes were also observed. Elevations of both systolic and diastolic blood pressure occurred, reaching statistical significance at 30 min, with the maximum changes noted within 1 hr. Blood pressure gradually returned toward normal during the 3-hr study period, the systolic pressure falling more slowly than the diastolic. Changes in heart rate were found to be biphasic. An initial bradycardia was noted, reaching a maximum at 45 min after caffeine and persisting for approximately 1 hr, coinciding with periods of greatest elevation of blood pressure. Afterward, a mild elevation in pulse rate occurred.

Other investigators have found the heart rate in response to caffeine to vary depending on dosage and time of day. Amounts of caffeine of less than 6 mg/kg usually result in bradycardia detectable within 30 min of ingestion and persisting up to 8 hr (11,12). Higher doses, however, may cause an increase in heart rate. Mathieu et al. (15) noted tachycardia to be present in 21% of 113 subjects who were heavy coffee drinkers, with bradycardia occurring in only 6%. Hawis (16) similarly found habitual coffee drinkers to experience tachycardia and extra systoles when their daily coffee consumption was doubled. Polonovski et al. (13) found the response of the pulse rate to coffee dependent on the time of day the beverage was ingested. Tachycardia rather than bradycardia was observed when coffee was taken with lunch, suggesting a moderating effect on increased gastrointestinal stimulation or on the absorption of caffeine in the presence of food.

Electrocardiographic Changes

Although the evidence presented about pulse rate is variable, one can hypothesize that excessive coffee consumption may exert a deleterious effect in individuals predisposed to ventricular ectopy. Prineas et al. (17), using a questionnaire technique, studied the association of coffee, tea, and alcohol intake, cigarette smoking, and sleep habits with the existence of ventricular premature beats. All 7,245 subjects screened were without a history of diabetes or heart disease. Serum electrolytes were all within normal limits. Ninety percent of subjects were coffee drinkers, averaging five cups per day. Sixty percent drank tea, on an average of four cups per day. On the basis of 2-min rest electrocardiograms (ECGs), the univariate analysis of data revealed a positive relationship between the amount of coffee or tea consumed and a negative relationship between average nightly hours of sleep time since last alcoholic beverage and the presence of 10 or more ventricular premature beats per minute. Of those persons consuming nine to 10 cups of coffee per day, 5% had frequent ventricular premature beats. Consumption of more than 11 cups daily was associated with a 6.5% frequency of ventricular premature beats. On multiple regression analysis, a significant relationship remained among the presence of ventricular premature beats, age of subjects, and average number of cups of coffee or tea ingested daily. The frequency of ventricular premature beats in persons 35 to 39 years of age compared to 55 to 57 years of age was 2.3 versus 6.6%, respectively. These findings were independent of either alcohol or cigarette intake, suggesting that excessive caffeine consumption in individuals in their sixth decade may be associated with an increased frequency of ventricular premature beats and possible detrimental effects.

The ability of caffeine to induce tachycardia and ventricular arrhythmias may be related to its action inhibiting cyclic AMP metabolism. Podzuweit et al. (18) have recently hypothesized a relationship between cyclic AMP accumulation and the onset of ventricular fibrillation and myocardial infarction. In animal studies, Rotenberg and DeFeo (19) have suggested that the threshold for induction of ventricular tachycardia by applied current is acutely decreased by the administration of caffeine. Validity of this hypothesis, its link with caffeine, and the relevance to the clinical setting, however, remain to be more clearly defined.

Persons With Coronary Artery Disease

Experimentally, evidence has accumulated that caffeine can dilate coronary arteries and increase coronary blood flow through a direct action on the vasculature musculature. However, this is accompanied by an increase in myocardial work and oxygen uptake as well as an increase in A-V oxygen difference. The effects of caffeine may differ considerably in normal persons as contrasted to those with preexisting coronary disease. Gould et al. (20) studied the hemodynamic response after drinking a strong cup of tea containing 140 mg caffeine in 12 patients with various forms of heart disease. After ingestion, a significant rise in cardiac index and stroke volume occurred without a change in cardiac rate. The mean oxygen consumption rose from 135 to 173 liters/min/m^2 ($p = 0.001$), and there was a small but significant increase in arteriovenous oxygen difference. Similar increases also occurred in mean pulmonary artery pressure as well as in right and left ventricular end-diastolic pressures (LVEDP). The average minute ventilation increased from 4.4 to 5.9 liters/min/m^2 ($p = 0.001$). No cardiac arrhythmias were observed. The small increases in LVEDP were offset by the large increases in cardiac output and stroke volume. The ability of both intravenous and orally administered caffeine to increase urinary catecholamine excretion in humans has also been observed (21).

Coffee as a Risk Factor in Coronary Artery Disease

Controversy exists about the role of caffeine as a risk factor in coronary artery disease. A number of epidemiologic studies investigating this relationship have been made during the past two decades. Many of these are subject to considerable criticism because of poor selection of case controls, sampling errors, biased data obtained from retrospective interviews, and incompletely defined variables. Failure to control for cigarette smoking, sucrose intake, or potency of coffee consumed may have considerably influenced the findings (9,22,23). Potency of brew can be most important and, unfortunately, is a subject that is least defined in most studies, with categorization of coffee drinkers based solely on a cup-per-day measurement.

Retrospective Surveys

Most of the studies performed have been retrospective, reporting conflicting findings (24–26). The most recent study was by the Boston Collaborative Drug Survey Program based on a population of 440 persons surviving a myocardial infarction. Controls consisted of persons without acute myocardial infarction, with two controls selected for each index case. A positive association between coffee intake and myocardial infarction was reported. The risk of infarction in those who drank less than or more than six cups per day was found to be increased by 60 and 120%, respectively, as compared to nondrinkers. The risk was independent of age, sex, past history of coronary heart disease, hypertension, diabetes, smoking, occupation, or use of sugar with coffee. These observations have been confirmed by other investigators (27,28). Mann and Thorogood (28), in a study of myocardial infarction in 64 women under 45 years of age, found a 2.5-fold increase in risk among women drinking six or more cups of coffee daily as compared to a group of matched controls. This risk was not altered when the effect of smoking was eliminated as a variable.

The existence of a positive association between myocardial infarction and coffee drinking, however, has been challenged by many other investigators. Hennekens et al. (29) reviewed multivariate risk analysis of data obtained from wives of 649 men succumbing to coronary heart disease. Control data were generated through interviews of neighborhood wives of the index cases. Matched pair and step-up multiple regression analysis techniques were utilized, and risk ratios for matched pair risk estimates were developed. The proportion of coffee drinkers between cases and controls was similar (77 versus 75%, respectively). Presence of diabetes, history of myocardial infarction, angina, or hypertension, cigarette smoking, congestive heart failure, physical activity, and weight were unrelated to coffee drinking. The risk of death of heart disease associated with coffee intake was found to be small; the maximum increased risk was estimated at 10%. However, the diagnosis of coronary heart disease was made on the basis of death certificates rather than autopsy reports. The accuracy of these diagnoses, therefore, is subject to question.

Prospective Surveys

Prospective studies, usually more difficult to initiate, have shown more uniform findings. The Framingham Heart Study (23), begun in 1949, drew from a cohort of 5,209 men and women, aged 30 to 62, admitted into the study between 1949 and 1952. Unfortunately, determination of coffee consumption was not made until 6 years into the study. Data, most recently reviewed by Dawber et al. (30), were recorded on 1,992 men and women. A statistically significant increase in risk with increasing coffee consumption was found only in the category of death from all causes. This risk, however, was attributed to the association between coffee drinking and cigarette smoking. The number of cigarettes smoked increased from 0.7/day in noncoffee drinkers to 21.8/day in those consuming more than seven cups ($p < 0.001$). The ratio of observed to expected deaths was not different at any level of coffee consumption, with mortality trends persisting after adjustment of cigarette intake.

Another early study was conducted by Paul in 1963 (31) at the Western Electric Company in Chicago (32). Men aged 40 to 55 and employed for at least 2 years at Western Electric were subjects in an 8-year trial. All were free of clinical coronary artery disease and had annual physical examinations. Input data included coffee and cigarette consumption, dietary information, and a complete medical history. A bimodal distribution of coffee consumption was noted in those subjects in whom coronary artery disease developed among those who either drank no coffee or consumed at least five cups per day. The initial data were inconclusive with respect to coffee drinking and association with myocardial infarction; later analysis, however, showed that when smoking habits were controlled, an association could not be found between coffee intake and risk of the development of coronary artery disease.

Heyden (33), utilizing a cross-sectional study design, reviewed the disease prevalence of heart disease and stroke in 3,102 adults, aged 40 to 75, in 1960 and in the same subjects between 1967 and 1969. Eighty-one percent were coffee drinkers, with 12% consuming at least five cups per day. No significant association was found between coffee consumption and cardiovascular disease. An analysis of the data suggested that the most important factor in determining an association between coffee drinking and coronary artery disease was the presence of cigarette smoking.

Confounding Variables

The prevalence of cigarette smoking among coffee drinkers is considerable. Data on 1,014 white men located in eight American cities, obtained by the

American Health Foundation, revealed heavy coffee consumption (more than four cups per day) to be directly associated with moderate to heavy cigarette smoking (more than 11 cigarettes per day). In each coffee category, coffee consumption increased as cigarette consumption increased. A reverse trend was observed among nonsmokers and cigar or pipe smokers.

The compounding effects that an increased sugar intake associated with an increased consumption of coffee might have on development of coronary artery disease have been reviewed by several investigators. Yudkin and Roddy (34) and Macmillan et al. (22) have suggested that dietary sucrose intake is an important variable. These findings have not been confirmed by other investigators. Paul (31,32) did not notice any significant association between heavy intake of sucrose and coronary artery disease. Howell and Wilson (35), in a comparison of sugar intake of 1,158 men without a history of heart disease and 170 men with confirmed or possible heart disease, were unable to show any significant correlation between sugar intake and coronary disease. The importance of an association between sucrose intake, in the absence of an actual diabetic state, and the development of coronary artery disease requires further clarification.

Summary

The evidence to date, based on prospective as well as retrospective studies, suggests the absence of a significant association between coffee consumption and coronary heart disease. This conclusion does not minimize the effects that excessive consumption of coffee might have on the coronary patient with respect to excessive stimulation, palpitations, and the production of an increased anxiety state. Restriction of coffee intake in patients with cardiac disease should be individualized, based on clinical findings relating to the presence of symptoms with respect to quantity of coffee consumed.

Other Caffeine-Containing Beverages

Tea

Tea is being consumed with increasing popularity. One reason for this is the assumption that while providing similar stimulative effects as coffee, it contains less caffeine and is associated with the production of less gastric irritation.

Although the varieties of commercially available tea are numerous, there are three basic types. Green tea is produced chiefly in China, Japan, and Taiwan, with the tea leaves steamed subsequent to picking to prevent fermentation. Black tea, produced mainly in India, Indonesia, East Africa, Sri Lanka, and China, differs from green tea in that it is changed chemically as well as physically in processing. The leaves are withered to remove moisture, then crushed and allowed to ferment. Oolong tea, produced mainly in Taiwan, is semifermented and in taste is midway between green and black tea.

The caffeine content of tea leaves is about 2%, which can actually be higher than coffee beans (0.7 to 2%). The final beverages, however, may contain almost equal amounts of caffeine, depending on potency of brew. Despite the controversies surrounding the association between coffee and coronary artery disease, a positive association with respect to tea consumption has never been documented. The reason for this may be related to several factors in addition to a greater caffeine content in a cup of coffee. Included among the other constituents of coffee is chlorogenic acid, a major nonvolatile acid. This substance is also found in the final product and has been shown to enhance coffee absorption in the gastrointestinal tract. Although in large doses chlorogenic acid has been shown to cause hypotension, the effect that this substance might have in heavy coffee drinkers has not yet been determined. At the least, it may result in a greater absorption of caffeine (9). The caffeine in coffee is bound by a protein and lipid-like substance. Roasting changes these substances into a tar-like material with an irritant action on the intestinal mucosa and may result in greater permeability and absorption of caffeine.

The caffeine in tea leaves is bound by carbohydrates and not usually subjected to high temperatures. In addition, other substances in tea, such as theophylline and tannins, may have a vasodilatory effect on the vasculature which may actually improve myocardial blood flow. The tannins have also been hypothesized to cause a decrease in absorption of cholesterol, bile acid, and neutral fat from the jejunum (36). These factors may tend to mitigate the effects of the caffeine. Cocoa contains a high tannin and theobromine content. Effects of cocoa-containing beverages on the cardiovascular system have not been well studied.

Cola Drinks

Cola beverages may contain up to 55 mg caffeine per 6 oz. Although this is less than one-half the amount of caffeine in a comparable cup of coffee, cola is usually consumed in a much greater quantity, which allows for the possibility of considerable caffeine ingestion. Consumption of large quantities of cola in an adolescent has been reported to be associated with insomnia and tachycardia (37).

Van Handel et al. (38) studied various physiologic parameters in subjects who ingested 10 oz of a cola-flavored soft drink containing up to 150 mg caffeine. Both urine volume and total catecholamine excretion increased with the amount of caffeine consumed. A moderate increase of circulating FFA was also noted. Heart rate and mean arterial pressure significantly increased during the ingestion of the 150-mg caffeine solution. Ingestion of lesser doses of caffeine resulted in nonsignificant increases. These results indicate that ingestion of reasonable amounts of cola-containing beverages is not associated with any significant effects on the cardiovascular system. It should be noted, however, that the sodium content of cola beverages may be as high as 30 mg. Consumption of unusually large quantities of cola might therefore be detrimental in patients with cardiac disease of a sufficient degree to be on severe salt-restricting diets.

Summary

The consumption of tea, cocoa, and cola-flavored drinks is not associated with any definite risk in individuals with cardiac disease. Nonetheless, these beverages are stimulants and, when consumed in excessive quantities, may have an adverse effect in those states where sedation would be an important factor, such as hypertension, uncontrolled angina, or essential anxiety states. Children are much more susceptible than adults to excitation by xanthines and may be particularly sensitive to excessive consumption. For this reason, although these beverages need not be proscribed in patients with cardiac disease, as in most instances, moderation is preferable to overindulgence.

NICOTINE

Nicotine probably follows alcohol and caffeine as the drug most frequently used by large numbers of the population. Although a warning is printed on each of the 30 billion packages of cigarettes sold annually, cigarette consumption continued to increase 2 to 30% each year until 1975. Subsequently, the prevalence of smoking adults started to decrease. In 1975, 32% of adults smoked cigarettes, as compared to 42% ten years earlier. The total number of adults who smoke cigarettes, however, is still impressive, estimated at 46.9 million. Unfortunately, the pattern of smoking among teenagers has not shown a similar trend. In 1975, 20% of 13 to 19 year olds smoked, as compared to 14% 10 years earlier (39). There has been an impressive increase in smoking among teenage girls within this group (40).

The total morbidity and mortality associated with cigarette smoking is impressive. It is estimated that smoking is responsible for 325,000 premature deaths annually, with total mortality rates twice as high in smokers as in nonsmokers. Of these deaths, 37% are believed to result from coronary heart disease and 19% from lung cancer (41).

Pharmacology

The percentage of nicotine in tobacco may vary from 0.5 to 0.8%, with cigarettes containing approximately 1.5% nicotine. Other known constituents include nicotinamine, nornicotine, and anabasine (42). The smoke from an average cigarette may equal 6 to 10 mg nicotine, from a cigar 15 to 40 mg, about 3 mg of which is taken into the mouth, the remainder being dissipated in side-stream smoke or the butt, or consumed by pyrolysis (43,44). Inhalation results in absorption of 90% of nicotine as compared to 25 to 50% of nicotine absorption when the smoke is taken into the mouth and then exhaled. Tobacco smoke is an aerosol-containing nicotine in its active levorotatory form, each puff containing 0.25 mg nicotine, with approximately 10 to 12 puffs per cigarette (45). Tobacco smoke also contains carbon monoxide and cyanide, as well as more than 200 other identifiable components, including pyridine, isoprenoids, volatile acids, tar, and phenolic substances.

During cigarette smoking, nicotine is absorbed rapidly from mucous membranes of the mouth, pharynx, and respiratory tract. Nicotine is also absorbed quite well from the gastrointestinal mucosa and even from the skin. Detoxification occurs predominantly in the liver (80 to 90%) but also in the kidneys and lungs. The major metabolites are cotinine, isomethylnictinium ion, γ-(3 pyridyl)-γ-oxybutyric acid, and 3 pyridylacetic acid. Excretion is through the urine at a rate dependent on urinary pH, with a much more rapid excretion of nicotine occurring in acid rather than alkaline urine.

With continued use, tolerance to many of the effects of nicotine may develop. Psychologic dependence and even a degree of physical dependence may occur, which may be accompanied by changes in autonomic system functioning when nicotine is withdrawn.

Hemodynamics

Experimentally, intravenous injection of nicotine in cats has been associated with a decrease in blood pressure followed by a sharp rise (46). Introduction of smoke into the lungs produces a similar response in one-third of animals. Although the precise mechanism remains to be determined, the evidence suggests a nicotine depressor response secondary to vagally mediated stimulation of sensory nerve endings in the lungs (47).

Commonly described clinical effects of smoking, occurring in both smokers and nonsmokers, include increases in blood pressure and heart rate (Table 3). These result from a stimulation of adrenal medullary tissue and sympathetic ganglions with a decrease in discharge from sympathetic nerve endings of the chromafin tissue in the heart (48). A direct stimulatory action of nicotine on the aortic and cartoid chemoreceptors also occurs, serving to produce additional adrenergic activity.

The use of either high- or low-nicotine cigarettes will produce this rise in systolic blood pressure and heart rate, although the magnitude of change differs. Tachmes et al. (49) found smoking high-nicotine cigarettes to be associated with a 38% increase in cardiac output, a 12% increase in systolic blood pressure, and a significant increase of 18 beats/min in heart rate. No change was observed in oxygen consumption and calf blood flow. Smoking

TABLE 3. *Effects of nicotine on the cardiovascular system*

Increase in blood pressure
Increase in heart rate
Electrocardiographic changes
Nonspecific ST and T-wave changes
Increased conduction velocity, propensity toward arrhythmias
Increased risk of development of coronary artery disease, myocardial infarction, and death
Increased incidence of angina in coronary patients
Diminished left ventricular performance in coronary patients
Increased prevalence of peripheral arterial disease

a low-nicotine cigarette was associated with a 16% increase in cardiac output, a 4% increase in arterial blood pressure, and an increase in heart rate of 4 beats/min. The hemodynamic alterations caused by nicotine are associated with measurable increases in plasma epinephrine and norepinephrine levels. Cryer et al. (50) have demonstrated significant deviations in plasma norepinephrine and epinephrine within 10 min of initiating smoking. These findings are associated with increments in the blood glycerol and blood lactate/pyruvate ratio. Elevations in serum FFA have also been observed.

Although the precise mechanisms of the cardiovascular effects produced by nicotine have not been clearly defined, the hypotheses include (a) increased sympathetic discharge, (b) elevation of plasma FFA, (c) tissue hypoxia secondary to increased levels of carboxyhemoglobin, and (d) increased platelet adhesiveness. The net clinically observable result of these effects relates to an increase in myocardial oxygen demand associated with a more rapid onset of angina in persons with coronary artery disease and a greater tendency toward myocardial infarction.

The studies described above were conducted in a laboratory setting under carefully controlled conditions. The effects of nicotine on the cardiovascular system of persons who are allowed free activity are therefore quite important. This has been studied by Cellina et al. (51) through continuous recording of heart rate and arterial pressure. During the first inhalation of cigarette smoke, a small fall followed by a rise in blood pressure was noted. This increase in both systolic and diastolic pressure has been observed in both normotensive and hypertensive patients.

Electrocardiographic Changes

Electrocardiographic effects of nicotine, consisting of minor T-wave changes and ST segment depression, have been reported (52,53). Electrophysiologic studies suggest that nicotine can cause alterations in conduction and automaticity of Purkinje fibers (54). Experimentally, the stimulation threshold for ventricular fibrillation has been shown to be decreased in laboratory animals inhaling cigarette smoke (54).

Belcheit and Fletcher (45), in a clinical study of 28 persons, found inhalation of only a few puffs of cigarette smoke to result in an increased conduction velocity and a diminished effective refractory period of the A-V node. Conduction velocity in the His Purkinje system was unimpaired. Two persons studied had the Wolf-Parkinson-White syndrome. Although conduction velocity of the A-V pathways was similarly affected, no changes were observed in the anomalous pathways. In eight of the patients with atrial fibrillation, the ventricular rate promptly increased by approximately 22% after one to three puffs. These effects, although immediate, were sustained and of sufficient intensity to antagonize the cholinergic actions of digoxin in those patients previously digitalized. The stimulant effect of nicotine was also sufficient to abolish induced pacing and spontaneous Wenckebach block. These actions of nicotine on the conduction system may be of considerable clinical importance in patients maintained on digitalis who have shortened ventricular filling, such as those with mitral stenosis and atrial fibrillation.

McHenry et al. (55), in an attempt to study the clinical effects of smoking on premature ventricular contractions, studied 586 healthy men utilizing maximal treadmill testing. In this group, 30% were nonsmokers, 46% smokers, and 24% former smokers. Although the duration of maximal exercise was significantly shorter in smokers ($p < 0.01$) and former smokers ($p < 0.005$) and maximal blood pressure during exercise greater in smokers than in nonsmokers ($p < 0.01$), no difference in the prevalence, frequency, or complexity of exercise-induced premature ventricular contractions was observed.

Chest Pain and Smoking

Chest pain, regardless of etiology, was found in a greater proportion of smokers than nonsmokers (1.6-fold) in 70,208 persons undergoing multiphasic health check-ups (56), being most prevalent in young smokers. Von Ahn (57) coined the term "tobacco angina" to describe these symptoms. Tobacco angina is considered to be chest pain of variable quality and location that occurs in smokers but is not directly related to the presence of cardiac disease or precipated by smoking, exertion, or emotion (58). There is no response to nitroglycerin. This pain may persist for years after total abstinence from tobacco. The value of this term is questionable, as up to nine distinct types of chest pain have been described in smokers.

Friedman et al. (56) have noted a positive correlation between the presence of pain and number of cigarettes smoked unrelated to alcohol or coffee consumption. Although one might expect chest pain in the presence of cough, shortness of breath, coronary heart disease, or musculoskeletal complaints, when all of these factors were excluded, the relationship between smoking and chest pain was only partially diminished. Unfortunately, the survey technique utilized was that of a questionnaire requiring yes or no responses. The smokers answered yes to most questions as compared to nonsmokers, even when the questions were related to symptoms clearly unrelated to smoking. Chest pain, however, did have the strongest association with smoking, suggesting that these symptoms are real, although the etiologic connection is not clearly defined.

Nicotine as a Risk Factor in Coronary Artery Disease

In persons with known coronary heart disease, most studies have shown that cigarette smoking increases the incidence of angina, although angina directly precipitated by smoking is rare (59,60). Angina, however, will also appear with less exercise following cigarette smoking. Physiologic studies have demonstrated an increased oxygen debt after moderate exercise and impaired endurance in smokers as compared to nonsmokers (61–64). Systolic time interval analysis following smoking of cigarettes in persons with coronary heart disease revealed an increase in preejection period/left ventricular ejection time ratio indicative of diminished left ventricular performance as compared to normal subjects, in whom an augmented left ventricular performance was suggested (65).

The relationship between cigarette smoking and coronary heart disease in humans has been extensively studied. Doll and Hill (66) have reported the mortality attributable to coronary heart disease between the ages of 35 and 44 to be increased five times and in those between ages 45 and 54 to be increased four times in smokers as compared to nonsmokers. A study of veterans in the United States reported an even higher risk, with the heavy smokers between the ages of 34 and 54 having a five- to 10-fold risk of death from coronary heart disease as compared to nonsmokers (67). Others have confirmed increased coronary heart disease mortality rates in smokers. Mortality ratios for smokers over nonsmokers have ranged from 1.43 to 3.50. averaging 2.08 for those smoking more than 20 cigarettes per day (68–71). This risk was independent of other known risk factors, such as serum cholesterol and hypertension, and was directly related to number of cigarettes smoked, the age at which smoking began, and the degree of inhalation. In addition, cigarette consumption enhances the chances of the development of coronary heart disease in the presence of other known risk factors (69).

The risk factor for coronary heart disease in premenopausal women is quite low, with mortality in women under 30 negligible; but the increase in smoking in young people, especially young women, raises the possibility of increasing the risk of coronary artery disease in this population. Mann et al. (72) reviewed smoking habits of 77 women sustaining a myocardial infarction. They found smoking 15 or more cigarettes per day to be associated with a relative risk of 4.0 after adjustment for the presence of other high risk states. This risk rose steadily with number of cigarettes smoked.

Slone et al. (73), in a larger study, surveyed the smoking habits of essentially healthy women under age 50 who sustained an acute myocardial infarction. These women were compared with a control group matched for age and geographic residence. The proportion of smokers in the study group as compared to controls was 89 versus 55% ($p < 0.001$). The rate of myocardial infarction in women smoking 35 or more cigarettes per day was 20-fold higher than nonsmokers. These findings were correlated to presence of other known risk factors, menopausal states, or physical activity. These data indicate a positive contribution of cigarette smoking to myocardial infarction in young women; when viewed along with the trend toward increased cigarette consumption among teenage girls, they suggest a probable increase in the future in myocardial infarction in premenopausal women.

Spain and Bradees (74) also reported a positive association between cigarette smoking and myocardial infarction and death. This relationship has been strengthened by pathologic findings demonstrating the degree of arteriosclerosis in the coronary arteries to be increased as a function of duration and intensity of cigarette smoking (68,71). It is of interest that this association has not been noted to be a significant risk factor in coronary heart disease in other countries, with the exception of Britain (75). These discrepant findings may relate to the method of data collection and statistical analysis as well as to the multiplicity of factors associated with coronary heart disease. In some areas where the population engages in a good deal of physical activity, and hypercholesterolemia and obesity are rare, the prevalence of coronary heart disease is extremely low, despite heavy smoking (70,75).

Effects of Stopping Smoking

Cessation of smoking has been followed by a reduction in risk of coronary heart disease of up to 50% in men under 65 years of age. The differential in mortality between former and current smokers was greatest when the group of former smokers included only those who stopped smoking for reasons other than doctors' orders (76,77). This improvement diminishes rapidly with advancing age and is no longer noted after age 65 (78,79).

The prognosis in men already experiencing a primary myocardial infarction and subsequently giving up cigarettes has been studied by Wilhelmsson et al. (80). In the study group of 564 men with primary myocardial infarctions, 89% of those aged 50 to 54 were smokers as compared to 56% in an age-matched control population. Three months postinfarction, 231 (53%) of the smokers had stopped smoking, 11 (3%) had died, and 21 (5%) were lost in follow-up; 174 (40%) continued to smoke. It is of interest that the nonsmoking infarction patients were shown to have larger infarcts and a more prolonged course than those who smoked, perhaps indicating a greater motivation toward changing lifestyles. Over a 1-year period, dyspnea with exertion unrelated to cardiac failure improved more frequently in those who had discontinued smoking, although mean systolic blood pressure was noted to rise. The rate of reinfarction was twice as high among those who continued to smoke as compared to those who stopped. A twofold incidence of cardiovascular deaths, as well as an increase in overall mortality, was noted in the persistent smokers.

Mechanism of Action

As described earlier, nicotine can act as both a stimulant and a depressant, depending on the phase of action (Table 4). Heart rate can be influenced by the action of nicotine on autonomic ganglia as well as by its influence on the carotid and aortic chemoreceptors in the medullary centers and the adrenal

TABLE 4. *Postulated mechanism of action of nicotine on the cardiovascular system*

Direct action on carotid and aortic chemoreceptors
Increased secretion of catecholamines
Increase in LDL-cholesterol
Decrease in HDL-cholesterol, resulting in enhanced atherogenesis
Increase in platelet adhesiveness
Carbon monoxide formation

gland. The increased secretion of catecholamines induced by nicotine results in a vasoconstriction of small blood vessels associated with an elevation in blood pressure, cardiac rate, and work load, all of which may increase myocardial irritability. In patients with coronary vascular disease, the vasoconstriction, tachycardia, and increase in blood pressure and oxygen consumption can have both immediate and long-term detrimental effects. Platelet adhesiveness may also be increased (81). When combined with the independent adverse response to carbon monoxide accumulation, these effects may result in myocardial infarction, ventricular fibrillation, and sudden death.

Atherogenesis

With chronic smoking, persistent structural arteriolar changes occur associated with anoxic damage to the arterial intimal lining or deposition of other atheromatous lesions. Epidemiologic studies have revealed a negative association between high density cholesterol and smoking in nondrinkers (82). This relationship was found to be related to the frequency of cigarettes smoked per day rather than duration of smoking. The depression in high density lipoprotein (HDL)-cholesterol was found to be reversible with a return to higher HDL-cholesterol values within a year of ceasing smoking. Since HDL-cholesterol in turn has been found to be negatively associated with a risk of coronary artery disease, the presence of low levels associated with reciprocal increase in low density lipoprotein (LDL)-cholesterol and very low density lipoprotein (VLDL)-cholesterol might promote an acceleration of the arteriosclerotic process.

Validity of this hypothesis has been suggested by Auerbach et al. (83,84), who performed postmortem examinations on 1,056 male veterans dying from causes other than coronary artery disease. Subjects with a history of diabetes and hypertension were excluded. Hyaline thickening of the coronary arterioles was noted in 90.7% of two-packs-a-day smokers, with fibromuscular thickening in the coronary arteries in 22% and advance arteriosclerotic lesions in 23%. In nonsmokers, there was no evidence of hyaline thickening, 8% of fibromuscular thickening, and 5% of advance arteriosclerotic disease. Although only 11% of exsmokers had advanced lesions, 97% had hyaline thickening of the coronary arterioles.

Role of Carbon Monoxide

It should be emphasized that although the use of nicotine-free cigarettes does not significantly affect heart rate or systolic blood pressure, in persons with coronary artery disease angina still develops sooner and with less work (85,86). This effect may be related to the production of carbon monoxide by the burning cigarette. Carbon monoxide levels in expired air increase with each cigarette smoked. The amount of carbon monoxide formed per volume in smoke may vary from 1% in cigarettes to 2% with pipes to 6% with cigars. No difference in carbon monoxide production exists between high-nicotine, low-nicotine, or nonnicotine cigarettes (86). Carboxyhemoglobin levels, which may represent 5 to 10% of circulating hemoglobin, have also been shown to increase. This can result in a decrease of oxygen extraction and in capillary oxygen tension secondary to a leftward shift of the oxyhemoglobin dissociation curve. An increase in ventricular work and oxygen demand, accompanied at times by an increase in coronary blood flow, may occur (87). Clinically, these changes result in a decreased amount of oxygen available to the myocardium. In patients with coronary heart disease and angina, this will result in a significant decrease in exercise performance with an earlier development of chest pain (85,86). Angina developing after exercise in smokers can therefore be related to two effects: (a) an increased myocardial oxygen demand secondary to nicotine, and (b) a decreased oxygen delivery to the myocardium, regardless of the presence of nicotine.

The role of carbon monoxide in contributing to coronary heart disease in smokers may be greater than previously realized. Experimentally, in rabbits exposed to carbon monoxide for 13 weeks, greater focal intimal and subintimal changes of their arterioles have been shown to develop than in animals not exposed. If cholesterol is added to the diet, the aortic cholesterol content increases two to five times (87).

Similar observations have been confirmed in primates. The effect of carbon monoxide on the endothelium appears to be increased permeability associated with subendothelial edema and increased formation of mucopolysaccharides. This may facilitate the precipitation of lipoproteins, culminating in fatty streaks or plaques (88). Ultrastructural myocardial changes, consisting of focal areas of necrosis of the myofibrils and degenerative changes of the mitochondria, have also been noted in animals maintained at carboxyhemoglobin levels of 16 to 18% for 2 weeks (89). As mentioned above, nicotine may even have a synergistic effect, with carbon monoxide enhancing accumulation of lipid in arterial walls and impairing oxygen supply to tissues already compromised by carbon monoxide-induced subendothelial edema.

Clinically, Wald et al. (90) have demonstrated carboxyhemoglobin levels in tobacco smokers to have a better correlation with coronary heart disease than the smoking history. Smokers with carboxyhemoglobin levels of 5% or greater had an incidence of atherosclerotic heart disease 21 times higher than smokers with values of 3% or less. Even in the absence of smoking, however, carboxyhemoglobin has been shown to exert a deleterious effect in coronary patients. Anginal patients breathing 50 ppm of carbon monoxide for 4 hr had a significant decrease in exercise performance as compared to breathing compressed purified air. Ischemic ST segment changes appeared earlier and were deeper with carbon monoxide inhalation (91,92).

The role of the more than 200 other compounds isolated from particulate and gaseous phases of tobacco smoke has yet to be evaluated with respect to cardiac effects.

Confounding Variables

All the studies quoted above indict nicotine as a definite risk factor in the production of coronary artery disease. There is, however, a factor closely related to smoking that may be considered a confounding variable. The role of stress as an inciting agent in acute myocardial infarction has only recently become prominent. It also is generally realized that a positive association exists between stress and smoking. Several investigators have documented this association, and some have even suggested that smoking might be an indication of "heightened and emotional tension rather than a predisposing causative factor in coronary heart disease" (93,94).

Russek (95), however, in a statistical survey of 12,000 professional men, found that although smoking was most frequent in stressful occupations, coronary heart disease was unexpectedly more common among nonsmokers and among persons who once smoked but subsequently ceased. This finding may be related to the association of high fat diets with emotional stress. King (96) found that among male adolescents, stress produced changes in behavior patterns, with nonsmokers responding by increasing their intake of food as compared to increasing cigarette consumption that occurred in the smoker. These data suggest that stress may exert a confounding influence on the association of nicotine in coronary disease and, whenever possible, should receive consideration in epidemiologic studies.

Other Vascular Effects

Smoking has been commonly observed to produce peripheral vasoconstriction in the clinical setting. The increased prevalence of smoking in persons with thromboangitis obliterans and Buergers disease is also well known. Recent analysis of data has convincingly connected cigarette smoking with the onset of peripheral arterial disease (86,97).

The effects of smoking in the production of chronic bronchitis and chronic emphysema are well known. These conditions can in turn produce pulmonary heart disease progressing to cor pulmonale and right-sided congestive failure.

Drug Interactions

Since nicotine is mainly detoxified in the liver, if cigarettes are smoked in sufficient quantity, induction of hepatic enzymes may occur, which can alter metabolic rates of substances detoxified by these enzyme systems. There is little evidence in the literature with respect to cardiac drug interactions with nicotine. Studies have been reported, however, about drug interactions with other mood-altering agents to suggest that this postulated effect may have some clinical relevance.

Keeri-Szanto and Pomeroy (98) found smokers to require greater doses of pentazocaine than nonsmokers to adequately supplement nitrous oxide anesthesia. Similarly, the analgesic effects of propoxyphene have been reported to be less in smokers, as have the CNS depressant effects of the benzodiazepines (99,100). Swett et al. (101) found the incidence of hypotensive reactions due to chlorpromazine administration to be indirectly related to the number of cigarettes smoked, with no heavy smokers, as compared to 10% of nonsmokers, experiencing hypotension. Since nicotine stimulates both epinephrine and norepinephrine release, the diminution of hypotensive reactions to chlorpromazine, an alpha blocker, suggests that the mechanism of this effect is related more to alterations in metabolism than nicotine-induced catecholamine release.

As discussed earlier, nicotine has been observed to antagonize the cholinergic effects of digitalis. Heavy smoking by persons maintained on digitalis may serve to diminish therapeutic effectiveness. This can be of special importance in persons with atrial fibrillation or other states characterized by reduced ventricular filling time.

Theophylline is metabolized in the liver by an enzyme system that is different from that induced by phenobarbital and related drugs. Recently, substances in cigarette smoke, mainly the polycyclic hydrocarbons, have been demonstrated to induce the cytochrome system responsible for theophylline biotransformation. Heavy cigarette smokers (1 to 2 packs/day) have been shown to have a shorter plasma theophylline half-life than nonsmokers, with a persistence of such alterations for an interval of 3 months to as long as 2 years following cessation of smoking (102–104). Proportionate alterations in plasma theophylline half-life, with a relatively more rapid return toward normal levels, were also noted in moderate and light smokers. These findings are believed to have clinical relevance. Larger theophylline doses will be required for heavy smokers. Upon cessation of smoking, dosage must be carefully monitored and gradually reduced to avoid theophylline toxicity (105).

Summary

In summary, all available statistical and biologic evidence demonstrates a strong association between smoking and cardiovascular disease. Cigarette smoking has been shown to be related to the occurrence of angina, myocardial infarction, and mortality due to coronary artery disease, especially sudden coronary death. Cigarette smoking is not only an independent factor but can act cumulatively with other major risk factors. It is encouraging that those studies reviewing risk in exsmokers have revealed a marked diminution in risk in patients under age 65 upon ceasing smoking. Patients who have experienced a myocardial infarction and subsequently stopped smoking experience half the rate of risk of death in coronary attacks when compared to those who continue to smoke. The evidence of a positive association of nicotine and peripheral arterial disease is similarly compelling. Cessation of smoking in this condition is associated with an increase in exercise tolerance.

The knowledge that cigarette smoking is an independent positive risk factor in cardiovascular disease has been put to practical use with the initiation of several multicenter studies utilizing the concept of risk factor intervention as an approach to chronic disease control (106). Two major projects in this country, The Multiple Risk Factor Intervention Trial (107) and the Stanford Heart Disease Prevention Program (108), have been developed recently to determine if habits could be influenced in a way to reduce the risk of premature heart disease and stroke. Initial data from Stanford are encouraging. Cigarette smoking decreased among community participants to a far greater extent than among control community members (7.24 versus 2.5%, respectively). Among those participants who received intensive instruction, the decrease in cigarette smoking reached 42%. The overall risk for coronary heart disease decreased 15 to 20% among the participant group as compared to an actual increase in risk of 5% for the control community, with the participant group receiving intensive instruction achieving a 30% decline in risk. It should be emphasized that these changes in risk of coronary heart disease cannot solely be attributed to change in smoking habits, as other risk factors also decreased in the participant versus the control groups.

Consumption of low-tar and -nicotine cigarettes, although reducing the amount of nicotine absorbed, still is associated with a risk due to carbon monoxide. A shift of the cigarette smoker to cigar and pipe smoking is effective only if the smoker does not inhale. As stated by the American Heart Association and the Ad Hoc Committee on Cigarette Smoking and Cardiovascular Disease:

> Although the smoker can reduce the health risk of smoking by smoking fewer cigarettes and switching to filtered, low tar and nicotine cigarettes and by taking fewer puffs and not inhaling, the only sure way is to abstain from smoking entirely.

There is little question that a marked reduction in mortality and morbidity due to cardiovascular disease would occur if this advice was heeded.

REFERENCES

1. Gilbert, R. M., Marshman, J. A., Schwieder, M., et al. (1976): Caffeine content of beverages as consumed. *Can. Med. Assoc. J.,* 114:205.
2. Nagy, M. (1974): Caffeine content of beverages and chocolate. *JAMA,* 229:337.
3. Martinek, R. G., and Wolman, W. (1955): Xanthenes, tannins and sodium in coffee, tea, cola. *JAMA,* 158:1030.
4. Bianchi, C. P. (1961): The effect of caffeine on radiocalcium movement in frog sartorius. *J. Gen. Pharmacol.,* 44:845.
5. Levi, L. (1967): The effects of coffee on the function of the sympathoadrenomedullary system in man. *Acta Med. Scand.,* 181:431.
6. Bellet, S., Kerschbaum, A., and Peck, E. M. (1968): Response of free fatty acids to coffee and caffeine. *Metabolism,* 17:702.
7. Bellet, S., Kershbaum, A., and Aspe, J. (1965): The effect of caffeine on free fatty acids. *Arch. Intern. Med.,* 116:750.
8. Sutherland, E. W., Robism, G. A., and Butcher, R. W. (1968): Some aspects of the biological role of adenosine 3′5′ monophosphate (cyclic AMP). *Circulation,* 37:229.
9. MacCormack, F. A. (1977): The effects of coffee drinking on the cardiovascular system: Experimental and epidemiological research. *Prev. Med.,* 6:104.
10. Colton, T., Gosselin, R. E., and Smith, R. P. (1968): The tolerance of coffee drinkers to caffeine. *Clin. Pharmacol. Ther.,* 9:31.
11. Grollman, A. (1930): The action of alcohol, caffeine and tobacco on the cardiac output (and its related functions) of normal men. *J. Pharmacol.,* 39:313.
12. Gilliland, A. R., and Nelson, D. (1939): The effects of coffee on certain mental and physiological functions. *J. Gen. Psychol.,* 21:339.
13. Polonovski, M., Donzelot, E., Brisicas, S., et al. (1952): The comparative effects of coffee and soluble extracts of coffee on normal persons and cardiacs. *Cardiologia,* 21:809.
14. Robertson, D., Frolich, J. C., Carr, R. K., et al. (1978): Effects of caffeine on plasma renin activity, catecholamines and blood pressure. *N. Engl. J. Med.,* 298: 181.
15. Mathieu, L., Hadot, S., and Hadot, E. (1962): Cardiac repercussions of coffee drinking. *Cardiol. Angiol. Int.,* 11:219.
16. Hawis, P. B. (1929): A study of the physiological and psychological reactions of the human organism to coffee drinking. *Am. J. Physiol.,* 90:380.

17. Prineas, R. J., Jacobs, D., Crow, R., et al. (1977): Coffee, tea and VPB. *Circulation* [*Suppl. III*], 55–56:15.
18. Podzuweit, T., Lubbe, W. F., and Opie, L. H. (1976): Cyclic adenosine monophosphate, ventricular fibrillation and antiarrhythmic drugs. *Lancet,* 1:341.
19. Rotenberg, F. A., and DeFeo, J. J. (1976): The effects of caffeine on cardiac irritability. *Fed. Proc.,* 34:384.
20. Gould, L., Goswami, M. J., Reddy, C. V. R., et al. (1973): The cardiac effects of tea. *J. Clin. Pharmacol.,* 13:469.
21. Atuk, N. O., and Westfall, T. C. (1973): Coffee and myocardial infarction. *N. Engl. J. Med.,* 289:977.
22. Macmillan, A., McKean, H., et al. (1968): Sucrose intake and coronary artery disease. *Lancet,* 2:1049.
23. The Framingham Study: Habits and Coronary Heart Disease (1966): United States Department of Health, Education and Welfare. PHS Publ. no. 1515, National Heart Institute, Washington, D.C.
24. Klatsky, A. L., Friedman, G. D., and Siegelaub, A. B. (1973): Coffee drinking prior to acute myocardial infarction. Results from the Kaiser Permanente epidemographic study of myocardial infarction. *JAMA,* 226:540.
25. Walker, W. J., and Gregoratos, S. G. (1967): Myocardial infarction in young men. *Am. J. Cardiol.,* 19:339.
26. Brown, A. (1962): Coronary thrombosis. An environmental study. *Br. Med. J.,* 2:567.
27. Jick, H., Miettinen, O. S., Neff, R., et al. (1973): Coffee and myocardial infarction. *N. Engl. J. Med.,* 289:63.
28. Mann, J. I., and Thorogood, M. (1975): Coffee drinking and myocardial infarction. *Lancet,* 2:1215.
29. Hennekens, C. H., Drolette, M. E., Jesse, M. J., et al. (1976): Coffee drinking and death due to coronary heart disease. *N. Engl. J. Med.,* 294:633.
30. Dawber, T. R., Kannel, W. B., and Gordon, T. (1974): Coffee and cardiovascular disease observations from the Framingham Study. *N. Engl. J. Med.,* 291:871.
31. Paul, O. (1963): A longitudinal study of coronary heart disease. *Circulation,* 28:20.
32. Paul, O. (1968): Stimulants and coronaries. *Postgrad. Med.,* 44:196.
33. Heyden, S. (1971): Coffee consumption, vascular diseases and risk factors in the Evans County, Georgia study. Presented at the Fifth International Coffee Research Conference, Lisbon, Portugal.
34. Yudkin, J., and Roddy, J. (1964): Levels of dietary sucrose in patients with occlusive atherosclerotic disease. *Lancet,* 2:6.
35. Howell, R., and Wilson, D. G. (1968): Dietary sugar and ischaemic heart disease. *Br. J. Med.,* 3:145.
36. Herbel, E. S., and Scala, J. (1973): Coffee, tea and coronary heart disease. *Lancet,* 2:152.
37. Silver, W. (1971): Insomnia, tachycardia and cola drink. *Pediatrics,* 47:635.
38. Van Handel, P. J., Burke, E., and Costill, D. L. (1976): Physiologic responses to cola ingestion. *Res. Q.,* 48:436.
39. Morbidity and Mortality Weekly Report (1978): Center for Disease Control, Atlanta, 26:160.
40. Teenage Smoking. National Patterns of Cigarette Smoking Ages 12 to 18 in 1972 and 1974 (1976): U.S. Dept. of Health, Education and Welfare, DHEW Publ. no. (NIH) 76–931.
41. AHA Report of Ad Hoc Committee on Cigarette Smoking and Cardiovascular Disease (1978): *Circulation,* 57:406A.
42. Kuhn, H. (1965): Tobacco alkaloids and their pyrolysis products in the smoke. In: *Tobacco Alkaloids and Related Compounds,* edited by A. Von Euler, p. 37. Macmillan, New York.
43. Larson, P. S. (1960): Absorption of nicotine under various conditions of tobacco use. *Ann. N.Y. Acad. Sci.,* 90:31.
44. Goodman, L. S., and Gilman, A. (1970): *The Pharmacological Basis of Therapeutics, Fourth Edition.* Macmillan, Toronto.

45. Bekheit, S., and Fletcher, E. (1976): The effects of smoking on myocardial conduction in the human heart. *Am. Heart J.,* 91:712.
46. Comroe, J. H. (1960): The pharmacological actions of nicotine. *Ann. N.Y. Acad. Sci.,* 90:48.
47. Armitage, A. K., and Hall, G. H. (1969): Mode of action of intravenous nicotine in causing a fall in blood pressure in the cat. *Eur. J. Pharmacol.,* 7:23.
48. Burn, J. H. (1960): Action of nicotine on the heart. *Ann. N.Y. Acad. Sci.,* 90:70.
49. Tachmes, L., Fernandez, R., and Sackner, M. (1977): Hemodynamic effects of cigarette smoking. *Circulation* [*Suppl. III*], 55–56:73.
50. Cryer, P., Haymond, M. W., Santiago, J. U., et al. (1977): Smoking, catecholamines and coronary heart disease. *Cardiovasc. Med.,* 2:471.
51. Cellina, G. U., Honour, A. J., and Littler, W. A. (1975): Direct arterial pressure, heart rate and electrocardiogram during cigarette smoking in unrestricted patients. *Am. Heart J.,* 89:18.
52. Von Ahn, B. (1954): The acute effects of tobacco smoking and nicotine on the electrocardiogram, especially during hypoxia. A clinical and experimental investigation. *Acta Med. Scand.* [*Suppl.*], 292:1.
53. Von Ahn, B. (1960): Tobacco smoking, the electrocardiogram and angina pectoris. *Ann. N.Y. Acad. Sci.,* 90:190.
54. Greenspan, K., Edwards, R. E., Knoebel, S. B., et al. (1969): Some effects of nicotine on cardiac automaticity, conductor and introphy. *Arch. Intern. Med.,* 123:707.
55. McHenry, P. L., Faris, J. V., Jordan, J. W., et al. (1977): Comparative study of cardiovascular function and ventricular premature complexes in smokers and nonsmokers during maximal treadmill exercise. *Am. J. Cardiol.,* 39:493.
56. Friedman, G. D., Siegelaub, M. S., and Dales, L. G. (1975): Cigarette smoking and chest pain. *Ann. Intern. Med.,* 83:1.
57. Von Ahn, B. (1965): Tobacco angina. In: *Tobacco Alkaloids and Related Compounds,* edited by W. W. Von Euler, pp. 253–262. Macmillan, New York.
58. Oram, S., and Sowton, E. (1963): Tobacco angina. *Q. J. Med.,* 32:115.
59. Aronow, W. S., Kaplan, M. A., and Jacob, D. (1968): Tobacco: A precipitating factor in angina pectoris. *Ann. Intern. Med.,* 69:529.
60. Aronow, W. (1973): Smoking. *Circulation,* 43:1169.
61. Fingell, W. H., Fischman, M. W., Schuster, C. R., et al. (1976): Cardiovascular effects of cocaine. *N. Engl. J. Med.,* 265:960.
62. Rappolt, R. T., Gay, G. R., and Inba, D. S. (1976): Propranolol in the treatment of cardiopressor effects of cocaine. *N. Engl. J. Med.,* 295:448.
63. Cooper, K. H., Gey, G. O., and Bottenberg, R. A. (1968): Effects of cigarette smoking on endurance performance. *JAMA,* 203:123.
64. Krumitolz, R. A., Chevalier, R. B., and Ross, J. C. (1965): Changes in cardiopulmonary function related to abstinence from smoking. Studies in young cigarette smokers at rest and exercise at 3 and 6 weeks of abstinence. *Ann. Intern. Med.,* 67:197.
65. Jain, A. C., Bower, A. F., Marshall, E. J., and Asata, H. (1977): Left ventricular function after cigarette smoking by chronic smokers. Comparison of normal subjects and patients with coronary artery disease. *Am. J. Cardiol.,* 39:27.
66. Doll, R., and Hill, A. B. (1966): National Cancer Institute, Monograph 19, p. 205, U.S. Government Printing Office, Washington, D.C.
67. Rosenman, R. H., Friedman, M., Straus, R., et al. (1966): Coronary heart disease in the Western Collaborative Group Study. *JAMA,* 195:86.
68. Doyle, J. T., Dawber, T. R., Kannel, W. B., et al. (1964): The relationship of cigarette smoking to coronary heart disease. The second report of the combined experience of the Albany, New York and Framingham, Massachusetts Studies. *JAMA,* 189:886.
69. Doyle, J. T. (1972): Cigarette smoking and coronary atherosclerosis. In: *Atherosclerosis and Coronary Heart Disease,* edited by W. Likoff, B. Segal, and W. Lusull, p. 35. Grune & Stratton, New York.
70. Ball, K., and Turner, R. (1974): Smoking and the heart. *Lancet,* 2:822.

71. Auerbach, O., Hammond, E. C., and Garfinkle, L. (1965): Smoking in relation to atherosclerosis of the coronary arteries. *N. Engl. J. Med.,* 273:775.
72. Mann, J. I., Doll, R., Thorogood, M., et al. (1976): Risk factors for myocardial infarction in young women. *Br. J. Prev. Soc. Med.,* 30:94.
73. Slone, D., Shapiro, S., Rosenberg, L., et al. (1978): Relation of cigarette smoking to myocardial infarction in young women. *N. Engl. J. Med.,* 298:1273.
74. Spain, D. M., and Bradess, V. A. (1970): Sudden death from coronary heart disease. *Chest,* 58:107.
75. Keys, A. (1970): Coronary heart disease in seven countries. *Circulation* [*Suppl. I*], 41:1.
76. Hammond, E. C., and Garfinkle, L. (1969): Coronary heart disease, stroke, and aortic aneurysm—Factors in the etiology. *Arch. Environ. Health,* 19:167.
77. Stamler, J. (1968): Cigarette smoking and atherosclerotic coronary heart disease. *Bull. N.Y. Acad. Med.,* 44:1476.
78. Gordon, T., Kannel, W. B., McGee, D. (1974): Death and coronary attacks in men after giving up cigarette smoking. *Lancet,* 1:1345.
79. Proceedings of the Third World Conference on Smoking and Health (1975): Modifying the risk for the non-smoker, vol. 1. U.S. Dept. Health, Education and Welfare, DHEW Publ. no. (NIH) 76–1221.
80. Wilhelmsson, C., Elmfeldt, D., Vedin, J. A., et al. (1975): Smoking and myocardial infarction. *Lancet,* 1:415.
81. The Health Consequences of Smoking (1975): A report of the Surgeon General. U.S. Dept. of Health, Education and Welfare. PHS CDC, U.S. Government Printing Office, Washington, D.C.
82. Garrison, R., Kannel, W. B., Feinleib, M., et al. (1977): Cigarette smoking and HDL-cholesterol. The Framingham Study, *Circulation* [*Suppl. III*], 55–56:44.
83. Auerbach, O., Carter, H. W., Garfinkel, L., et al. (1976): Cigarette smoking and coronary artery disease. *Chest,* 70:697.
84. Auerbach, O., Carter, H. W., Garfinkel, L., et al. (1977): Smokers heart. *Arch. Intern. Med.,* 137:435.
85. Aronow, W. S., and Rokow, S. N. (1971): Carboxyhemoglobin caused by smoking non-nicotine cigarettes. Effects on angina pectoris. *Circulation,* 44:782.
86. Aronow, W. S., Dendinger, J., and Rokaw, S. N. (1971): Heart rate and carbon monoxide level after smoking high, low, and non-nicotine cigarettes. *Ann. Intern. Med.,* 74:697.
87. Ayres, S. M., Giannell, S., and Mueller, H. S. (1970): Effects of low concentrations of carbon monoxide. Myocardial and systemic responses to carboxyhemoglobin. *Ann. N.Y. Acad. Sci.,* 174:268.
88. Astrup, P., Kjeldsen, K., and Wanstrup, J. (1967): Enhancing influence of carbon monoxide on the development of atheromatosis in cholesterol fed rabbits. *J. Atheroscler. Res.,* 7:343.
89. Astrup, P. (1973): Carbon monoxide, smoking and cardiovascular disease. *Circulation,* 43:1167.
90. Wald, N., Howard, S., Smith, P. G., and Kjeldsen, K. (1961): Association between atherosclerotic disease and carboxyhaemoglobin levels in tobacco smokers. *Br. Med. J.,* 1:761.
91. Anderson, E. W., Andelman, R. J., Strauch, J. M., et al. (1973): Effects of low level carbon monoxide exposure on the onset and duration of angina pectoris. A study in ten patients with ischemic heart disease. *Ann. Intern. Med.,* 79:46.
92. Aronow, W. S., and Isbell, M. W. (1973): Carbon monoxide effect on exercise-induced angina. *Ann. Intern. Med.,* 79:392.
93. Russek, H. I., and Zohman, B. L. (1958): Relative significance of heredity, diet and occupational stress in coronary heart disease of young adults. Based on an analysis of 100 patients between the ages of 25 and 40 years and a similar group of 100 normal control subjects. *Am. J. Med. Sci.,* 235:266.
94. Pincherle, G., and Williamson, J. (1971): Smoking and neuroticism. *Lancet,* 3:981.
95. Russek, H. I. (1965): Stress, tobacco, and coronary disease in North American

professional groups. Survey of 12,000 men in 14 occupational groups. *JAMA,* 192:189.
96. King, A. J. (1971): Stress, cigarette smoking and snacking behavior in adolescent males. *Can. J. Public Health,* 62:297.
97. Feinlieb, M., and Williams, R. R. (1975): Relative risks of myocardial infarction, cardiovascular disease and peripheral vascular disease by type of smoking. In: *Proceedings of the Third World Conference on Smoking and Health,* vol. 1. U.S. Dept. of Health, Education and Welfare, DHEW Publ. no. (NIH) 76–1221.
98. Keeri-Szanto, M., and Pomeroy, J. R. (1971): Atmospheric pollution and pentazocine metabolism. *Lancet,* 1:947.
99. Boston Collaborative Drug Surveillance Program (1973): Decreased clinical efficacy of propoxyphene in cigarette smokers. *Clin. Pharmacol. Ther.,* 14:259.
100. Boston Collaborative Drug Surveillance Program (1967): Clinical depression of the central nervous system due to diazepam and chlordiazepoxide in relation to cigarette smoking and age. *N. Engl. J. Med.,* 288:277.
101. Swett, C., Cole, J. D., Hartz, S. C., et al. (1977): Hypotension due to chlorpromazine. *Arch. Gen. Psychiatry,* 34:661.
102. Jenne, J., Nagasawa, I. T., McHugh, R., et al. (1975): Decreased theophylline half life in cigarette smokers. *Life Sci.,* 17:95.
103. Hunt, S. N., Jusko, W. J., and Yurchak, A. M. (1976): Effect of smoking on theophylline disposition. *Clin. Pharmacol. Ther.,* 19:546.
104. Powell, J. R., Thercelin, J. F., Vozek, S., et al. (1977): The influence of cigarette smoking and sex on theophylline disposition. *Ann. Rev. Respir. Dis.,* 116:17.
105. Rafsky, K. M., and Ogilvie, R. I. (1975): Dosage of theophylline in bronchial asthma. *N. Engl. J. Med.,* 292:1218.
106. Breslow, L. (1978): Risk factor intervention for health maintenance. *Science,* 200:908.
107. Multiple Risk Factors Intervention Trial Group (1976): *JAMA,* 235:825.
108. Maccoby, N., Farquhar, J. W., Wood, P. O., et al. (1977): Reducing the risk of cardiovascular disease: Effects of a community based campaign on knowledge and behavior. *J. Comm. Health,* 3:100.

Subject Index